CURED

81 NATURAL CURES

FOR CANCER, DIABETES, ALZHEIMER'S AND MORE...

NUTRITION & HEALING

Additional orders and inquiries can be directed to *Nutrition & Healing*, NewMarket Health, L.L.C., P.O. Box 913, Frederick, MD 21705; tel. (443)353-4204.

600B0009C6

Table of Contents

Part I: Cancer

Chapter 1: Prevent and beat prostate cancer with
this powerful—and proven—plant pigment 3

Chapter 2: Hybridized mushroom extract destroys
cancer cells and provides powerful immune protection 7

Chapter 3: Natural 4-ingredient "herbal cocktail"
could be the key to avoiding THIS deadly cancer 11

Chapter 4: New science proves you can make your
body cancer-proof! 17

Chapter 5: Fight aging, cell damage, Alzheimer's and
even cancer with this powerful plant secret 21

Chapter 6: Become practically invincible to major
diseases like cancer, Alzheimer's, and shingles 33

Chapter 7: Survive pancreatic cancer—and feel
better—with this century-old nutritional therapy 39

Chapter 8: The cancer-fighting mineral you can't afford to ignore 47

Part II: Alzheimer's and Brain Health

Chapter 1: ICT Protocol for reversing and
even curing Alzheimer's 55

Chapter 2: Alzheimer's breakthrough reveals an all-natural
nutritional solution to protect your precious memories 71

Chapter 3: The mineral breakthrough helping
terminal patients defy death: and why you should
be taking a little of it too 77

Chapter 4: "Clean" your brain and stop dementia
and Alzheimer's with this simple sleep trick 83

Chapter 5: Is this weird-looking mushroom the
key to preventing and reversing dementia? 89

Chapter 6: This secret virus can give you Alzheimer's—
and there's a good chance you're carrying it. 95

Chapter 7: Head trauma from decades ago can wreck
your brain now—but it's never too late to repair the damage! 101

Chapter 8: This toxic crud could be hiding in your
home, attacking your brain and making you sick!.............. 107

Part III: Heart Health

Chapter 1: Five blood-flow secrets to slash your
risk of heart attack and stroke............................ 115

Chapter 2: Beware of the statin drug trap.
Lower cholesterol is making us old and sick 119

Chapter 3: Two signs on your body that may
point to heart trouble.................................... 123

Chapter 4: OPCs: What are they and how do
they help your heart? 125

Chapter 5: How to drop your cholesterol level by
as much as 134 without drugs or deprivation 129

Chapter 6: Red yeast rice drops LDL cholesterol 35 points........ 135

Chapter 7: The ONE number that can really predict
your heart attack risk (Hint: it's not your cholesterol count!) 137

Chapter 8: How to drop your blood pressure by
20, 30, or even 40 points—naturally 141

Chapter 9: Can this one "hero mineral" keep you
from ever having a heart attack? 151

Chapter 10: Don't touch that next dose of aspirin
until you've had this important test 157

Chapter 11: Could this "blacklisted" treatment end
up saving your life?...................................... 163

Chapter 12: The "broken heart syndrome" that could
kill you—and that lots of doctors miss 167

Chapter 13: A contaminant in your water may be
clogging your arteries 171

Chapter 14: The No. 1 heart-protecting mineral................ 173

Part IV: Chronic Pain and Arthritis

Chapter 1: Drive down your inflammation and
relieve arthritis with these natural pain busters!.............. 177

Chapter 2: Natural substance stops crippling
arthritis pain—without the risks! 183

Chapter 3: Catch the culprit behind your arthritis pain 189

Chapter 4: Quit the limping and hobbling and
banish knee pain with this time-tested treatment 197

Chapter 5: Feds order crackdown on prescription painkillers!
Here's what it means for you—and your doctor 201

Chapter 6: In pain? Nowhere to turn? Send even the
worst pain packing... without drugs!. 209

Chapter 7: Banish pain, inflammation—and even
asthma—with this "suction secret" 215

Part V: Diabetes

Chapter 1: The hidden link between digestion and diabetes 221

Chapter 2: Maintain "perfect" blood sugar,
blood pressure and cholesterol levels naturally 225

Chapter 3: Warning: Could you get diabetes just
from drinking water? 229

Chapter 4: Get your type 2 diabetes under control
without a single drug 235

Chapter 5: Is it Alzheimer's—or is it "Type 3 diabetes"?
Learn the three ways diabetes is costing you
your precious memories 243

Part VI: Anti-Aging, Hearing and Vision

Chapter 1: Put the brakes on aging—and jumpstart
your body's natural healing process—with the world's
simplest antioxidant 249

Chapter 2: The vitamin that erases 20 years of aging in 90 days 255

Chapter 3: Stop vision loss in its tracks with these 6 "super herbs" . . 261

Chapter 4: Five ways to avoid that hearing aid 267

Chapter 5: Don't go deaf, blind or lose your mind!
Natural strategies for keeping your hearing, vision,
and thinking sharp well into old age. 271

Part VII: Digestion and Weight Loss

Chapter 1: The "youth hormones" that make weight loss nearly effortless! 285

Chapter 2: Is this hidden illness leaving you tired, bloated and in pain? Cure it for good with a simple diet trick! 293

Chapter 3: Cure THIS weird digestive disorder and watch years of brain fog vanish 297

Chapter 4: Powerful protein extract fights chronic GI disorders... and you won't believe how much better you'll feel! 303

Chapter 5: Indigestion... colitis... IBS... Can this one "super probiotic" tackle them all? 309

Part VIII: Immune System and Autoimmune Diseases

Chapter 1: Six simple steps to make your body flu-proof—no shot required!. 317

Chapter 2: Everyday exposure to hidden parasites could be making you sick 321

Chapter 3: Stunning research reveals gut bug balance causing everything from diabetes to colon cancer!. 327

Chapter 4: Fight infections... eliminate toxins... and stop disease with your body's "secret system" 331

Chapter 5: 5 ways to make sure you've had your last bout with the common cold. And 3 cures you never knew could work so well. 337

Chapter 6: Tired of the sneezing... sniffling... and sinus pain? Relieve stubborn seasonal allergies with these all-natural cures 345

Chapter 7: Get control of your Parkinson's symptoms with these simple (and fun) programs. 349

Chapter 8: Real cause of dozens of autoimmune diseases revealed: Simple three-step plan treats everything from rheumatoid arthritis to Crohn's disease. 355

Chapter 9: Allergies, asthma, and autoimmune diseases are exploding. Here's why your immune system is broken— and how to fix it. 363

Part IX: Energy and Thyroid Health

Chapter 1: Stomp out chronic fatigue and get back your old get up and go 373

Chapter 2: Keep your energy levels from sagging with this (seriously) misunderstood vitamin fix. 375

Chapter 3: Sluggish and suffering? Doc says you're fine? Take a closer look at your thyroid function with this commonly overlooked test!. 379

Part X: Women's Health

Chapter 1: Ladies: Losing your head over your thinning hair? My "Halt the Hair Loss" plan can help! 387

Chapter 2: Warning: Unsightly varicose veins could be sending you a warning sign. Try these 4 simple steps to send them packing 393

Chapter 3: Say goodbye to those dreaded "cottage cheese" thighs with my "Beat the Cellulite" plan. 399

Chapter 4: Forget your annual mammogram! New tool offers better, earlier breast cancer detection (and it's pain free, too!) 405

Chapter 5: The natural secret to great sex after menopause 411

Chapter 6: Breast cancer—stop the most feared disease among women from happening to you. 413

Part XI: Men's Health

Chapter 1: Become "King of the Bedroom" again! Powerful three-part combo helps reverse erectile dysfunction 425

Chapter 2: This dangerous sleep disorder could be the real reason for your "overactive bladder" 431

Chapter 3: Was your last testosterone number dead wrong? Here are the 4 tests that give you the real story 437

Chapter 4: Turn back the hands of time with testosterone. Powerful hormone helps you lose weight, lower blood sugar, and build strength...in and out of the bedroom! 443

Chapter 5: Feeling fat? Irritable? No sex drive? "Female" hormone is wrecking your health—here are 3 ways to beat it 449

Chapter 6: Detect and reduce your prostate cancer
risk with these simple steps 457

Part XII: Essential Health Secrets

Chapter 1: Keep killer stress at bay for mere pennies
a day using this one simple vitamin secret 465

Chapter 2: Hidden heavy metal exposure could be killing you! 469

Chapter 3: Soothing Solutions for Anxiety 471

Chapter 4: No more needles, no more waiting...
Four life-saving health tests you can do at home! 473

Chapter 5: That supplement or detox may be making
you miserable—but don't panic! Power through the
darkest hours to get to the dawn of good health 477

Chapter 6: Stop marinating in your own toxins!
Cleanse your system... and look and feel better...
with this crazy bedroom trick 483

Chapter 7: Send UTIs packing with this simple sugar secret 489

Chapter 8: Medical foods: The natural health revolution
that even the mainstream can buy into 493

Chapter 9: Send those winter blues packing with
this amazing vitamin cure 497

Alternative Health Resources 503

References 505

PART I

Cancer

Chapter 1:

Prevent and beat prostate cancer with this powerful— and proven—plant pigment

Prostate cancer is on the rise. More men are being diagnosed with it, and more men are dying from it. In 2014 it was responsible for an estimated 29,480 deaths in the U.S. alone.

But today, I want to share with you my research on a remarkable, yet common, natural substance that can both *treat* and *prevent* prostate cancer.

Quercetin is a plant pigment that belongs to a group of compounds called flavonoids. Flavonoids are a type of polyphenol, the most prevalent group of substances found in the plant world. Polyphenols give plants their bright colors, fragrances and unique tastes.

Polyphenols put up a fight against cancer

While *all* of nature's polyphenols have shown some anti-cancer (and cancer-fighting) activity, you no doubt have heard of only a few of them. Curcumin (turmeric), resveratrol and plant tannins—which have been found in a number of studies to help prevent diseases, including cancer—

often make splashy headlines. But among the polyphenols, quercetin has been one of the *most* studied, and yet somehow overlooked.

Polyphenols protect plants from the harmful effects of ultraviolet radiation from the atmosphere, environmental pollutants and diseases. They all share a chemical structure in common called a benzene ring that can ward off or interfere with the growth and spread of these environmental dangers. And the souped-up activity of these rings (known as "volatility" in the chemistry world) is exactly what gives the plants their unique flavors, odors and colors.

Quercetin causes cancer cells to commit suicide

In March of 2015, a review published in the journal *Oncology Reports* chronicled the dozens of published studies on quercetin and prostate cancer. The researchers concluded that both in vitro and in vivo studies have proven that quercetin "effectively inhibits prostate cancer via various mechanisms."

They noted that human clinical trials have shown promising results, and that animal studies even suggest that the powerful flavonoid has a "chemopreventive effect." In other words, quercetin may be able to prevent, or slow, the development of prostate cancer.

So let's take a look at how this plant pigment accomplishes this incredible feat.

Our immune systems react to cancer cell invasions by sending out messages that promote inflammation. Inflammation gets a bad rap, but it's not *all* bad. Its purpose is to bring immune cells to the area where they're needed. Unfortunately, however, it *also* promotes tissue damage. And in the cancer cell, pro-inflammatory messengers stimulate growth, and slow down their natural death process.

Much like the Borg of old *Star Trek* shows, cancer cells need to be in constant communication with one another, and there are signaling pathways within the cancer cells to accomplish this. One of the main growth stimulating signals used by cancer cells triggers a pathway called STAT3 (signal transducer and activator of transcription 3). Many flavonoids and other natural polyphenols fight cancer by blocking this STAT3 pathway, but few do this as effectively as quercetin.

According to a March 2015 study, quercetin blocks an important messenger called IL-6 (Interleukin 6). IL-6 is a good guy or a bad guy depending on the situation. But in the case of cancer IL-6 is *generally* a bad guy since (among other things) it activates the STAT3 pathway which encourages tumors to grow.

This study showed that quercetin inhibits IL-6, which in turn shuts down the STAT3 pathway. The result? The cancer cells can't grow, and instead they essentially commit suicide in a process in medicine known as apoptosis!

Another inflammatory messenger that helps stimulate prostate (and other) cancer growth is called NF kappaB. A number of studies have shown that quercetin, and its polyphenol relatives, *block* NF kappaB, but one in vitro study is particularly exciting. This 2011 study used an extract of Brazilian propolis, that nearly magical nutrient-rich substance produced by bees to repair their hives. (I'm an amateur beekeeper so anything involving these fascinating creatures captures my attention). Quercetin extracted from the propolis had inhibited the NF kappaB in prostate cancer cells causing them to… you guessed it… commit suicide.

Nutrients in produce partner up against cancer

Our immune systems are constantly vigilant against cells which might be turning cancerous. Your body uses the nutrients and chemicals found in fresh fruits and vegetables, quercetin among them, to fight against cancer. They turn off inflammation, block the growth and development of potential cancer cells, and trigger the apoptosis of existing cancer cells before they can do damage. In one 2014 study using a rat model of prostate cancer, quercetin was shown to slow down or stop the growth of prostate cancer cells by FIVE different mechanisms!

Quercetin doesn't occur by itself in nature. Flavonoids and other polyphenols work as partners to supply those captivating tastes and smells, as well as cancer-fighting activity.

Several recent studies have demonstrated that quercetin with green tea extract can be even more effective than either alone, and others have looked at quercetin combined with the soy flavone genistein. All combinations have shown positive activity against prostate cancer.

Beef up cancer-fighting benefits with a supplement

One of the great things about quercetin, and other polyphenols, is how abundant in nature they are. If you eat a diet rich in fresh fruits and vegetables (as you should, for many reasons) you're already consuming quercetin.

Foods particularly rich in this miraculous substance include...

- capers
- berries
- onions
- various salad greens
- quinoa and
- buckwheat

Grapes and red wine are good sources too, but even an apple contains about 10 mg of quercetin if you leave the skin on.

In order to get the *full* health benefit, though, it's probably necessary to take a quercetin supplement. Most studies use levels of the flavonoid that are higher than we can get with diet alone. And when you're taking polyphenols as supplements (whether it's quercetin, resveratrol, green tea extract etc.) it's especially important to choose a high quality product and not just the cheapest one available.

Remember, these are highly active antioxidant and anti-inflammatory compounds, and if they're not processed properly they will easily break down in the capsule and not give you the full benefit of their amazing cancer-fighting powers.

Chapter 2:

Hybridized mushroom extract destroys cancer cells and provides powerful immune protection

By: Michele Cagan, Health Sciences Institute

Until now, the only way to get access to this remarkable immune booster was to live in Japan. For the last five years in Japan, people with cancer, AIDS, and other life-threatening illnesses—as well as healthy people who want to stay that way—have been revving up their immune systems, destroying tumor cells, and preventing cancer and other illnesses with a powerful extract called AHCC (activated hexose correlate compound). Now, AHCC is available to consumers in the United States.

AHCC is an extract of a unique hybridization of several kinds of medicinal mushrooms known for their immune-enhancing abilities. On their own, each mushroom has a long medical history in Japan, where their extracts are widely prescribed by physicians. But when combined into a single hybrid mushroom, the resulting active ingredient is so potent that dozens of rigorous scientific studies have now established AHCC to be one of the world's most powerful—and safe—immune stimulators.

In vitro animal and human studies confirm that AHCC effectively works against and, in some cases, even prevents the recurrence of liver cancer, prostate cancer, ovarian cancer, multiple myeloma, breast cancer, AIDS, and other life-threatening conditions, with no dangerous side effects. In smaller doses, AHCC can also boost the immune function of healthy people, helping to prevent infections and promote well-being.

Calling up your first line of defense

Our immune systems stand between us and the rest of the world. Without it, our bodies would be overrun by bacteria, viruses, parasites, fungi, and other invaders, infections would rapidly spread, and cancer cells would proliferate. Like a highly responsive and well-coordinated army, our immune systems are composed of a variety of specialized immune cells that identify, seek out, and destroy microbes, pathogens, and tumor cells.

First on the scene of possible trouble are the phagocytes and natural killer (NK) cells, which respond quickly to potential threats. Often referred to as the body's "front-line of defense," these cells are constantly on the lookout for any suspicious substances. NK cells latch onto the surface of substances or the outer membranes of cancer cells and inject a chemical hand grenade (called a granule) into the interior. Once inside, the granules explode and destroy the bacteria or cancer cell within five minutes. Itself undamaged, the NK cell then moves onto its next victim. In its prime, a NK cell can take on two cancer cells at the same time, speeding up the process.

Recent research shows that as we age, our immune systems function less efficiently. In particular, the ability of our NK cells to respond quickly and effectively declines with age and illness. When NK cells lose their ability to recognize or destroy invaders, health can deteriorate rapidly. Moderately low to dangerously low NK cell activity levels have been found in people with AIDS, cancer, immune deficiency, liver disorders, various infections, and other diseases. Because measurements of NK cell activity are closely correlated with one's chances of survival, anything that helps increase NK cell activity may help people treat, recover from, and/ or prevent these illnesses.

Research finds remarkable immune system boost in multiple ways

Scientific studies of the extract AHCC, published in respected peer-reviewed journals such as *International Journal of Immunology*, *Anti-Cancer Drugs*, and *Society of Natural Immunity*, have established the health benefits and safety of AHCC more conclusively than nearly any other natural supplement. What is especially remarkable about AHCC is that it consistently and effectively boosts immune system function. Specifically, AHCC:

- Stimulates cytokine (IL-2, IL-12, TNF, and INF) production, which stimulates immune function.

- Increases NK cell activity against diseased cells as much as 300 percent.

- Increases the formation of explosive granules within NK cells. The more ammunition each NK cell carries, the more invaders it can destroy.

- Increases the number and the activity of lymphocytes, specifically increasing T-cells up to 200 percent.

- Increases Interferon levels, which inhibits the replication of viruses and stimulates NK cell activity.

- Increases the formation of TNF, a group of proteins that help destroy cancer cells.

These dramatic immune effects translate into profound health benefits. A 1995 clinical trial reported in the *International Journal of Immunotherapy* showed that 3 grams of AHCC per day significantly lowered the level of tumor markers found in patients with prostate cancer, ovarian cancer, multiple myeloma, and breast cancer. This study documented complete remissions in six of 11 patients and significant increases in NK cell activity in nine of 11 patients. T- and B-cell activity levels also rose considerably.

AHCC now available in the United States

After years of successful use in Japan, AHCC is available in the United States as the active ingredient in a product called ImmPower. Distributed by The Harmony Company, ImmPower comes in gelatin capsules containing 500mg of AHCC (proprietary blend).

ImmPower can be taken in preventive or therapeutic doses and should be discussed with your personal physician. For prevention, the recommended dose is 1 gram per day taken as one 500mg capsule in the morning and again at night. This dose will help increase NK cell activity and support immune system functioning for good health and general well-being. For those with cancer, AIDS, or other life-threatening conditions, the research indicates a therapeutic dose of two capsules in the morning, two at mid-day and two at night for a total of 3 grams per day to jump start NK cell activity. After three weeks, the dose can be reduced to 1 gram per day (one capsule in the morning and one at night), to maintain the increased NK cell activity level.

Chapter 3:

Natural 4-ingredient "herbal cocktail" could be the key to avoiding THIS deadly cancer

If there's one thing I've learned throughout my career, it's that inflammation is one of the most significant causes of literally hundreds of diseases.

And that's why when a patient comes to see me, I always start by testing their immune systems, which is where inflammation begins. I've always run these tests to get a better picture of my patients' overall health. But along the way, I've discovered something remarkable.

A common immune system test can produce an early warning signal that you may be about to develop multiple myeloma, a dangerous type of bone cancer. But here's the good news—once you learn you're at risk, you can use my powerful, four-ingredient herbal cocktail to help prevent the cancer from ever taking hold.

Antibodies hold a cancer secret

Before I tell you about the test I'm using—and how it may help predict multiple myeloma—it's important to understand how your immune system works.

Your immune system kicks into action whenever a harmful substance (known as an antigen) enters your body. Some common antigens are viruses, parasites and bacteria.

Plasma cells, lymphocytes in your bone marrow, start producing proteins called antibodies or immunoglobulins in response to the antigen.

These immunoglobulins are like the first responders at an accident. They neutralize the invading antigen, attach themselves to it to identify what the antigen is, and trigger your immune system to take additional steps.

Every antigen has a specific corresponding antibody or immunoglobulin. And each of those immunoglobulins falls into four basic types...

- *Immunoglobulin M* (IgM) is the first to respond to illness.
- *Immunoglobulin G* (IgG) is the main antibody of the immune proteins.
- *Immunoglobulin A* (IgA) is the immune protein that covers the mucous membrane linings including the digestive tract, sinuses and breathing passages.
- *Immunoglobulin E* (IgE) is the main responder in allergic reactions.

The immunofixation (or immunoglobulin) assay blood test measures the levels of the individual *components* in these antibody proteins, making it a great place to start when evaluating a person's health and immune system response.

Because I run the immunofixation test on most of my patients, I tend to spot some abnormalities that other doctors often don't.

One of those abnormalities is when a plasma cell produces one immunoglobulin out of proportion to the others, a condition known as monoclonal gammopathy of undetermined significance, or MGUS for short.

Up to 25% of MGUS sufferers develop cancer

MGUS isn't common, but it's not rare either. It occurs in around 1 percent of the general population, and increases to 3 percent in people over age 70. MGUS doesn't cause any symptoms, so unless you were tested you'd never know you had it.

But in 20-25 percent of people with MGUS, the plasma cell protein continues growing until it begins to interfere with the production of *other* cells in the bone marrow. This is called multiple myeloma, and it's one of the most insidious and dangerous of all cancers.

Many doctors—hematologists and oncologists included—will tell a patient with MGUS not to worry about the finding and to simply "watch and wait." Well I don't know about you, but sitting around waiting for an accident to potentially happen just isn't my style.

I'm more of an action kind of guy, which is why I began researching ways to slow down or halt the development of multiple myeloma. And as a result I've developed a natural, four-ingredient protocol designed to react to MGUS and help mount a defense against the development of this deadly cancer.

Herbal ingredient #1: *Berberine* is a powerful multitasking herb that can help control blood sugar, fight off bacteria and, it appears, help fight off cancer. In fact, there are literally hundreds of scientific articles in the literature documenting the effects of berberine on malignant cells.[1]

This remarkable compound interferes with the signaling mechanisms of cancer cells, triggering the cells to essentially commit suicide in a process known as apoptosis. In one in vitro study using myeloma cells, berberine was found to hasten cell death by actually changing the DNA of the cancer cell, causing an important form of metabolism in the cells to slow down.[2]

Berberine supplements are available online and in health food stores.

Herbal ingredient #2: *Proteolytic enzymes* such as bromelain which comes from pineapple, and enzymes derived from papaya and the mold aspergillus (as well as the pancreatic enzymes trypsin, chymotrypsin and papain) are proven cancer fighters with a growing stack of research behind them. In fact there's so much evidence for their use in preventing and treating cancer that an entire issue of the journal *Integrative Cancer Therapies* was devoted to the topic.[3]

However research has shown that one enzyme preparation in particular, Wobe-Mugos which combines the proteolytic enzymes papain (100 mg), trypsin (40 mg), and chymotrypsin (40 mg), could help increase survival times, slow the spread of cancer and lead to fewer cancer symptoms overall.

The supplement has also been shown to have a positive effect on patients undergoing chemotherapy or radiation. In one randomized study multiple myeloma patients who received Wobe-Mugos with their chemotherapy treatments lived almost twice as long as the group on chemotherapy alone.[4]

The evidence behind Wobe-Mugos is so impressive that the FDA actually began the process of licensing the supplement as an orphan drug for treating multiple myeloma. But licensing negotiations with the German manufacturer broke down (with I suspect some heavy pressure from the U.S. drug industry), and the planned study... and the FDA's endorsement... were soon squashed.

But the fact remains that enzyme therapies are highly effective and they have become a standard treatment in my own practice for MGUS and multiple myeloma. If you find it difficult to find Wobe-Mugos here in the US talk with your doctor about other proteolytic enzyme preparations that would make a good substitute.

Herbal ingredient #3: There are literally thousands of published studies on using curcumin—extracted from the common kitchen herb turmeric—to prevent and treat cancer. In one randomized, double-blind, crossover study published in the *American Journal of Hematology*, researchers gave MGUS patients, or patients with a related condition called SMM (smoldering multiple myeloma), either 4 gm of curcumin or a placebo for four months.[5] Some patients were then studied for longer, using 8 gm of curcumin.

There were significantly fewer cases of the condition turning into multiple myeloma in those who received the curcumin, as well as an improvement in other factors like bone resorption and kidney function. The authors concluded that "… curcumin might have the potential to slow the disease process in patients with MGUS and SMM."

You can pick up curcumin supplements just about anywhere.

Herbal ingredient #4: *Baicalin*, an extract of scuttelaria (skullcap) is a flavonoid, and comes from the large group of plant-derived chemicals called polyphenols. Research shows that the herbal extract can interfere with cancer cell growth.

Baicalin seems particularly effective at targeting blood-based malignancies such as multiple myeloma. A recent review of baicalin's effects on myeloma cells highlighted the herbal extract's ability to slow the growth of myeloma cells and hasten their death.[6] Baicalin powders are available online and in some health food stores.

Put the brakes on cancer

While more clinical research is needed, there's already plenty of evidence that the four safe, natural ingredients in my "MGUS Cocktail" could put the brakes on this condition, helping to prevent it from ever turning into a full-blown case of multiple myeloma.

If you've been diagnosed with MGUS, or if you're *already* fighting cancer and want to enhance your treatment, talk with your own doctor about how these herbal interventions might be able to help.

Chapter 4:

New science proves you can make your body cancer-proof!

Is everything the mainstream has been telling us about cancer *completely wrong?*

For years we've been told that getting cancer was a matter of bad luck of bad genes—just an unfortunate roll of the dice. And the mainstream's answer has been to make billions by trying to detect cancer early, instead of stopping it in the first place.

But an amazing new study is setting the entire cancer industry on its ear—and it just may hold the key to saving your life.

In the December edition of the journal *Nature,* researchers from Stony Brook University confirmed that almost all cancers are caused by outside factors that you can CHANGE or even FIX.

That means that you don't ever have to be doomed to a cancer diagnosis or sickening and dangerous treatments like radiation and chemotherapy. And by understanding—and eliminating—some common causes of cancer, you can actually stop the disease from ever taking hold.

The avoidable toxins that are giving you cancer

The Stony Brook researchers' conclusion that the majority of cancers are caused by "external factors, such as environmental toxins, behaviors, and infections" shouldn't come as too big of a surprise.

The mainstream has sung its old song forever about how only a handful of cancers—like lung cancer caused by cigarette smoking—are triggered by external toxins. But if you do the research, the shocking truth is that almost every major chemical or heavy metal that we are exposed to is definitively linked to some type of cancer. Multiple medical studies have been published that link each of the hundreds of toxins that you can be exposed to a respective cancer or cancers.[1, 2, 3]

In fact, in May of 2010, the President's Cancer Panel warned President Obama in a letter along with a comprehensive report that "the true burden of environmentally induced cancers has been grossly underestimated."[4]

So with so much evidence, how can such a discord still exist?

Because the carcinogenic toxic exposure is almost always at a low level over a prolonged period of time—and not a high contamination state of emergency.

According to these reports, there is growing scientific evidence that exposure to LOWER levels of chemicals in the general environment is contributing to society's growing cancer burden.

Of course, this should come as no shock to you—the story of low level toxic burdens has even hit the Hollywood studios. Ever seen the movie *Erin Brockovich* about cancer caused by hexavalent chromium in water? A documentary film from 2013, *Unacceptable Levels*, also explores this issue—and watching it can be a good wake-up call, if you're not already worried about what the environment is doing to your body.

Cancer can be brought on by a nasty bug

The *Nature* study also admitted that infections can be a root cause of cancer. We already know that Human Papilloma Virus (HPV) can cause cervical cancer AND some head and neck cancers. The Hepatitis C virus can cause liver cancer, and the Epstein-Barr virus can cause some forms of lymphoma, a type of blood cancer that develops in the body's lymphatic system. And the *Helicobacter pylori* bacteria (H. pylori) has been shown to cause stomach cancer.

Because these are known and accepted root causes of cancer, your conventional doctor is probably willing to screen and treat you for these infections. But the somber truth is: there are many OTHER stealth bacterial and viral infections that can bring on that dreaded "C word" diagnosis...that doctors AREN'T testing for...or treating.

A wonderful synopsis of this topic published in the *Journal of Translational Medicine* in 2006 shines light on the various studies that show the multitude of cancers with infectious causes, including:[5]

- Some gallbladder cancers and salmonella

- Lung cancer and Chlamydial pneumonias

- Colon cancer and at least three different bacterial infections

In fact, a study published in a urology journal showed a strong connection between the inflammation caused by a certain virus in certain patients and prostate cancer.[6]

There are even reports about certain PARASITES causing bladder and bile duct cancer.[7]

You've got to be strong enough to fight what ails you

So it sounds pretty obvious, right? Identify the cancer-causing bacteria and viruses (or parasites), treat the infection when it occurs, and avoid cancer. But conventional doctors continue to miss the boat and ignore infections as a potential sources of cancer because they actually need to look *beyond* the infectious agents themselves when identifying the true root cause.

It's most likely the strength of your immune system—and not the infection itself—which is the root cause of the cancer.

That means that while killing the infection is important, it might quickly return and continue to wreak havoc...*if your immune system is weak*. Holistic cancer regimens therefore focus on bolstering the patient's immune system—which is the opposite of mainstream protocol, chemotherapy, which is guaranteed to LOWER your immune system.

That's why garlic can be an amazing food and supplement. Its germicidal properties can help boost your immune system[8]—which is probably why it's been touted for so many generations to be a potent treatment for cancer and other diseases.

And now there's scientific data to back up what might be dismissed as just a "wives' tale"—that a high intake of dietary garlic lowers the rate of stomach and colon cancers. Even the National Cancer Institute has gotten on the garlic bandwagon and recommended the pungent vegetable for its anti-cancer properties.[9] (Not to mention it tastes great when mixed into your stir-fry or rubbed on your favorite meat.)

Cancer isn't something that just happens to you

Despite the overwhelming evidence that cancer is NOT just a matter of "*C'est la vie*," many doctors aren't screening for environmental factors like toxins OR heavy metals in your body. They also aren't screening for most of these infectious agents or even treating you if you do come up with a hint of an infection.

If you want to make sure the odds are stacked in your favor to remain cancer-free, change your "luck" by switching to a holistic doctor. He'll work with you to reduce your toxic load in your home or work environment, find and reduce the toxins that have worked their way into your body, strengthen your immune system, and test and kill potential infections that you could be harboring—and keep them from coming back.

Chapter 5:

Fight aging, cell damage, Alzheimer's and even cancer with this powerful plant secret

Imagine, you're home after a long day of hitting the links. You've got a glass of red wine in your hand and a bowl of peanuts in front of you.

Well, it turns out that while you're kicking back and enjoying some well-deserved "me" time, you're also doing something incredibly important for your health.

You're protecting yourself from cancer...sharpening your brain against Alzheimer's...turning back the clock on your heart health...and even managing your weight.

No, your imagination isn't playing tricks on you. It's all true—and it's all thanks to a remarkable compound called resveratrol.

Resveratrol first came to popular attention in the 1980s because scientists had noted that French people had particularly low rates of cardiovascular disease—despite their habit of "living the good life," like eating high saturated fats and drinking lots of Bordeaux and Burgundy.

They called this phenomenon the "French paradox."

So, scientists began to credit a compound in red grapes, wine, and nuts called resveratrol for protecting the people of France from heart disease—and since then, this amazing substance has been investigated thoroughly.

Resveratrol is produced by certain plants in nature to protect them from stressors—fungus growth, disease, weather events—much like how our immune system protects us. Therefore, it has both antifungal and antibiotic properties—but it's resveratrol's antioxidant and anti-inflammatory activities that gives it such broad-ranging functions.

It's classified as a polyphenol, which means it's responsible for taste, color, and smell in the plant world.

And there's lots that resveratrol can do for *humans*, too.

Based on scores of studies and some enlightening research, resveratrol can protect your heart, kidneys and brain...work throughout your central nervous system...and even zero in on your DNA.

And best of all, it can even keep you younger—longer!

Ten times the protection

Recent experiments on mice have shown that resveratrol can trigger protective activity in cardiovascular cells by stimulating the production of a protein called SIRT1.[1] Just one of the "Sirtuins" group of proteins, SIRT1 is responsible for keeping cells working longer and better.

And resveratrol can stimulate the production of SIRT1 by *up to 10 times!*

Other animal studies have shown that resveratrol can lower blood pressure and improve cholesterol levels, heart function, and blood flow.

In one rat study, resveratrol was shown to a lower blood pressure and slow the progression of hypertension by affecting the genes involved with angiotensin II production—which is exactly the target for most blood pressure medications.[2]

In other rat studies, high-dose resveratrol has also improved blood pressure as well as cholesterol levels, ventricular function,[3] and even cardiac hypertrophy, a condition in which the heart muscle thickens and shrinks the size of the heart's chamber.[4]

In patients who'd had a heart attack, resveratrol was found to improve the strength by which the heart pumps its blood and to reduce dangerous LDL cholesterol levels.[5]

Resveratrol has also been shown to reduce the size and density of the plaques that harden the arteries, in a condition known as atherosclerosis. Based on those same animal studies, scientists have theorized that this miracle substance suppresses the molecules that help substances in the blood stick to each other (like cholesterol, fat, and calcium)—and to the artery walls.

This is exciting research, since the lessening of platelet stickiness and clumping is a goal of many cardiovascular treatments in humans. Even more encouraging is that in one population study, resveratrol had a significantly positive effect on platelet clumping even in high-risk cardiac patients with aspirin resistance.[6]

Banish inflammation and prevent kidney damage

Traveling down the body from the heart, we reach another area where resveratrol also has a remarkable role to play: the kidneys.

A number of studies involving different kidney-related illnesses—from diabetes to chemical damage to the kidneys—have demonstrated antioxidant and anti-inflammatory activity of resveratrol. And this brings us back to that protective protein I mentioned earlier, SIRT1. By activating the production of SIRT1, resveratrol can also reduce inflammation, which can ward off kidney damage AND kidney failure.

Resveratrol seems to work by lowering the levels of two inflammatory markers, TNF-alpha and TGF-beta. That, in turn, reduces the production of the dangerous molecules that are associated with oxidative stress, known as "reactive oxygen species" (or ROS for short).

It's that oxidative stress that can damage your kidneys and even cause them to fail.

Amazingly, resveratrol's kidney benefits don't end there. In animal models, resveratrol has been shown to protect kidney function in cases of acute injury through fibrosis by lowering the effect of certain proteins—called ECM (for "extracellular matrix")—which can deteriorate the kidney tissue.[7]

The lessening of those ROS molecules and ECM proteins also seems to diminish the damage from kidney stones. Not only that, but it also seems to help prevent kidney stones from forming in the first place!

That may be enough reason to raise a glass to resveratrol, but I'm not done yet.

Keep your blood sugar—and your weight—from spiking

What resveratrol can do for parts of your body, such as your heart and kidneys, is downright remarkable. But equally as impressive is its apparent effect on the *processes* of your body.

Take, for instance, metabolism. Multiple studies of animals (and some on humans) have demonstrated that resveratrol can improve insulin sensitivity...and even promote weight loss.

In one double-blind, placebo-controlled study, a small dose of resveratrol—just 10 mg—was given to patients with type 2 diabetes. Amazingly, their blood glucose was lowered—and their blood sugar spiked (say, after a meal) to a lesser extent than the control group.[8]

Results from other clinical trials have suggested a lower average blood sugar by reducing levels of hemoglobin A1c, which binds to glucose in the blood. So, less hemoglobin A1c means lower blood sugar.

As you know, controlling your blood sugar goes hand-in-hand with managing your weight and preventing diabetes damage—so it's no surprise that resveratrol can actually reduce belly fat (in one study on mice, by as much as 33 percent) and even improve metabolic syndrome.[9]

Resveratrol has even been shown to boost metabolism, right in your brain cells![10]

Keep your brain cells intact and your mind razor sharp

Resveratrol's ability to control and squelch free radical activity is largely responsible for all its positive effects in the body, however, nowhere is this more important than the central nervous system.

The structures of your central nervous system—that is, your brain and spinal cord—have a particularly high rate of metabolism and oxygen needs. The faster the metabolism, the more reactive oxygen species are produced. In addition, heavy metals like iron can store in the brain and act as irritants to create ROS as well.

The central nervous system is particularly susceptible to oxidation because of its high fat content—and as we age, we're exposed to more and more ROS.

And the older you are, the harder your brain needs to work to counteract that oxidative stress.

Sometimes, your brain just can't work hard enough on its own to completely avoid damage and disease. It needs a little help.

Perhaps the most exciting therapeutic application of resveratrol is its effect on neurodegenerative diseases—particularly ALS, Parkinson's, and Alzheimer's disease—since they're thought to be the result of oxidative stress on the brain, leading to the development of senile plaques and neurofibrillary tangles.

Although we're not clear yet on the *exact* mechanisms involved, we know this process it has *something* to do with tau proteins. Tau proteins are found in abundance in the neurons of everyone's brains; but when they undergo a process called "acetylation," they begin to collect and "stick" together (much like the sticky platelets as found in atherosclerosis, as mentioned earlier).[11] In aggregate, these proteins can lead to the development of the neurofibrillary tangles (or NFT's) that are commonly found in the brains of Alzheimer's patients.

Resveratrol can actually counteract the acetylation of those tau proteins in the brain. It can prevent the degeneration of the nervous system by activating the anti-inflammatory SIRT1 proteins and reducing the activity of the cell-damaging ROS.[12]

Yes, this same process also occurs in the brain—with *equally protective* benefits!

And this doesn't only apply to Alzheimer's disease. Parkinson's disease, for example, is an illness in which inflammatory messengers seem to be involved, leading to:

- increased activity of the "glial cells" that surround and support neurons,

- deposits of a protein called alpha synuclein,

- and eventual damage to dopamine-containing brain cells.

In all, there are at least SEVEN known pathways of messaging that can go awry, leading to Parkinson's-like symptoms and full-blown Parkinson's disease—and resveratrol is known to have a modifying effect on ALL of them.

For instance, resveratrol has been found to quiet down the glial cell activation and inflammation in animal studies[13] and improve function—even after Parkinson's-like symptoms had already emerged.[14]

Of course, human studies are still lacking in the field, but the body of evidence from animal and laboratory studies is fairly strong.

The same goes for ALS, a.k.a. Lou Gehrig's disease. In this fast-progressing disease, motor nerves are lost throughout the nervous system.

There's no cure, but findings from animal studies suggest that resveratrol might be useful in its prevention and treatment—especially since ALS is associated with:

- high levels of oxidative stress,

- aberrant calcium metabolism

- elevated levels of the neurotransmitter glutamate in the brain.

Resveratrol has been shown to work on all three of these mechanisms, by:

- preventing and reducing oxidation

- keeping calcium down

- buffering the damage caused by a glutamate buildup and the resulting flood of messages that overwhelms and damages brain cells.

And, as previously noted, the SIRT1 that's activated by resveratrol also decreases the brain damage associated with ALS symptoms.

Kill and shrink tumors, and stop them from forming

The power of resveratrol extends beyond those diseases of the brain—because this remarkable molecule also seems to fight cancer.

Now, this is true for many of the micronutrients known as polyphenols. As a class—particularly with their anti-inflammatory properties—they seem to limit the growth and spreading of cancerous cells and therefore limit the development of cancer.

While there aren't a great many human studies yet to support this theory, there are a lot of *in vitro* and animal studies which outline and support a role for resveratrol in cancer therapy and prevention.[15]

In both human and animal studies, resveratrol has appeared to stop colon cancer in its tracks—before it even starts! For example, in one rat study, resveratrol appeared to stop colon cells from developing into cancer by preventing the formation of abnormal glands called aberrant crypt foci (ACF) in the lining of the colon and rectum.[16] ACF can appear even before colorectal polyps—which are usually the first sign of colon cancer that patients (and doctors) ever notice.

ACF can be particularly scary—and dangerous—because, like tumors, they're resistant to the natural cycle of cells dying off (or, committing "suicide"), called apoptosis.

Finally, in a human study, the group treated with resveratrol was found to have a reduced gene expression of the type that leads to cancerous transformation of cells.

This cancer-preventing compound has also been shown in the laboratory to slow down the formation of other gastrointestinal tumors—and by *as much as 70 percent* in one mouse study![17] It does this partially by maximizing the power of the body's immune system—for example, by activating the body's own cancer-killing cells, called cytotoxic T cells.

Lab studies has shown that resveratrol has antitumor effects, anti-inflammatory effects, and apoptosis-promoting activity in cases of pancreatic cancer[18] and liver cancer, where laboratory mice showed a 25 percent decrease in tumor cell content of their livers as a result of resveratrol therapy.[19]

Resveratrol even slows the progression of hepatitis B to liver cancer.[20]

In the case of prostate cancer, resveratrol seems to help prevent it by regulating the enzymes involved in its development, called extracellular regulating kinases (ERK).[21]

Resveratrol has also been shown to slow the growth of prostate cancer cells, and multiple animal studies have demonstrated that it also can stimulate the suicide of cancer cells...and only cancer cells.

That's like the holy grail of cancer therapy research!

Even more encouraging is that an increase in apoptosis has been seen in breast tumors treated with resveratrol as well.[22]

In fact, resveratrol has shown much promise in both the prevention AND the treatment of breast cancers. It seems to interfere with the ability of cancerous cells to form new blood vessels to carry supplies and nourishment to the tumor—which can stop tumor growth in its tracks. This process, known as anti-angiogenesis, is a valued activity of an anti-cancer medication.

But the proof, as they say, is in the pudding: Breast tumors decreased both in SIZE and in NUMBER in experimental laboratory mice that were given resveratrol. They also showed a downregulation of the HER2 gene mutation that promotes cancer cell growth and can develop into more aggressive types of breast cancer.[23]

Resveratrol has also been shown to lower levels of two enzymes involved in the metastasis of tumors in cases of breast cancer, called MMP-9 and COX-2.[24]

Some study authors have also suggested that resveratrol may act similarly to the estrogen-blocking medications often prescribed to breast cancer patients receiving hormone therapy, like tamoxifen.[25] Blocking estrogen can be an important part of the treatment of breast cancer, since some breast cancer tumor cells NEED estrogen to grow.

That's not to say that resveratrol could replace mainstream cancer therapies *altogether*—but some research does suggest that resveratrol could be used with other treatments.

In studies of non-small cell lung cancer (with a very poor prognosis), resveratrol actually enhanced the value of radiation therapy by stimulating apoptosis and slowing the formation of dangerous oxidizing substances in the tissues.[26]

When resveratrol has been combined with the chemotherapy drug 5-fluorouracil in mice, it helped prevent the onset of severe side effects.[27]

Find your fountain of youth in a bottle of red

Now, resveratrol can do something else, too...that you can't see or feel...deep inside your cells.

Studies show it can actually protect your DNA—and that, my friend, can help you live longer.

Longevity is generally associated with a substance at the end of your chromosomes called "telomeres." You want those telomeres to stay long, because the shorter your telomeres, the shorter your lifespan.

Our bodies have some protective mechanisms to ensure that telomeres don't become shorter—including producing an anti-aging substance called "telomere maintenance factors." And guess what? In a lab, resveratrol has been shown to stimulate the production of it.[28]

Shorter telomeres don't just mean you won't live as long. In the nervous system, they're associated with age-related diseases like Alzheimer's because of an abnormally increased apoptosis of nerve cells.

Now, while *some* cell death is normal by the body's natural processes, too many nerve cells dying off can be a sign of damaged DNA. Your telomeres specifically can be damaged by ROS and environmental toxins—but resveratrol can protect against that damage by transferring electrons to free radicals and rendering them harmless.

Believe it or not, these aren't even ALL the benefits that we can derive from this blessing given to us by the plant world! I've seen it prevent arthritis pain and lessen the pain of fibromyalgia.

Live your own "French paradox"

Resveratrol is actually produced in nature by a variety of plants, including grapes, peanuts, and berries.

Because it's present in greater concentrations in the rigid parts of a plant (like stems, bark, and shells), the process of mashing everything up like you would in producing wine leads to a higher concentration of resveratrol than peanuts. But it's only present in wines made from *red* grapes (and that include the grape skins in the winemaking process), so uncorking that Chardonnay won't do you much good.

Fortunately, wine isn't your only option when it comes to getting the age-defying, cancer-preventing, heart healthy benefits of this remarkable natural cure.

Instead, you could sip on some unsweetened, organic red or purple grape juice...or even grab some red grapes. A cup of red grapes has about the same amount of resveratrol as about three glasses of red wine—but with more fiber, and no alcohol.

You could also snack on some *boiled* peanuts, which contain even more resveratrol than red grapes—and more than raw peanuts or sugary peanut butter. (That's because they're cooked with the shells, where resveratrol is found in highest concentrations).

And finally, to take advantage of that "French paradox" for yourself for just pennies a day, you can pick up resveratrol supplements pretty affordable just about anywhere.

Chapter 6:

Become practically invincible to major diseases like cancer, Alzheimer's, and shingles

What if I told you that you could ward off cancer, Alzheimer's, shingles, and potentially many more diseases by doing something that takes just seconds and costs just pennies a day?

It's becoming incredibly apparent that weakened immune systems are the root cause of many diseases, and that supporting your immune system with daily supplements can prevent them.

But conventional doctors are so focused on treating the symptoms of diseases rather than their root causes that they're "missing the boat"!

And as a result, you're getting sick, when you don't have to.

Back in the late 1800's, there was a famous debate between two heavyweight scientists that, to me, clearly illustrates the divide between the conventional and integrative medical communities.

The famous chemist and microbiologist Louis Pasteur waged a scientific debate with another famous physiologist, Claude Bernard, that still continues between the integrative medical and conventional medical doctors.

Pasteur argued that infectious organisms from the outside world attack and infect humans as foreign invaders, while Bernard felt that we "house" these bugs inside of us and that infection is a result of the immune system becoming weaker and allowing these bugs to "come out of hiding" and turn "evil."

Of course, Pasteur's germ theory is what's taught in medical school and what ultimately drives the *business* of medicine. The killing of these "foreign invaders" has become a trillion-dollar industry.

Thus, the bad news for Bernard—and the integrative medical world that agrees with him—is that Pasteur's idea is much more profitable and "headline-grabbing."

And that means there's no way that modern medicine is going to change their minds anytime soon about this debate.

But before you think that it's a lost cause, there's a fascinating twist in this story. On his deathbed, Pasteur made a profound statement: "Bernard is right. The microbe is nothing. The environment is everything."

In the end, it really doesn't matter how many bugs you have or what bugs you've been exposed to.

What really matters is how strong your immune system is... and how your body can provide an inhospitable place for infections to thrive or to replicate.

The enemy is already inside your body

We're all exposed to many infections as we live our lives—from having been around hundreds of different bacteria and viruses in our childhood school days... to our own children and grandchildren bringing infections back home from their schools.

There's also the risk of getting type 1 herpes (HSV-1) from kissing... and the multitude of sexually-transmitted diseases (like HPV) from having unprotected intercourse.

And then you may travel to foreign countries or even get bitten by different insects—and if you do get infected, the antibiotics you're given can destroy your healthy gut bacteria and leave you vulnerable to all sorts of OTHER illnesses.

It's up to our immune systems to keep all of these infections in check!

I like to think of it as keeping infectious agents behind bars. When your immune system gets weak, the tiny convicts can break out of their jail cells, run amok, and wreak havoc in the body.

When we were younger, we'd get exposed to these infections and—most of the time—our immune systems would have been strong enough to wall them off and "lock" them away for good. But as we age... or are under stress... that padlock on the jail cell door starts to loosen.

Why YOU get sick, when others don't

Believe it or not, the conventional medical community doesn't believe that we really have "jail" cells... or that the majority of infections that we've been exposed to in our lives could be locked away in those jail cells.

They still believe in the Pasteur philosophy that most of the infections are in-and-out of the system and could not reside in the body for longer than we are "sick."

They're only willing to admit to *just a handful* of viruses that can live in our bodies for our whole lives—herpes, HIV, and HPV—as well as one bacteria, H. pylori (a stomach infection).

Of course, if you ask me, Bernard *should* have been the more famous figure from that era—because it is becoming obvious that there "could" be other infections that live a long time and thus other infections that could cause other serious diseases.

But now, the data is becoming too obvious for the conventional community to ignore that simple chronic infections can cause SERIOUS diseases down the road.

The fact is, a simple case of chicken pox when you were a little kid can stay dormant in your body for many, many years—and come back as shingles, a disease that can cause permanent horrific nerve pain.

Being innocently exposed at a young age to HPV (Human Papilloma Virus) is clearly linked to cervical cancer later in life.

And as discussed earlier, new data about Alzheimer's being caused by cold sores (HSV-1) is another nail in the coffin on the Pasteur "germ" theory... and another feather in Bernard's cap.

If close to 100 percent of the current non-vaccinated adult population has had chicken pox[1]... 90 percent of Americans have been exposed to HSV-1[2,3]... and roughly 80 million Americans are currently infected with the HPV virus[4].. then how is it that only some of those people get shingles, Alzheimer's, or cervical cancer?

Isn't it obvious that the main determining factor is the health and the strength of the immune system of the person who's been exposed?

It is a known medical fact that the human immune system weakens as we age[5]—and thus, without some outside intervention, the resurgence of these infections to some degree later in life is almost inevitable.

Be good to your body, and it'll be good to you

As an integrative medical doctor on the front lines, I take care of some very "sick" patients—and I've found almost all of them to have damaged or "weak" immune systems.

Every day that goes by and the older I get, I cannot believe how true Bernard's theory was... and how far we as a medical community have diverged from it.

But I'm still optimistic. Even though Pasteur got all the headlines, I feel that Bernard's immune system philosophy will win in the long run and become the treatment of the future.

I really hope that the conventional doctors can look back upon history and consider that Bernard could have been right—and that an ounce of prevention truly is worth a pound (and maybe MORE) of cure philosophy.

But I'm not holding my breath. The answer to these issues... and the way to prove Bernard correct... doesn't really grab headlines because the modern medical world hasn't found a way to patent ways of improving the immune system.

And they probably never will.

One of the ways to get these patients better, of course, is to kill these infections—but, more importantly, we must improve their bodies' internal environments (what Bernard called the *milieu intérieur*) and bolster their immune systems.

Unfortunately, there are so many ways to improve the immune system that it would be impossible to list them all here. But the reality is that anything that you do "good" for your body will bolster your immune system... and everything you do bad for your body will weaken it.

Since a large percentage of the immune system is housed in the organs of the gut, colostrum and probiotics are big ticket items in this fight.

If I want to use the "big guns" for the immune system, I am a fan of a product called "Transfer Factor."[6]

Two oldies-but-goodies for the immune system are zinc and vitamin C. A low dose of zinc (even as low as 10 mg a day) and 1,000 mg of vitamin C should be the backbone of most peoples' regimens.

And finally, as boring as it sounds, getting good healthy sleep is paramount to allow your immune system to recharge.

Chapter 7:

Survive pancreatic cancer— and feel better—with this century-old nutritional therapy

As a doctor, I have to have difficult conversations with patients. And one of the most difficult conversations we doctors can have is when a patient has got pancreatic cancer.

It's hard to treat and hard to detect. In many cases, patients only experience symptoms *after* it's already spread—which is too late.

It's not just serious; it's one of the most lethal diseases out there. Famously, it took down *Dirty Dancing* movie star Patrick Swayze in 2009 and Apple CEO Steve Jobs in 2011.

As the third leading cause of cancer-related death, only 20 percent of pancreatic cancer patients make it past a year.[1]

And while the best way to beat pancreatic cancer is to never get it in the first place, that doesn't turn out to be very good advice if you've already got it and you've been given just months to live.

The mainstream medical community has thrown its hands up in the air when it comes to late-stage (and end-stage) pancreatic cancer, often "treating" it with toxic chemo that will only significantly worsen the patients' quality of life.

The truth is, there's really no conventional method of treating pancreatic cancer. Surgery to remove the pancreas is risky and won't do much good if the cancer has already spread. Pumping your body full of poison has not been shown improve your survival rate and will only add to your symptoms.

The integrative medical community has made tremendous strides in fighting multiple forms of cancer naturally with therapies like intravenous vitamin C, but there's another protocol that hasn't gotten much attention in recent times.

It's called enzyme therapy, and it's actually been used by physicians for over 100 years!

Long forgotten, it was reintroduced and pioneered in modern times by the late Dr. Nicholas Gonzalez as a nutritional regimen that could be used to treat advanced forms of cancer—including pancreatic.

Although studies of it have been funded by Fortune 500 companies like Procter & Gamble and Nestle,[2] it's still relegated to "new and experimental" status in the US and Britain (although it's more common in Europe and around the world).

But if you ask me, I'd rather "experiment" with nutrition—namely, diet, supplements, enzymes, and detox—than with toxic chemicals that kill everything in their wake.

The "Gonzalez Protocol" remains as an option for you if you've got cancer and—as many other cancer patients—have exhausted all other options.

The stem cell secret to cancer's spread

In brief, the theory is that enzymes called "proteases" are missing from some patients, leading to a growth of certain stem cells into cancer cells. But to really grasp it, you've got to go back to its beginnings—all the way back to the early 1900s and Dr. John Beard.

By training, Dr. Beard was an embryologist and studied stem cells called "trophoblasts" that occur in the developing fetus. Trophoblasts go on to form the placenta.

He observed that the placenta stem cells not only had an anatomical makeup that was similar to cancer cells (called anaplastic), but they also exhibited certain behaviors that are also associated with cancer cells. For example, they:

- invade the uterine tissue (to make the connection to the uterus)

- build up a vigorous blood supply to support growth (of the placenta)

- will very rapidly reproduce

- produce the hormone human chorionic gonadotropin (hCG).

And many of these conditions have been proven since![3]

As a result of his observations, Dr. Beard came to believe that cancer cells were actually trophoblast stem cells that have gone awry (in his words, cancer is "an irresponsible trophoblast").

He also noted that around day 56 of gestation, the trophoblast cells lost their "malignant" characteristics and began to behave like mature fetal cells. At the same time, the fetal pancreas began to show evidence of pancreatic enzymes being produced.

Since there seemed no reason for a fetus to develop pancreatic enzymes so early (the nourishment to the fetus has no need of digestion), he proposed that there was another reason for pancreatic enzymes: They were responsible for down-regulating the malignant nature of the trophoblast cells.

This led to his theory that pancreatic enzymes, particularly one called trypsin, could control malignancy in OTHER circumstances.

Dr. Beard's ideas about the similarity between trophoblast and cancer cells were largely forgotten after his death in 1923.

Recently, however, scientific groups (including one at the University of North Carolina and several in Europe) have actually started using placental trophoblasts as a wonderful model for the study of cancer and molecular biology.[4]

What Dr. Beard could not have known in his time was that cancer cells and placental trophoblasts use the same mechanisms to alter gene expression. They also use the same signaling mechanisms and the same substances, called "matrix metalloproteinases," to invade tissue around them.

And furthermore, researchers have been demonstrating that cancer develops from stem cells gone awry[5]—much like Dr. Beard predicted. This is contrary to the long-held belief that cancer cells are *mature* cells that have gone haywire and degenerate!

The second part of Dr. Beard's theory is also slowly being validated. We now know that, in fact, the fetal pancreas does become active at the same time as the trophoblast begins maturing into a placenta.[6]

A forgotten therapy gets a second— and third—life

So how did Dr. Gonzalez come to discover the work of Dr. Beard and decide to pursue it further?

Well, you can thank a dentist named Dr. William Kelley for that.

In the 1960s, Dr. Kelley had developed a four-part program based on Dr. Beard's ideas, which consisted of:

1. A whole foods diet

2. Nutritional supplements and glandular extracts

3. Detoxification, including daily use of coffee enemas

4. High doses of pancreatic enzymes

In the early 1980s, Dr. Gonzalez began a student project at Cornell University Medical College to review over 450 cancer patients who had done unexpectedly well on Dr. Kelley's program, under the direction of Sloan-Kettering President Dr. Robert Good (widely considered the father of modern immunology).

In 1987, he and a colleague Dr. Linda Isaacs began practicing in New York City, utilizing his own version of the four-pronged approach developed by Dr. Kelley, which included:

- pancreatic enzymes in quantity to replace the missing proteases

- animal glandular extracts and nutrients, and

- detoxification including dietary management and coffee enemas daily.

Dr. Gonzalez did make a few adjustments to Dr. Kelley's protocol, including in the type of enzyme being used. He'd discovered that it was not necessary—and, in fact, was counterproductive—to use too strong of an enzyme. He also felt that the fat content of the enzyme was critical in adding some cofactors that were synergistic to the pancreatic enzymes.

In addition, he helped to counteract the commonly held belief that proteolytic enzymes would be broken down in the stomach by hydrochloric acid and therefore not absorbable.

Dr. Beard himself felt that enzymes had to be injected to be effective; but Dr. Kelley's successes with oral enzymes convinced Dr. Gonzalez that the oral route was ultimately superior, and that the enzymes enter the body intact.[7]

In the years that followed, Dr. Gonzalez published lots of case histories showing positive effects of the protocol, even in advanced cancers[8]—and that convinced the National Cancer Institute (NCI) to perform a randomized controlled trial (RCT) comparing the Gonzalez protocol to standard chemotherapy for pancreatic cancer.

In the study, the chemotherapy drug gemcitabine was used on 126 patients with pancreatic cancer, none of whom lived beyond 19 months.

Of the 11 patients with very severe stage IV pancreatic cancer or slightly less advanced cancer receiving the Gonzalez protocol, nine lived for one year, four of them for three years and two lived beyond four years, which was unheard of in conventional treatment circles at that time.[9]

Several animal studies have also shown possibilities with this unique therapy, particularly in pancreatic cancer. In one study, utilizing the enzyme therapy on mice with pancreatic cancer, the principal investigator concluded that "PPE (porcine pancreatic enzyme) is the first experimentally and clinically proven agent for the effective treatment of pancreatic cancer."[10]

Dr. Gonzalez continued to publish case histories and develop research models up until his death in July 2015, including 36 patients with advanced cancer who survived way beyond what was predicted for them, as published in the peer-reviewed journal *Alternative Therapies in Health and Medicine*.[11]

Hope against hope

One of the most encouraging things about this protocol from Dr. Gonzalez is that although he developed it and published research relating to its application to pancreatic cancer, he actually used it in his own practice on all types of cancers.

He even used it to treat autoimmune disorders like chronic fatigue and multiple sclerosis.

Because the protocol is ideally customized for each individual, you'll need to work with a doctor to create the regimen of diet, supplements, enzymes, and detox. In terms of diet, Dr. Gonzalez's recommendations will sound familiar to you if you've read my writings on the Paleo diet—including eating organic foods, and avoiding packaged foods and refined flour and sugar.

Dr. Gonzalez's protocol also recommends that you make and drink fresh vegetable juice, which certainly sound like a healthy dietary habit to me.

The supplements can also vary, but you can expect a mix of vitamins, minerals, trace elements, and antioxidants to complement the accompanying nutritional eating plan.

As I mentioned earlier, Dr. Gonzalez unfortunately passed away last year—and his death has tragically taken away one of our biggest proponents of integrative oncology.

Although Dr. Gonzalez's loss is deeply felt in our field, the important nature of his work and that of his predecessors continues.

If you've been given such a dire prognosis that conventional therapy seems futile, visit www.Dr-Gonzalez.com for more information on this protocol that's given so many people hope and relief.

Chapter 8:

The cancer-fighting mineral you can't afford to ignore

If someone had predicted 30 years ago that iodine would become one of the most important breast cancer treatments, I doubt many people would have believed it. And they would have been right—it *isn't*. In fact, it's hardly used at all. But it should be.

Iodine kills breast cancer cells without killing off normal cells in the process. In other words, it's ideal for both the treatment *and* prevention of breast cancer.

Chances are your doctor hasn't heard of this. (I'll tell you why in just a minute.) So if you want the treatment—and believe me, you should—it's up to you to share this information with your doctor.

Solid research conveniently ignored

In the 1960s and 70s, pioneering iodine researcher Benjamin Eskin, M.D., reported time and again that iodine is a key element in breast health.

In one of his studies, Dr. Eskin demonstrated that deliberately blocking breast cells from access to iodine resulted in precancerous changes—changes that were aggravated when those same cells were exposed to either estrogens or thyroid hormone. Surprisingly, in the absence of iodine, thyroid hormone appeared to be more likely than estrogen to produce abnormalities in breast cells.[1]

In another report, he noted that when breast tissue cells are lacking in iodine, the cells are more likely to be abnormal, precancerous, or cancerous. He said, "Iodine-deficient breast tissues are also more susceptible to carcinogen action and promote lesions earlier and in greater profusion. Metabolically, iodine-deficient breasts show changes in RNA/DNA ratios, estrogen receptor proteins." He concluded that: "[Iodine] presents great potential for its use in research directed toward the prevention, diagnosis, and treatment of breast cancer."

Despite its obvious potential, not much has been done with this treatment over the past 30 to 40 years—at least not in these United States. Since iodine isn't patentable (and is therefore unlikely to be "approved" for use to prevent or treat breast cancer), Dr. Eskin's work has been ignored. Patent medicine companies simply looked elsewhere for profits. Sadly, since most mainstream doctors are dependent on patent medicine company reps, the doctors have been kept in the dark regarding this potential use for iodine.

Over the past two years, though, researchers in Mexico and India (where low-cost, unpatented medicine is a necessity) have begun further investigations into iodine's potential as a breast cancer treatment. So far, all of their results confirm Dr. Eskin's original research: Iodine directly kills many types of human breast cancer cells, and it doesn't kill healthy cells in the process.

Traveling beyond the border for natural cancer cures

In 2005, researchers from the Autonomous National University in Juriquilla, Mexico, reviewed evidence showing that iodine supports breast health by slowing or preventing the spread of cancerous cells. They said, "In animal and human studies, molecular iodine [I(2)] supplementation exerts a suppressive effect on the development and size of both benign and cancer neoplasias… Iodine, in addition to its incorporation into thyroid hormones, is bound into antiproliferative iodolipids [iodinated lipids with anti-cancer activity] in the thyroid called iodolactones, which may also play a role in the proliferative control of the mammary gland." They concluded that breast cancer patients should consider supplementing with I2 in addition to their traditional breast cancer therapy.[2]

In June 2006, a group from the Sanjay Ghandi Institute of Medical Sciences in Lucknow, India, found that iodine is cytotoxic (deadly) to several human breast cancer cell lines, including (for the technically inclined) MCF-7, MDA-MB-231, MDA-MB-453, ZR-75-1, and T-47D. When iodine was applied to human blood cells (monocytes), it inhibited growth and proliferation, but it didn't kill the cells.[3]

Then, in December 2006, the group in Mexico tested the effect of iodine on the MCF-7 form of human breast cancer cells. They found that iodine (but not iodide), along with an iodinated fatty acid, inhibited the MCF-7 cancer cells. At the same time, the iodine neither harmed nor inhibited fibroblasts—normal human connective tissue cells that help to support breast tissue and other tissues throughout the body. Other technical details led the researchers to suggest that iodine may become active against cancer cells when it is bound to certain lipids or proteins that are normally present in the breasts.[4]

A safe adjunct treatment to conventional cancer therapies

These recent research reports give new hope and an added tool for breast cancer patients. It's true that the research isn't conclusive at this point, but you don't need to wait for academic and scientific certainty—which will likely take many more years—to try out the benefits for yourself.

If you have breast cancer and are undergoing regular treatment, adding iodine to your treatment plan will only increase your odds of a favorable outcome—and it's perfectly safe. Numerous studies have proven that iodine (and its iodide form) are among the safest of all the elements.

In one case, a 54-year-old man mistakenly drank 600 ccs (over 20 ounces) of a saturated solution of potassium iodide—100,000 times the recommended daily allowance. The initial reaction was a bit scary: He developed swelling in his neck, mouth, and face, and he experienced transient heart rhythm abnormalities—but he recovered uneventfully.[5]

In another instance, a researcher had 2,400 patients with asthma take 5,000 milligrams of potassium iodide daily on a cycle of four days on followed by three days off. Only 12 of the individuals (1/2 percent) became hypothyroid as a result, and four developed swollen thyroid glands. There was no report of any adverse reaction among the rest.

Even though it's generally safe, some individuals are sensitive to iodine and/or iodide. There have been anecdotal reports of iodide's causing auto-immune thyroiditis, hyperthyroidism, and hypothyroidism. Too much iodine in a few individuals has caused iodism—an acne-like rash, a runny nose, and a bad taste in the mouth, all of which went away when the dosage was reduced or eliminated.

But the possible consequences of unchecked breast cancer are considerably more likely—and, of course, much worse—than experiencing a negative reaction to iodine. So if I were you, I'd give it a try.

Rub away your breast cancer?

A suggestion for you and your doctor to consider: Put the treatment right onto the problem! Mix a solution of 50 percent iodine/50 percent DMSO and rub it directly onto your breast as near as possible to where the cancer is (or used to be). The DMSO will ensure penetration deep into the tissue. A 70-percent DMSO solution is widely available, and iodine is available by prescription as Lugol's Iodine and in natural food stores as Triiodide (from Scientific Botanicals). If you're worried about the breast cancer spreading, you can also rub the mixture into the area under the arms that is rich in lymph glands (nodes) where breast cancer spreads first.

But please don't do any of the above without consulting a physician skilled and knowledgeable in the use of high-dose iodine!

You should also be sure that your physician monitors your thyroid function and gives you other nutrient suggestions while you use iodine as an adjunct to your regular breast cancer treatment. (To find a physician, see the Alternative Health Resources section on page 485 or check with the International College of Integrative Medicine, www.icimed.com, (419)358-0273.)

PART II

Alzheimer's and Brain Health

Chapter 1:

The ICT Protocol for reversing and even curing Alzheimer's

If you or a loved one suffers from Alzheimer's, you're about to discover a simple, proven, 10-step program to reverse—and even cure—this frightening disease.

It's an all-natural, at-home treatment known as the ICT Protocol.

ICT (Individualized Combination Therapy) is an individualized program tailored to suit each person. No more generic treatments…or one-size-fits all remedies that fail for most people.

And the ICT Protocol is specifically designed to target multiple causative factors in Alzheimer's instead of only focusing on one potential factor. Patients undergo a number of clinical tests, including blood analysis, to determine what deficiencies and imbalances may exist.

So far, researchers have identified 36 deficiencies, sources of inflammation and hormonal imbalances that all play a part in decreasing memory function in Alzheimer's.

Dr. Dale Bredesen, the director at UCLA's Mary S. Easton Center for Alzheimer's Disease research, explains that every deficiency is like a piece of a puzzle. And they all fit together to create the memory problems in Alzheimer's.

As he explains, some people may have a larger deficit in one area, such as a deficiency in vitamin D, but smaller deficits in another, such as estrogen. But when both of these deficiencies are combined together, they can cause the cognitive function to decline.

As the author of one of the most important studies into Alzheimer's disease, Dr. Bredesen has identified a program that covers all of the deficiencies…instead of simply treating one. This study was very small, only involving 10 patients, yet the results were extremely promising. You see, 9 out of the 10 participants showed a remarkable improvement in just 3-6 months. And the 1 participant who did not show an improvement was in the late-stages of Alzheimer's dementia, which shows it's best if you can catch Alzheimer's in its early stages.

How the Study Was Conducted

Each of the participants came in with a wide range of dementia symptoms, from mild memory loss to the more severe. They were aged between 55 and 75, and were put through a variety of tests. These included brain scans, blood tests, and other assessments. The results of the testing showed that the study participants had a range of between 10-24 deficiencies and imbalances, including vitamins, hormones, glucose metabolism and lifestyle factors that could be corrected.

Once the deficiencies and hormonal imbalances were identified, each participant was given a tailored program to follow. Some of these treatments included optimizing the health of the gut. Others included repairing Vitamin D deficiencies, fasting from meals to balance insulin levels in the blood and the use of DHA (omega-3 fatty acids) to improve any faulty connections in the brain.

Within a few months, 9 of the participants were showing an improvement. Some had returned to a normal level. Six of the participants in the study had previously had to either give up work or were struggling to stay in employment due to their symptoms. Within 6 months of starting the program, all 6 had managed to either go back to work or showed a large improvement in their ability to do their job.

Although this study was small, it's a big step forward in the treatment of Alzheimer's disease. The ability to restore memory and cognitive function to the point where the patient can return to work and do their job well is a huge result.

Until now, people with Alzheimer's would continue to deteriorate until they needed full-time care. Instead of Alzheimer's disease being considered a death sentence, and the 3rd highest killer in the United States, this study shows promising results that could turn that situation around completely.

10 Simple Steps to Eliminate Alzheimer's: The ICT Protocol in Action

For the ICT protocol to be successful, the participant must follow each stage step by step, starting at the first step and working their way down. Completing the steps out of order won't create the same results, so it is very important to follow them carefully.

Here are the steps, how to take yourself through them, and the reasoning behind them:

Step 1: Reduce Inflammation and Stabilize Blood Sugar Levels

Alzheimer's disease is often referred to as Type 3 Diabetes, because of insulin resistance in the brain. A research team at Brown Medical School discovered that not only was insulin produced by the pancreas, it was also produced in the brain. This is why those with Type 2 Diabetes have a higher risk of developing Alzheimer's disease. High levels of glucose in the blood are accepted as one of the main causes of Alzheimer's disease.

Treatment: Diet

Many medical problems can be treated by following certain diets, and this is also true in Alzheimer's disease. A diet that is low in grains, simple carbohydrates, sugars and on the low glycemic index are recommended for this step. Suitable diets include the Paleo diet, Bulletproof and low-carbohydrate Mediterranean diet. Instead of processed foods, you should consume plenty of fresh foods, like vegetables, and good quality meats and fish.

Also, you shouldn't eat later than 3 hours before bed. A fasting period of 12 hours between dinner and breakfast should be followed each day. Fasting has a superb effect on the production of insulin and the body's sensitivity to it—and can make all the difference when it comes to preventing Alzheimer's.

Treatment: Supplements

Recommended supplements for this step are DHA (docosahexaenoic acid—an omega-3 fatty acid), EPA (eicosapentaenoic acid—also an omega-3 fatty acid), and curcumin. According to research studies, both DHA and EPA can reduce the risk of a decline in cognitive function, possibly due to the effect of omega-3's on the blood circulation. Curcumin is naturally found in turmeric, and research has shown that it helps to reduce the amyloid plaques in the brain, therefore enabling better function.

Treatment: Other

The final recommendation for this step is to improve oral care. It is essential to look after your teeth, gums and mouth, as swelling and infection in the gum can cause an inflammatory response through the body. Regular dental check-ups and the use of electric toothbrushes and dental floss are highly recommended.

Step 2: Optimize Hormones

As we age, different hormones that are produced by the body can be affected, leading to imbalances. When there is an imbalance of a hormone, it can greatly affect how different organs function...and this includes the brain. The most common hormonal problems are related to the thyroid and decreasing estrogen production. Hormone replacement therapy can be used to balance out the levels of each hormone, optimizing their performance in the body—but isn't necessary to restore cognitive function.

Stroke prevention in one easy-to-follow outline

Here's what you need to do:

- eat more vegetables and fruits
- eat whole grains (not refined flour products)
- eat more fish (and reduce animal protein)
- quit smoking
- cut alcohol consumption to no more than one drink daily
- exercise!

And here's what you need to take:

- vitamin C: 1,000 milligrams twice daily (more for optimal health)
- cod liver oil: 1 tablespoonsful daily always with
- vitamin E: 600 IU daily
- ginkgo (standardized extract): 80 milligrams twice daily
- hawthorne solid extract: one teaspoonful daily
- centella asiatica (standardized extract): 60 to 120 milligrams daily
- turmeric: 20 (or more) milligrams daily (or put turmeric into your cooking regularly)
- magnesium: 250-400 milligrams daily
- copper: 2 milligrams daily
- nattokinase: 138 milligrams three times daily

Treatment: Test Your Hormone Levels

A full hormone assessment needs to be carried out to determine if there are any imbalances that may be present. This includes thyroid hormones and the steroid hormones such as cortisol, estrogen and testosterone. Simple blood tests ordered by your doctor can identify the levels of certain hormones in your blood. You can't test your own hormones at home; it needs to be done by a laboratory. You should ask your doctor about conducting a hormone test during your next check-up.

If tests show you have a hormonal imbalance, hormone replacement treatments should be introduced by your doctor to correct any hormonal imbalances.

Treatment: Stress Reduction

Finding methods to help you relax and remove stress is important at this step. Stress can have a major impact on your body, due to anxiety symptoms and tightening of your muscles. Uncontrolled stress can lead to a number of dangerous medical conditions including heart disease… and can even lead to cognitive decline. Daily meditation, yoga, or using music to relax are all recommended treatments for stress. You don't have to go to special classes to learn how to meditate; there are numerous books and instructional videos you can learn from. Yoga is easier if it is learnt in a class, but once you have the basics, you can do this at home.

Treatment: Supplements

The recommended supplements at this step include vitamin D3 and Ashwagandha. Research is ongoing at the moment, but what is known so far is that those with a deficiency in vitamin D are twice as likely to develop Alzheimer's disease. Supplementing vitamin D3 can therefore help to reduce the risk. Ashwagandha is known to prevent beta-amyloid plaques from forming in the brain, and therefore reduce the symptoms of Alzheimer's.

Step 3: Optimize Antioxidants

Antioxidants are important because research has shown that when fats oxidize in the brain there is a strong relationship with Alzheimer's disease. The results of a study published in the Journal of Alzheimer's Disease showed that people with a deficiency in antioxidants like beta-carotene and vitamin C had a higher rate of Alzheimer's disease. Therefore, they came to the conclusion that supplementing the antioxidants could prevent or slow down the development of Alzheimer's. And I recommend adding foods high in beta-carotene and vitamin C to your diet as soon as you can.

Treatment: Diet

As well as the recommended diets in step 1, including the Paleo, Bulletproof and low-carb Mediterranean diet, a cup of organic blueberries each day is a good addition to your diet. Also spinach, kale, oranges—and other foods high in beta-carotene or vitamin C. Researchers believe that blueberries can help with memory decline due to their antioxidant properties.

Treatment: Supplements

The supplements used in this step include tocotrienols, tocopherols, selenium, vitamin C, N-Acetyl cysteine and alpha-lipoic acid. Tocotrienols and tocopherols are types of vitamin E, and Swedish researchers found that people with low levels of vitamin E were more likely to suffer from Alzheimer's. Selenium helps to protect the nerve cell function in the brain, preventing memory loss. N-Acetyl cysteine protects the nerve cells by acting as an anti-inflammatory agent in the brain. And alpha-lipoic acid is a powerful antioxidant that can slow down the Alzheimer's process.

Step 4: Optimize Gut Health

Researchers have discovered that there is a very strong link between the number of healthy flora in the gut and brain function. In fact, gut health is essential for managing many different medical illnesses—especially Alzheimer's.

Treatment: Diet

Again, the diets mentioned in step 1, including the Paleo, the Bulletproof and the low-carb Mediterranean, should help to improve the health of your gut. They help to balance out the flora and bacteria that lives in the gut, which greatly improves the digestive system. This is because these diets are based on whole, healthy foods, and eliminate grains, carbohydrates and sugars, which can all upset the balance of flora in the gut.

Treatment: Supplements

The main supplement used in this step for promoting a healthy gut is a probiotic. A probiotic that also includes a prebiotic is even better. Probiotics break down glutamate, which produces gamma-amino butyric acid (GABA). GABA is a neurotransmitter in the brain, and research has shown that a deficiency in GABA results in memory decline and dementia. Therefore, probiotics are essential in ensuring the level of GABA is optimal.

Step 5: Plenty of Healthy Fats

Although we should stay away from harmful fats, there are some which are essential for our health. Healthy fats are needed to keep our brain functioning well. Unhealthy fats include trans and saturated fats, such as eggs, dairy and meat. Healthy fats are those that are polyunsaturated and mono-unsaturated, and include avocados, olives, seeds and nuts. Healthy fats help towards the production of acetylcholine, which is a vital chemical for learning, concentration and memory—which is why you should add some of these delicious healthy fats to your diet immediately.

Treatment: Fats

As well as DHA and EPA that were mentioned in step 1, another recommended fat to consume is MCT oil, which is derived from the oil of coconuts. This has been shown in research to be very good for improving Alzheimer's disease symptoms. MCT oil, or coconut oil, is readily available these days and can be used the same way as other cooking oils. This type of oil can also be used in many different types of recipes, including baking, instead of using unhealthy oils. The best way to tell if a fat is unhealthy is to look at the ingredient list. Watch out for anything labelled as partially hydrogenated, as this is referring to a trans-fat.

Step 6: Enhancing Cognitive Performance and NGF (Nerve Growth Factor) Levels

This step is made up of supplements that should be taken to boost the speed of your cognitive function and regenerate the cells of the brain by stimulating the nerve growth factor. When the cells are healthy and regenerated, they function more effectively, thus improving memory. Many of these supplements are found in natural sources, particularly in mushrooms. These supplements also include an herb that has been used by Indians medicinally for generations.

Treatment: Supplements

Recommended supplements for this step include Lion's Mane (Hericium Erinaceous), mushroom extract, Bacopa Monnieri and citicoline. Lion's Mane is a type of mushroom that research has shown it contains 2 types of NGF. Multiple studies have shown it to have positive effects on how the brain works. Bacopa is an herb that has been used in traditional Indian medicine to treat memory problems. A trial on humans has shown an improvement in the areas of maintaining attention and verbal recall. Citicoline is a chemical that is naturally found in the brain. It has long been known that it increases the production of another chemical called phosphatidylcholine which is very important for brain function.

Step 7: Boost Mitochondrial Function

A contributing factor in Alzheimer's disease is when there is a decline of activity in certain brain cells. This may seem obvious, but here's *why* your memory starts slowing down:

It all has to do with mitochondria. Mitochondria regulate the metabolism of energy in the cells of the brain, which is vital for cell health and function. When there is a mitochondrial dysfunction, the ability of the brain to work effectively in areas of memory declines. You can treat this quickly, and easily, by adding a supplement to your daily routine.

Treatment: Supplements

The supplements recommended for this step are PQQ and CoQ10. In Alzheimer's there is often an accumulation of a protein called amyloid in the brain, and PQQ has been shown to reduce the amount of amyloid from forming. The use of CoQ10 in mice studies has shown it can help with improving memory and learning capabilities in the mice. I recommend you take a PQQ or CoQ10 supplement daily, in addition to the steps above.

Step 8: Mental and Physical Exercise

Mental and physical exercise is essential for everyone to stay healthy. Mental exercises keep the brain alert, and help to improve thought processes and memory. Physical exercise is vital to the health of your body, as it stimulates the circulation of blood throughout the body, making tissues and cells healthier.

Treatment: Mental Exercise

Any type of mental exercises is helpful at this step, including those that can be found on websites such as BrainHQ.com. Some suggestions are crossword puzzles, Sudoku, or any type of activity that requires memory and recall. It has been shown that simply exercising your brain helps to keep brain cells active—and prevent cognitive decline.

Treatment: Physical Exercise

You should try to do at least 30 minutes of physical exercise every day…preferably up to 1 hour if possible. Strength training or low impact cardio exercise should be undertaken between 4- 6 times each week. Low impact cardio and strength training are less strenuous on the body, but still increase the blood flow to vital organs such as the brain.

Step 9: Ensure Nocturnal Oxygenation

Nocturnal oxygenation refers to the amount of oxygen your brain receives during the night while you are sleeping. Not only do you need a good night's sleep, more importantly you need a good quality sleep. Some medical problems can interfere with your breathing while you are sleeping, which can lead to your brain being starved of vital oxygen.

Treatment: Sleep

Your brain needs plenty of oxygen to function correctly, and a disorder called sleep apnea can prevent this from happening. Sleep apnea causes multiple episodes during sleep where the breath is held, or stopped, and it starts again after a pause. When this occurs, your brain gets less oxygen, which can damage the cells of the brain. Treating apnea will allow your brain to get the oxygen it needs to keep the cells healthy and working properly. If you think you have sleep apnea, your doctor will refer you to a sleep clinic for a sleep study, and you may need to use a machine to keep you breathing while you sleep. This is called a CPAP machine, and you have to wear a mask which forces air into your lungs. A good hint that you may have sleep apnea is excessive snoring.

Step 10: Detox Heavy Metals

We are often exposed to heavy metals in our environment, and these have been linked to the development of Alzheimer's disease. Research has shown that getting rid of heavy metals in the blood can prevent Alzheimer's disease symptoms from worsening.

Treatment: Detox

Chelation therapy is the only method for removing heavy metals from the blood and the body. A chemical is injected into the bloodstream which removes any heavy metals and some minerals. It must be done by a medical professional in a clinical setting, as it can have dangerous side effects.

Case Studies—How the ICT Protocol Works on Real Patients

Patient 1

A 67 year old female presented with increasing loss of memory over a period of 2 years. Her job was very technical and demanding, where she needed to travel a lot and also had to prepare documents and reports. She was starting to struggle doing the reports, and she couldn't analyze data properly anymore. She was considering leaving her job.

Whenever she read a document, by the time she got to the bottom of the page, she couldn't remember what she had already read, and would have to start all over again. Her ability to recall numbers was also affected. She would often get lost driving along roads that she used to know very well. Other effects included forgetting where the light switches were in her home, and confusing the names of her pets.

Her mother had suffered a severe decline in her cognitive function in her early 60s. By the time she passed away in her 80s, she was seriously demented and had spent many years in a nursing home. Concerned she was suffering the same problem, the patient discussed her issues with her doctor who told her she did have the same problem as her mother and there was nothing that could be done. Unfortunately, because the doctor only documented 'memory problems' in her medical notes instead of a diagnosis of Alzheimer's, she did not qualify for long-term care if it was needed.

The thought of ending up like her mother, and knowing she couldn't get the care she needed, made the patient depressed and she thought about suicide. Thankfully a friend managed to get her an appointment to be assessed.

She began the protocol, and although she couldn't follow all of the steps, she still experienced a great improvement in her symptoms. Her memory improved dramatically, and she no longer got lost easily and was able to continue her work. In fact, she was still able to work full-time 2 ½ years later and at the age of 70.

Once during the protocol, the patient developed a viral illness, and had to stop following the program. Almost straight away she noticed her cognitive function and in particular her memory were starting to decline again, but once she restarted the protocol, the symptoms disappeared.

The parts of the protocol the patient was able to complete included:

- Eliminating simple carbohydrates from her diet

- Weight loss of 20 lbs.

- Removed processed food and gluten from her diet

- Increased her intake of fruit, vegetables and wild fish

- Began studying yoga
- Meditated for 20 minutes 2 times a day
- Used melatonin to help her sleep better
- Increased the amount of sleep to 7-8 hours per night
- Took 1 mg of methylcobalamin each day
- Supplemented with vitamin D3 each day
- 2000 mg of fish oil tablets every day
- She took 200 mg of coenzyme Q10 each day
- Began using an electric toothbrush and flosser
- Restarted hormone replacement therapy
- Fasted for 12 hours between dinner and breakfast
- Had her evening meal 3 hours before bed
- 30 minutes of exercise for 4-6 days each week

Patient 2

A 69 year old professional man had presented with memory loss that was getting worse over a period of 11 years. During the last 2 years before presentation, the loss had been increasing at a much faster rate. A scan of his brain in 2003 showed typical patterns for early Alzheimer's disease. Similar to patient 1, patient 2 also had difficulty recalling numbers, and forgetting what had been read previously by the bottom of the page.

Within 6 months of starting the protocol, patient 2 had improved a lot, and he was able to remember his schedule each day. He was also able to recognize faces again. His wife and co-workers noticed the dramatic improvements, and he was able to perform his work a lot easier than he had previously. Once again he was able to add up several numbers in his head quickly, a skill he had lost. Not only had he improved, but the speed he had been declining had been stopped.

For patient 2, the protocol involved the following:

- Fasting for at least 3 hours before bed

- Fasting for 12 hours between dinner and breakfast

- Eliminating simple carbohydrates and processed food from his diet

- Increased consumption of fruit, vegetables, wild fish, grass-fed beef and organic chicken

- He took probiotics

- Took 1 tablespoon of coconut oil twice a day

- Increased exercise to swimming 3 or 4 times each week, running once a week, and cycling twice a week

- He took melatonin to help him sleep

- Increased his sleep to 8 hours per night

- Took 250 mg of Bacopa, 500 mg of Ashwagandha and 400 mg of turmeric each day

- Took 1 mg of methlycobalamin, 0.8 mg of methyltetrahydrofolate, and 50 mg of pyridoxine-5 phosphate each day

- Also took 500 mg of citicoline twice a day

- Supplements of vitamin C, vitamin D3 and vitamin E each day

- 200mg of coenzyme Q10 daily

- Zn picolinate 50 mg per day

- DHA and EPA

Patient 3

A 55 year old female attorney had suffered progressive loss of memory over a 4 year period. She often left the stove on when she left the house. She also forgot about meetings that were scheduled and often overbooked meetings because she couldn't remember she already ones to attend. She started using an iPad to record meetings. Her children noticed she would sometimes forget what she was talking about mid-sentence, and she was much slower in responding. Also, she would think she had asked them do so something, when she hadn't.

Patient 3 spent 5 months following the protocol and had a huge improvement. She could finally go back to work, and no longer needed to use the iPad or recording device during meetings. Not only was she able to return to her previous working standards, she was also able to go on to do more study.

The treatment for patient 3 on the protocol included the following:

- Fasting for at least 3 hours before bed

- Fasting for 12 hours between dinner and breakfast

- Eliminating simple carbohydrates and processed foods from her diet

- Increased her intake of fruits, vegetables, and wild fish

- Exercise 4-5 times each week

- Took melatonin to help her sleep

- Tried to get at least 8 hours sleep each night

- Used meditation and relaxation techniques to reduce stress

- Took 1 mg of methylcoalamin 4 times per week

- 20 mg of pyridoxine-5 phosphate per day

- 200 mg of citicoline each day

- Supplements of vitamin D3

- 200 mg of coenzyme Q10 per day

- DHA and EPA

- Hormone replacement

- Reduction of bupropion prescription

How to Make the ICT Protocol Work for You

As you can see, the steps of the ICT Protocol include diet, exercise for your body and brain, correction of hormone and antioxidant levels, and improving the gut flora. When gut flora become imbalanced, it can have a wide range of effects on the health of your brain and your body.

As shown in some of the case studies, stopping the protocol can result in a return of mental and memory problems. Yet restarting the protocol can reverse this trend. This may seem like the protocol is going to be difficult for some people to manage long term. However, it is just about changing your diet, and managing your vitamin and hormone levels.

Alzheimer's disease is a terrible disease, and the decrease in cognitive function can stop anyone from being able to take care of themselves. The development of the ICT protocol is exciting, and the potential it has to return people with Alzheimer's back to their normal state is a tremendous breakthrough. No longer does Alzheimer's disease have to be a death sentence.

If you believe you are suffering from early Alzheimer's disease, talk to your doctor to find out whether or not the ICT protocol is a possibility for you. The results of the studies completed to date are staggering, and the sooner you start the protocol, the sooner you can reclaim your cognitive function.

Chapter 2:

Alzheimer's breakthrough reveals an all-natural nutritional solution to protect your precious memories

Dementia runs in my family. My grandfather had severe Alzheimer's disease, which is why when my father misplaces his keys (which should be acceptable in a 91-year-old!) we all glance nervously at one another.

I've always been interested in neurological illness, and have treated many patients with Alzheimer's disease—and similar neurological conditions—over the years. People often come to see me looking for an "out of the box" alternative to the litany of drugs conventional medicine has tried to shove down their throats.

And then 10 years ago it happened. I developed Parkinson's disease. It came out of the blue, launching me on a 10-year journey investigating the causes and treatments of neurological conditions. And through that investigation I've discovered the critical factors that cause neurological illnesses like Alzheimer's disease (and Parkinson's), and uncovered natural ways of preventing and treating them.

This knowledge has kept me drug-free and physically active for the past decade, enabling me to help countless others as well. But, shockingly, the root causes of these diseases are already known. This life-saving knowledge is readily available and entirely supportable by medical literature—for those who just bother to look.

Unfortunately few doctors do. And this is a BIG problem because the standard treatments for Alzheimer's just flat out don't work. Like most modern drugs used to treat chronic ailments, those used to "treat" Alzheimer's, Aricept and Namenda, at best slow the progression of this disastrous disease. They're really nothing more than band-aids that you have to take forever. And the reason why is simple, they don't address the root cause of memory loss and Alzheimer's.

Toxins target your vulnerable brain

It turns out toxins in our environment are a leading cause of these neurological illnesses. You see, the human body is actually built to protect our brain from these toxic assaults by eliminating them when we're exposed. But every once in a while these built-in protection systems come with a defect and this bug in the system keeps your body from effectively eliminating the toxins. With virtually nothing standing between your vulnerable brain and these poisons severe neurological consequences and damage can develop.

The sad reality is that we live in a toxic world. These poisons surround us. Our brains are being marinated in them daily, and this constant low level of exposure over time is slowly killing us and robbing us of our precious memories. And to make matters even worse, we're not going to be able to stop this onslaught anytime in the foreseeable future.

The evidence that these toxins have deep and devastating effects on a cellular level continues to stack up. A recent study published in the journal Current Alzheimer's Research is just one example among many. Researchers reviewed the available data linking environmental toxins to Alzheimer's disease, and revealed the frightening path these toxins take, literally altering the metabolic pathways associated with the development and progression of the disease.

In other words, they confirmed the root cause of this terrible disease! These incredible findings should have been splashed across the front page of every single newspaper and website in the world. And yet, chances are you've never even heard about this study before.

Why? Well the short answer is that some pretty powerful people like it that way. The big industries, specifically those that produce the toxins that are slowly poisoning us, have a stake in keeping us from learning the truth. And that's especially true of the heavy metals industry, which is unleashing a wave of Alzheimer's and other neurological diseases.

Heavy metal mayhem destroys memories

Heavy metals—mainly mercury, aluminum and copper—have been clearly linked to memory loss. But of the three, mercury is by far the biggest culprit. High levels of this heavy metal in the brain lead to two brain abnormalities connected to Alzheimer's disease, neurofibrillary tangles and amyloid plaques. And mercury levels in the brains of Alzheimer's patients are typically at least three times that of the rest of the population.

While you may already be aware of the dangers of high mercury levels in certain fish and seafood, what you may not realize is that no matter how pristinely you eat you're still being exposed to this metal. That's because the coal-burning industry is pumping out a staggering 48 tons of mercury into the air every year.

Another frequently overlooked heavy metal, aluminum, has been linked to Alzheimer's disease for over 20 years now. According to the CDC, we ingest 7-9 mg of the stuff every single day. When you add that to the exposure that comes from lathering on antiperspirants, cooking with aluminum utensils, and taking aluminum-containing drugs and vaccinations, the effects can be devastating.

And then there's the growing threat of copper. The amount of this heavy metal in our environment is skyrocketing, which is alarming since it's been shown to have toxic effects on the neurological system and has been specifically linked to Alzheimer's.

In addition, high copper levels have been found to destroy essential detoxifying nutrients including vitamin C, B vitamins and zinc. If you're a woman taking birth control pills you need to be especially careful, since these drugs can raise your copper levels.

An integrative medicine doctor can test your levels of these heavy metals, and if they're found to be dangerously high can help you get started on an effective detoxification plan.

"Master antioxidant" could be the key to beating Alzheimer's

Day in and day out you're being bombarded by neurotoxins. And while your body does its best to fight back that assault, eventually, like continuing to stuff garbage into a trashcan until it's overflowing, the toxic debris starts leaking over the sides and builds up in places like your brain. This can lead to a variety of troubling symptoms including the types of brain and memory issues we've been talking about today.

But despite this onslaught we don't all succumb to Alzheimer's or other degenerative toxin-related diseases. That's because our individual genetic makeup comes into play. While the human body is an amazing vessel, and the brain has an incredible built-in protection system (more on this in a moment), in the end we're all individuals and our bodies respond to the toxic assault differently. Some of us reach the point of toxic overloaded sooner than others.

Your brain has a natural method of protecting itself against the onslaught of mercury, aluminum, copper and other toxins... it enlists the help of the amino acid glutathione. Glutathione—often referred to as the master antioxidant—is a powerful detoxifier and immune system enhancer that serves as the main antioxidant protectant of the entire body.

Glutathione is produced and regenerated in a powerful process called methylation that's responsible for immune system function, brain chemical (neurotransmitter) production, organ protection and detoxification. During the methylation process enzymes, which are controlled by our genes (one in particular, MTHFR, is critical in the methylation process), use B vitamins and other nutrients to churn out an almost endless supply of the master antioxidant.

Well, when the process works correctly that is.

And here's where things get REALLY interesting. I've discovered that an alarmingly high percentage of patients have slight genetic blips in their DNA that hamstrings their ability to make the amount of glutathione they need to effectively tackle those toxins we've been talking about. Even worse, some unfortunate people have far more than just genetic blips in their ability to produce glutathione… instead they practically have gaping holes. And without sufficient glutathione protection they're prone to significantly more neurological damage.

In other words, that "minor" memory loss you or a loved one have been experiencing—the forgetfulness you may have already chalked up to normal aging—could actually be an outward sign of a slow buildup of toxins, along with a slow loss of glutathione. It's a basic supply and demand problem, but with devastating consequences.

But it's not all bad news because knowledge is power. Now that we know that methylation and the production of glutathione are the key to unlocking the mysteries of Alzheimer's, we can focus on bypassing these potential defects with nutrients. An approach that, unlike current Alzheimer's drugs, targets the true root cause of the neurological damage.

Tackle toxins using this powerful triple-nutrient combo

Cerefolin NAC is a powerful nutraceutical brain supplement aimed at helping to prevent Alzheimer's and memory loss. This, prescription only, natural treatment (known as a medical food) was created to address problems with methylation and to target the toxic damage that's linked to memory loss. Cerefolin NAC contains sophisticated "activated" versions of B12 and folic acid, as well as the potent amino acid NAC (a well-known glutathione producer).

This triple-threat combo of powerful nutrients aids the liver in genetically bypassing methylation defects so your body can generate generous amount of glutathione. This smart medicine approach not only helps the body process the onslaught of new toxins that we're exposed to every day it also helps with detoxification, purging the old toxins out of the body.

Covering the cost of a breakthrough

Unfortunately, there is one downside to Cerefolin NAC. Despite being an incredibly effective treatment, some insurance plans refuse to cover this natural solution. It can be quite expensive... but for good reason. Despite not having the resources that a traditional drug company would have at their disposal, the holistic company that created this breakthrough nutraceutical took one for the team. They forked over the cash and man hours that were needed to complete the studies proving that raising glutathione does indeed combat memory loss.

And frankly, their considerable investment has given us a priceless gift. They not only introduced the world to the methylation and glutathione connection to Alzheimer's and provided us with an effective solution to combat this devastating condition, but they simultaneously proved to the conventional medicine community that supplements and natural remedies are the real deal. And for that they should be applauded.

If your doc refuses to write you a script for Cerefolin NAC, or if you just find the medical food is simply too pricey for your pocket book, I've got good news. Although Cerefolin NAC is available only by prescription, you can get a similar memory-saving effect by combining natural glutathione-enhancing ingredients that are readily available at your local vitamin shop, or online, including B vitamins, NAC, alpha lipoic acid, zinc and selenium.

By combining these powerful natural ingredients you can unlock the ability to produce a continuous supply of glutathione and protect your valuable brain cells and invaluable memories.

Chapter 3:

The mineral breakthrough helping terminal patients defy death: And why you should be taking a little of it too

Between the lack of any media coverage at all about the hundreds of encouraging lithium research papers, and the general impression that lithium is a prescription "drug" used "only" for bi-polar disease, even the most dedicated anti-aging enthusiasts are seldom taking advantage of the brain-protective and brain anti-aging effects of low-dose lithium.

If you're one of the many people not using supplemental low-dose lithium yet, you may want to take another look at it—especially since some very recent research reports have added even more weight to the already heavy mountain of evidence in favor of lithium's brain-protective benefits. In fact, a groundbreaking study appeared in the *Proceedings of the National Academy of Sciences* journal showing that lithium may help halt the progression of a degenerative disease even more deadly than Alzheimer's.

But before I tell you about the new lithium breakthrough, let's review a bit.

Just for the record: Lithium is a mineral element in the same "family" as sodium and potassium. It's not a drug, and definitely not patentable, which is very likely why you haven't read or heard much in the media about its enormous potential for protecting and improving brain health, despite truly abundant and all-positive research.

Below are titles of some studies on lithium and the brain, along with descriptions of what each article reported.

More brain power—literally

"Lithium-induced increase in human brain grey matter"[1]

"Lithium stimulates progenitor proliferation in cultured brain neurons"[2]

Using MRI scans, the researchers in the first study found that lithium actually increases the numbers of brain cells in older individuals. The second headline explains at least part of how lithium does this. This study found that lithium stimulates "progenitors," which promote the growth of new nerve cells.

Three-pronged protection against the most common brain-destroyers

"Neuroprotective effects of chronic lithium on focal cerebral ischemia in rats"[3]

"Lithium at 50: Have the neuroprotective effects of this unique cation been overlooked?"[4]

"Lithium exerts robust neuroprotective effects *in vitro* and in the CNS in vivo: Therapeutic implications"[5]

These studies explain more about how lithium protects the brain. There are lots of research articles showing that lithium protects against both internally produced molecules toxic to nerve cells (such as glutamate) and external toxins (including aluminum). But the first group of researchers above reported that lithium not only protects brain cells against toxins, but also against lack of blood flow.

The second article explained that one way lithium protects neurons is by increasing levels of a major neuroprotective protein called "bcl-2." Bcl-2 also increases regeneration of neural axons, the "branches" that project out from the main bodies of nerve cells and contact other neurons.

And the third study headline shows just how impressive these results are: "Robust" is a term rarely seen in the titles of research articles. Basically, scientific publications use it as a restrained code word for "Wow! That really works!"

The best—and least used—treatment for Alzheimer's

"Lithium inhibits amyloid secretion in COS7 cells transfected with amyloid precursor protein C100"[6]

"Lithium protects cultured neurons against beta-amyloid-induced neurodegeneration"[7]

Amyloid and beta-amyloid are byproducts of nerve cell metabolism that, in excess, contribute to Alzheimer's disease. These two studies showed that lithium inhibits amyloid production and protects nerve cells against damage from excess beta-amyloid. Other researchers have reported that lithium also prevents the formation of "neurofibrillary tangles," another contributor to Alzheimer's disease.

And here's another encouraging study "headline" that came out very recently:

"Lithium: A novel treatment for Alzheimer's disease?"[8]

This research review from the Indiana University School of Medicine cites some of the evidence noted above and considerably more, and came to the following conclusion: "One intriguing clinical application is in the treatment of Alzheimer's disease."

But after reading all the other research evidence that came before this, I think its potential goes well beyond "just" treatment of Alzheimer's disease. After all, "a milligram of prevention may be worth a kilogram of cure." And since low-dose lithium is so safe, it really should be a part of everyone's supplement program—especially if you have a family history of Alzheimer's disease, senile dementia, Parkinson's disease, any other neurodegenerative disease (or if you just want to "keep all your marbles").

I generally recommend 10 to 20 milligrams of lithium (as aspartate or orotate) daily. Of course, like any other substance, lithium can be dangerous in high doses, so please be sure to read the box on above about using lithium safely.

Battling inner demons with an all-natural weapon

"Lithium in drinking water and the incidence of crimes, suicides, and arrests related to drug addiction"[9]

"Lithium and the treatment of alcoholism: A critical review"[10]

They may seem unrelated to the previous studies listed, but both of these articles show lithium's potential to protect against a different type of disease—addiction. One study also shows that even very low levels of lithium have a measurable effect: In the first study, researchers found that levels of lithium less than 200 parts per million in drinking water are associated with significantly fewer arrests for crimes committed as the result of drug addition: Homicide, robbery, rape, suicide, and drug trafficking.

The second study was a review of lithium treatment for alcoholism. These researchers concluded that lithium significantly improves mood and behavior in alcoholics, and is even associated with fewer repeat hospitalizations for alcohol intoxication.

New hope for a "hopeless" disease

Unfortunately, despite all of these proven benefits, the mainstream still basically ignores lithium. But when the following research paper was published in February, the title alone was so shocking and such a potential breakthrough against an otherwise rapidly fatal disease that I thought for sure—finally—there would be some mention in the "mass media world" of newspapers, radio, and television.

There wasn't!

So unless you've been actively searching "online" because you have a loved one dying of this disease, you'll probably be reading the following "headline" for the first time:

"Lithium delays progression of amyotrophic lateral sclerosis"[11]

You may know amyotrophic lateral sclerosis by its more common names, ALS and Lou Gehrig's disease. This "nickname" came after the disease struck home-run-hitting major-league baseball player Lou Gehrig back in 1939. After his diagnosis, Gehrig deteriorated very rapidly: Less than two years after his initial symptoms of weakness and stumbling appeared, he suffered a helpless, totally-paralyzed death. The same has happened to nearly all other ALS victims. So anything at all which "delays progression" of this terrible disease should receive major media attention—even if just a brief notice to "get the word out" to ALS sufferers.

Actually, the term "delays progression" used in the study's title is quite conservative. Lithium treatment definitely did much better than that.

Quoting from the summary: "ALS is a devastating neurodegenerative disorder with no effective treatment…we found that daily doses of lithium…delay disease progression in human patients affected by ALS. None of the patients treated with lithium died during the 15 months of the follow-up, and disease progression was markedly attenuated when compared with age-, disease duration-, and sex-matched control patients treated with riluzole for the same amount of time." Riluzole is one of several patent medications used to "treat" ALS, with practically no effect.

The researchers observed two groups—16 patients who took lithium along with "routine" riluzole treatment, and 32 who took just the riluzole. The patients in the riluzole-only group experienced an average symptom worsening of 50 percent in just the first three months, and 30 percent of the "riluzole-only" patients died within the 15-month study period. In stark contrast, none of the patients who took lithium died within the 15 months. In fact, none of them even got significantly worse.

This is a fantastic breakthrough, and hopefully it will revive interest in clinical trials—and clinical usage—of lithium for nearly <u>any</u> disease in which brain cells and nerve cells are degenerating.

<u>But don't try this for a loved one on your own</u>! The lithium dosages the researchers administered to the ALS patients in the study were considerably larger than the typical brain anti-aging doses. While they can be safely tolerated by most adults, they definitely require close and careful monitoring by a physician skilled and knowledgeable in nutritional and natural therapy.

Chapter 4:

"Clean" your brain and stop dementia and Alzheimer's with these simple sleep trick

Imagine being able to boost your immune system, improve your memory and even ward off devastating diseases like Alzheimer's—all while lying flat on your back.

You know how important sleep is to your memory and your health. And we've all experienced the brain fog after a rough night tossing and turning in the sack.

But researchers are now claiming that too many sleepless nights could cause dangerous toxins to accumulate in your brain, triggering inflammation, dementia and even Alzheimer's. And just a few simple sleep tricks could be all it takes to keep your brain "clean" from these poisons and razor sharp in your golden years.

Poor sleep linked to brain disease

As we age, the ability to remember becomes more of a challenge. And diseases such as Alzheimer's—which frequently starts with the forgetting of names, facts and basic orientation—may have an overlooked connection to sleep. Much of our ability to remember things depends on good quality sleep—and that means that while a lack of sleep doesn't cause Alzheimer's, it could make it show up decades earlier.

We also know from current research that good sleep is critical for proper immune system function. T cells (the large family of lymphocytes that form the cornerstone of our immune response) plummet when we're sleep deprived. Even healthy people with robust immune systems experience a loss of immune system function when they don't get enough good quality sleep. This can lead to colds and flu, an inability to ward off chronic conditions such as shingles and may even make us less able to fight off cancer cells.

In addition to its effects on lymphocytes and other white blood cells, sleep deprivation raises the level of inflammatory messengers in your body. Several studies have shown that sleep deprived people have higher levels of inflammatory cytokines such as IL-6 (interleukin-6) and inflammatory markers such as CRP (C-reactive protein). And unchecked this inflammation can have dire health consequences contributing to heart disease, cancer and brain diseases such as Alzheimer's.

Get more shuteye for a sparkling clean brain

But as important as memories and immune function are, we're just beginning to understand the critical function sleep plays in maintaining our health. Dr. Maiken Nedergaard, a sleep biologist who runs the sleep laboratory at the University of Rochester, has been doing exciting research into the role of sleep in proper brain function. And in time her team uncovered a tantalizing new idea: Sleep is your body's way of cleansing your brain.

Our bodies have a built in method for cleaning out toxins called the lymphatic system. Lymph, a colorless fluid that contains white blood cells, courses throughout our bodies using an intricate system of lymph channels. The lymph weaves between cells carrying macrophages and other immune cells that can move into body tissues engulfing debris and the toxic products of metabolism.

But cleansing lymph cells are unable to reach the brain, which is encased behind a protective blood-brain barrier. Your brain uses an incredible 20 percent of your body's total energy to perform its critical functions, and all of that energy expenditure naturally creates a lot of waste products. Some of those waste products, like tau protein and beta-amyloid plaques, can be toxic to your brain, leading to Alzheimer's and similar dementias if they aren't removed.

When we're awake, our brains are too busy and active to be heavily involved in cleansing. We do have "clean-up" units called glial cells whose job it is to move through the fluid spaces of our brains during the day. But the glial cells only clean up the surfaces of the brain while we're awake. That's where Dr. Nedergaard's discovery, derived from mouse studies, comes in.

A "dirty brain" is linked to Alzheimer's

Tagging markers were injected into the cerebrospinal fluid of mice and tracked. They were found to follow specific pathways through the brain and out again. When the mice were asleep, however, the fluid exchange increased by 20 times!

It turns out that while we sleep our brain cells actually shrink. This shrinkage allows the channels between the cells to swell and fill up with cerebrospinal fluid, providing a medium for the cleansing glial cells to move in and around each cell, removing any debris they discover.

The researchers measured a 60 percent increase in the flow through the interstitial fluid, the channels around and between the brain cells which were inactive when the brain was busy in activities of wakefulness. This finding was so shocking that at first the researchers thought they must have calculated wrong. But on repetition it became obvious that the sleeping brains were clearing out twice as much waste as the waking brains. And much of that waste was identified by the researchers as beta-amyloid, the toxic substance linked to the development of Alzheimer's disease.

Much like the white blood cells found in lymph, the glial cells move throughout the brain gobbling up waste products and washing them through the channels of the cerebrospinal fluid. Dr. Nedergaard coined the term "glymphatic system" to describe the brain's cleansing process that's remarkably similar to the lymphatic system of the rest of the body. Similar studies in dogs, goats and baboons have confirmed the presence of this sleep-induced cleansing system, and human studies are being planned.

Get control of this hidden condition for better sleep

While it's clear that adequate sleep plays a critical role in protecting us from the build-up of damaging dementia-linked toxins, frighteningly, a stunning 50-70 million Americans are currently suffering from insomnia and other sleep disorders such as sleep apnea.

Sleep apnea is a condition that causes you to literally stop breathing repeatedly throughout the night for several seconds at a time. Sleep apnea sufferers may snore loudly or simply have periods of silence followed by a gasping for air, and they're often unaware they even have the condition until a spouse or roommate brings it to their attention. Extreme fatigue and unexplained high blood pressure are other signs of sleep apnea and either, or both, could cause your doctor to suspect you have the condition.

A sleep apnea diagnosis is made by scheduling a "sleep study," during which you spend a night in a sleep lab attached to electrodes that monitor your oxygen level and sleep rhythms.

Sleep apnea is usually caused by one of three things: 1. extra fatty tissue in the adenoids or back of the throat, 2. too much weight in the neck and facial areas, or 3. swelling of the adenoids and sinuses.

Losing weight can often help reverse the condition for many sufferers. Since allergies can be responsible for sinus and adenoid swelling, treating allergies can help relieve apnea as well. And in the most extreme cases surgery may be required.

CPAP and BiPAP machines that push air through the obstructions at night are often prescribed as well. These machines have become less obtrusive in recent years, but they still aren't tolerable for many. As a first step I often have my own patients try a small non-invasive devise that slides into the nostrils. Provent (www.proventtherapy.com) can help provide just enough of an increase in breathing passages to improve sleep for some sufferers.

Six shuteye tricks to try

Insomnia, trouble either falling asleep or staying asleep (or both), is another common sleep problem. But today I'm going to reveal my six secret tricks for beating insomnia and finally getting some quality shuteye.

Shuteye trick #1: Try to go to bed at the same time each night. We are creatures of habit, and our bodies can essentially be trained to begin winding down and preparing for sleep at a specific time if we stick to the same routine.

Shuteye trick #2: Try elevating the foot of your bed a few inches. Believe it or not, there are multiple reports and some scientific data suggesting that elevating the foot of the bed increases circulation into the brain at night.

Shuteye trick #3: Turn off any blue light screens in the room, including tablets, laptops, phones and computer screens at least an hour before bed. Studies show that these devices send our brains mixed messages if we use them while we're trying to settle down for sleep.

Shuteye trick #4: Don't do work, or any type of heavy problem solving, in bed. Choose another room in the house to be the room for cerebral activity, and leave your bedroom for intimacy and sleep ONLY.

Shuteye trick #5: Try taking a warm bath before bedtime. Epsom salts, containing the valuable sedating mineral magnesium, will assist in the relaxation process.

Shuteye trick #6: If waking up during the night is your main issue, try eating a very light snack before bedtime. Low blood sugar is one of the most common causes (next to frequent urination) of waking in the middle of the night. A couple almonds, a few spoons of full-fat yogurt or even a bit of almond butter on a cracker can frequently do the trick.

Skip the sleep drugs and go natural instead

Of course, if you still need a little extra help, Big Pharma will be more than happy to supply you with pills to drug you to sleep. But taking them can be disastrous. Many of these heavy duty meds are addictive, and some can even be life-threatening. In addition, studies show that users often get very little extra quality sleep using them.

Instead of putting yourself at risk with questionable drugs, I suggest you try some safe alternatives. My fa-vorite natural sleep remedies include: valerian, skullcap, magnesium, melatonin, 5-hydroxytryptophan (5- HTP) and/or L-Tryptophan, Jamaican Boxwood, L-Theanine, GABA and GABA-promot-ing nutrients, phosphatidylserine, and curcumin.

One of these natural sleep remedies, or a combination of them, could be the key to finally getting the quality sleep you need to stay healthy and hold on to your precious memories.

If you find you're still having trouble sleeping I suggest you make an appointment to see an integrative medicine doctor who can help get to the bottom of your sleep problems, and personalize a plan to get you the critical shuteye you need. Pleasant dreams!

Chapter 5:

Is this weird-looking mushroom the key to preventing and reversing dementia?

There's an old saying among natural healers that for every disease out there, Mother Nature has provided a cure. And if you want proof of that, you don't have to look any further than the humble mushroom.

There are thousands of varieties of mushrooms growing all over the world—and many have been used for centuries to treat everything from infections to cancer.

But now scientists say that a weird-looking mushroom—one that may be growing right near where you live—may be the most impressive we've ever seen.

And if you're battling mood disorders, dementia, or even Alzheimer's, it may be the key to protecting your brain—and saving your precious memories.

Together, these tiny troops are as mighty as a lion

This miracle (and quite edible) mushroom is *Hericium erinaceus*, commonly called "lion's mane." It grows in North America, Europe and

Asia, and it doesn't really look like a mushroom at all. It has no "cap" like the Portobello, crimini, and white mushrooms you see the produce aisle. Instead, it's got long shafts (called "spines") that hang down, which have earned it some pretty colorful other nicknames like "Bearded Tooth" and "Pom Pom" mushroom.

Now, while lion's mane wouldn't be out of place in a gourmet meal (or starring in a "B" horror movie!), there's somewhere very important that this versatile mushroom SHOULD be a staple: in the prevention and treatment of neurological illnesses like dementia and Alzheimer's.

For centuries, traditional Chinese medicine has been using lion's mane for its antioxidant effects, treating anything from stomach ailments to cancer.

But it's only relatively *recently* that we've begun to understand how important it is for your brain. And it all comes down to a group of compounds called hericenones, first isolated by Japanese researchers in the early 1990s.

And now, at least eight different hericenones (classified with letters A through H) have been discovered in total, with remarkable potential for the neurological system.

It turns out that hericenones can stimulate the production of Nerve Growth Factor (NGF), a protein produced by the body that is critical in communication between nerve cells and the brain.

NGF is necessary for brain cells to function and to heal, and it has an important role in the activity and survival of spinal cord sensory neurons and cholinergic neurons of the brainstem.

NGF is so essential that depriving mice of it in a lab resulted in an increase in beta amyloids AND in cell death—as well as the development of Alzheimer's-like dementia.[1]

Now, because NGF doesn't cross the blood-brain barrier, no attempts to administer it orally or by injection ever succeeded in getting the protein into the brain cells where it needed to be. That meant we needed to find something else...something that could promote the production of NGF in the brain and neurological system...that could be given orally or by injection...and that would be small enough to pass the blood-brain barrier.

The compounds found in lion's mane fit in the bill on all counts—and that's not where their benefits end.

Protecting your brain, one cell at a time

Not only have they been shown to promote NGF synthesis, but hericenones also lower the cell damage caused by beta amyloid peptide, one of the presumed culprits of Alzheimer's). They also appear to lessen the apoptosis (cell death) of neurons and other brain cells.

The first lab study to show that lion's mane could stimulate NGF synthesis was published in 1991. Using beta amyloid, Japanese researchers induced a dementia state in laboratory mice and then fed them a powdered extract of lion's mane mushroom (containing hericenones C, D, and E).[2] This was an important study, whose results suggested that hericenones could prevent the damage that leads to Alzheimer's and similar dementias.

It also overcame a very basic obstacle, demonstrating that hericenones could, in fact, be taken orally and pass through the blood-brain barrier.

A human study published in 2009 demonstrated intriguing results as well. Thirty men and women aged 50 to 80 with mild cognitive impairment from dementia were studied in a double-blind, placebo-controlled trial. Half the group was given powdered lion's mane and half placebo. When tested at eight, 12, and 16 weeks, the cognitive function of the treated group improved significantly, compared to the placebo group.[3]

Interestingly, when the lion's mane therapy was halted after 16 weeks, the effects wore off within a month.

Your recovery could be downright miraculous

But there's even more magic to be had from these mushrooms—because the hericenones turned out to be just the FIRST of several phenolic substances to be extracted from lion's mane mushrooms.

A fat-soluble phospholipid molecule with a tongue-twister of a name (called *dilinoleoyl-phosphatidylethanolamine*, or DLPE for short) can also be extracted from lion's mane—and it's yet ANOTHER component that appears to protect the brain cells from the kind of oxidative damage that could lead to cell death in a variety of neurodegenerative diseases such as Alzheimer's, Parkinson's, and even Bovine spongiform encephalopathy (a.k.a. "Mad Cow Disease").

Natural combinations of hericenones and DLPE, called amyloban, have popped up in several animal studies, which have produced encouraging results. In one rat study out of China, for example, a preparation containing 9.5 percent hericenones and 6 percent amyloban was compared to a prescription drug used to treat Alzheimer's, called donepezil. When each were given to a respective group of dementia-induced rats, the lion's mane extract proved superior in memory tests.[4]

In fact, the combo almost completely REVERSED the effects of the dementia.

Clear the dark clouds and feel sharp as a tack

The applications of this amazing fungus almost seem endless, as studies have also suggested that people with mood disorders and mental illness might also reap its benefits.

In one study of 30 women with depression and/or anxiety—some who received the powdered extract, and others who didn't—the treated group scored significantly lower on standardized tests for depression and anxiety after just four weeks.[5]

In another small study, schizophrenic patients who were given a lion's mane extract for several weeks showed improvement in a standardized test of symptoms.

But you don't have to be experiencing ANY health issues at all to have reason to start loving this 'shroom.

In one small study, healthy subjects with no prior cognitive issues experienced a measurable improvement in their well-being, energy and mood after just two months on the lion's mane extract.[6]

Obviously larger studies must be conducted to further support these other potential benefits. But to me, the findings so far are enough to suggest that this tasty and versatile mushroom should be added to the growing list of natural therapies for preventing and treating neurodegenerative diseases...and to your stir fry, while you're at it.

Just don't try to go foraging for them on your own. Many types of fungi in the forest are NOT edible and are actually quite toxic. You can find safe, natural, and effective lion's mane supplements in the form of a pill, liquid extract, or a powder that you can add to your smoothie or even cook with.

Choose a high quality supplement from a maker you trust, like Mushroom Matrix. Their products are certified 100% organic, gluten-free, and raw, and they come from mushrooms grown right here in the U.S. For more information, visit www.mushroommatrix.com.

Chapter 6:

This secret virus can give you Alzheimer's—and there's a good chance you're carrying it

I am constantly on the lookout for the latest, cutting-edge medical research—and I'm always excited when I can share something new with you.

Well, a month or so ago, I stumbled upon an article that really got my attention.

A psychiatrist from Colorado named Theodore Henderson, MD, PhD wrote a brilliant piece about the overwhelming data linking Alzheimer's disease to a virus that may shock you: herpes simplex 1 (HSV-1).[1]

In fact, it turns out that just having one simple cold sore... at _any time in your life_... gives you a higher chance of Alzheimer's.

This is incredible news because Alzheimer's is becoming an epidemic. There are about five million Americans with Alzheimer's[2]—and that does not include the many more millions of people with mild memory loss (mild cognitive impairment) that could be looked at as "pre-Alzheimer's."

On top of that, most conventional doctors will admit that the current drugs for Alzheimer's are clearly not working... and there's really no hope in sight for a new blockbuster drug to cure this disease any time soon.

Therefore, the conventional community should be as excited as I am by this article—because this data can really help focus our attack against this disabling disease!

And, as you know, we doctors in integrative medicine are always focusing on addressing the root cause of a disease... and if the root cause of Alzheimer's is an *infection*... or, more specifically, a *virus*... then there's a target we can zero in on.

Is a dormant virus stealing your memories?

While the link between herpes and Alzheimer's may surprise you, it actually makes perfect sense to me.

It's a well-known fact that stealth viruses like HSV-1 hide and live in the nerves and nervous system.

The chicken pox virus, for example, lives in the nerves—and it will only resurface along the root of the nerve that stems from the spinal cord in which it was hiding.

Some genital herpes sufferers tell me that before they get an outbreak, they feel a tingle in their tailbone or back area, which is where the virus is residing most of its time.

Since we know that the HSV-1 virus is living in the nerves of the face and head, it's not a stretch to think that this virus could make the short trip to the brain if it were to "wake up."

And according to Dr. Henderson's article and the several studies he references, if someone's immune system isn't strong enough to keep this pesky virus dormant, then it can slowly but surely cause permanent damage to the brain—and thus cause Alzheimer's.

In total, the article listed too many prior studies to discuss here—but needless to say, they all made a strong connection between the HSV-1 and Alzheimer's.

To summarize:

- Multiple studies show a positive correlation between HSV-1 showing up in blood work and the incidence of Alzheimer's.

- At least three studies show that autopsies have found the DNA of HSV-1 in the tangles and plaques in the brains of both humans and animals with Alzheimer's.[3]

- HSV-1 is more prominently found in the places of the brain that are damaged (the frontal and temporal lobes).[4]

- Three studies show HSV-1 induces the formation of the classic plaques seen in Alzheimer's patients when injected into tissue in a laboratory petri dish.[5]

And to cap it all off, one blockbuster (yet overlooked) study from 2011 that he shared showed that when antiviral medication was placed in test tubes with nerve cells that had the classic plaque and sticky proteins of the disease, the medications actually slowed down, stopped the production of, or even erased the classic signs of Alzheimer's in those tissues.[6]

Believe it or not, this could be good news

There are two ways of looking at this revelation: The glass is either half-empty, or half-full.

If you're a pessimist, this is pretty darn scary stuff. *At least* 34 percent of the population has antibodies to this pesky virus, although some data sources quote the statistic to be much higher—up to 90 percent of the population—because you could've easily been exposed to HSV-1 and have it in your system but never know it.

When you first acquired this virus (probably from something like sharing a cup with someone or kissing your high school sweetheart), your immune system was robust and strong enough to lock up the infection and throw away the key.

If you haven't had any symptoms despite having been exposed, you could be a carrier of the virus and not even know it.

But I'm a "glass half-full" kind of guy—and if you're like me, you'll remember that the integrative medical community has been treating chronic infections for many years and has found safe and effective ways of fighting these villainous viruses and strengthening the immune system to keep them in check.

Integrative medicine is a "take-the-bull-by-the-horns" kind of medicine. While we treat patients offensively, the conventional medical community sits back and waits for the horrible disease to occur. When it does, they then try to save the day with a rescue therapy... or cover the symptoms with a dangerous medication.

Fortunately, most of the success that we've had has been with natural and holistic approaches, so you may not even need the help of a closed-minded conventional doctor.

But imagine if the scientists behind these studies were to get what they're requesting: that is, for antiviral medications to be used in the treatment of Alzheimer's.

Now, that would be something!

You can fight it, even if you can't see it

I have written in previous articles about the B vitamins and glutathione for memory loss and Alzheimer's—and these supplements still provide amazing benefit, and I still use them widely in my office.

But I feel that all of this research will change the way that I treat patients who are experiencing even a moderate amount of memory loss. I might even start checking HSV antibodies on some patients as a screening tool.

You can ask your doc to test you for the presence of HSV-1 antibodies if you've never been tested before—but, in the meantime, it's a good idea to start some natural supplements that tend to slow viruses as well as improve the immune system.

I will be honest with you: I don't claim to cure viruses in my clinic, but I would assert that it is very possible to _slow them down_ and to at least get into a virtual stalemate between your immune system and the virus or viral infection.

There are actually _many_ supplements that slow viruses down. I do like the use of garlic, grapefruit seed extract, oil of oregano, and olive leaf extract... but I usually start with the simple, safe, and effective amino acid called lysine for HSV and the other herpes viruses.

This amazing supplement has been very effective in many of my patients, and I really consider it the best way to slow down the herpes virus. I usually recommend 1,000 to 3,000 mg a day.

But slowing down the virus is only one part of this two-pronged attack. The second prong to keeping this virus from replicating and damaging your brain is to strengthen the immune system.

I do feel that this is the "elephant in the room"—not just in this scenario, but also with many other diseases, including shingles, cervical cancer, and even all of the other versions of cancer.

The issue that everyone is missing is that it's not about the bug/infection itself. Rather, it's really about how strong your immune system is in keeping these bugs where they belong—locked up.

Just ask anyone who suffers from cold sores. Most of them will admit that physical and mental stress, poor sleep, and poor diet (i.e. too much sugar) are the main culprits of their outbreaks.

Now, if you're one of those chronic cold sore sufferers... or if you're having a few too many "senior moments"... DON'T PANIC.

As simple as it seems, taking just 20 mg of zinc and 1,000 mg of vitamin C over a long period time can be a huge "An-apple-a-day-keeps-the-doctor-away" approach to keeping your immune system strong enough to fight off all kinds of infections... and maybe even beat back Alzheimer's!

Chapter 7:

Head trauma from decades ago can wreck your brain now—but it's never too late to repair the damage!

When I was younger, it wasn't uncommon for me to "see stars" after a bang on the head.

I remember lifting my head too fast when exiting a basement once... and getting clocked by the bulkhead door.

At age 12, I got hit in the teeth by a baseball bat that had been swung by a boy who mistook my face for the ball.

And as a young teen, my uncle knocked me out when I walked straight into a punch he had pulled while we were horsing around (thus cementing my reputation as the "glass jaw" of the family.)

In all cases, I was knocked out or close to it, but I shook it off and popped back up.

Now decades later, I thought about those times as I watched the juxtaposition of the end-of-life version of Muhammad Ali shuffling and freezing with the last stages of Parkinson's Disease with the youthful Ali, employing his "Rope-a-dope" strategy. He became somewhat infamous for taking as many punches as he could to tire out his opponent.

Common wisdom says—and I believe—that the multitude of punches to his head was the cause of his Parkinson's. Traumatic Brain Injury (TBI) is now known to lead to a condition called Chronic Traumatic Encephalopathy (CTE), a progressive neurological disease that's the result of head trauma earlier in life.

And now we know that CTE can mimic Parkinson's, Alzheimer's, and other neurodegenerative diseases in which the brain literally "shrinks."

On a molecular level, there seem to be a number of similarities between CTE and these known brain illnesses:

- chronic inflammation of the brain, leading to disruption of intracellular and intercellular messengers

- a damaging of the glucose metabolism in the nervous system, leading to an underproduction of energy, and

- a disruption of the cerebrospinal fluid circulation, an activity that is critical in clearing toxins from the brain.

So it turns out that the "dings" that we might have experienced when we were younger, even if they were fleeting at the time, may have disabling neurological effects much later in life.

Protects before and after your lights get knocked out

CTE (and TBI) is very much in the media today, primarily because of the former NFL players who've been posthumously diagnosed with CTE... but also because of the recently-released movie Concussion starring Will Smith (who also happened to have portrayed "The Greatest" in the movie Ali).

Fortunately, we are becoming more aware of the ways we can use natural medicines—so-called "neuro-prophylactic compounds"—to prevent the results of concussion, even decades after the fact.

According to a recently published "meta-analysis" of the many studies already published of these neuro-prophylactic compounds,[1] many of them are antioxidants. This isn't surprising, since there's an inflammatory and oxidative component to CTE.

One such antioxidant compound is resveratrol, is an example of a flavonoid, the very metabolically active portion of the plant kingdom that gives plants their unique smells, colors, and taste as well as their potent anti-inflammatory and antioxidant properties.

While there haven't been any human trials as yet, multiple in vitro and animal trials have shown that it crosses the blood-brain barrier and improves the outcomes in situations that stem from TBI (and stroke, spinal cord injury, etc).

Some animal studies have shown that resveratrol can improve both behavior and neurological activity when given after head trauma; and other animal studies have demonstrated that resveratrol can slow the progression of neurodegenerative diseases like Alzheimer's.

It can lessen fluid on the brain (cerebral edema) and anxiety, and it can improve functional performance and memory. Even movement is enhanced!

While it is thought that the anti-inflammatory effects of resveratrol are responsible for its activity, there are suggestions that it has other neuroprotective effects as well.

Another natural product that has been shown to have remarkable neuroprotective effects is green tea. Green tea actually has three components that are known to protect the brain:

1. Epigallocatechin-3-gallate (EGCG), a flavonoid like resveratrol. EGCG readily crosses the blood-brain barrier and into the brain where it has been shown to improve cognitive function after neurological traumas. In addition, animal studies have demonstrated protection in ALS, PD, and AD.

2. L-theanine, a unique amino acid that's thought to give green tea its relaxing qualities. Like EGCG, theanine has been shown to be anti-inflammatory to nerve tissue and to protect it from injury.

3. Methylxanthine, best known as caffeine. Caffeine actually acts as a so-called "nonselective adenosine receptor antagonist," which enables it to model and modify cell signals in the nerves, as well as enhance nerve healing after injury. Multiple studies using experimental injury to nerve tissue have shown that, over time, caffeine intake is neuroprotective. Intracranial swelling has been shown to decrease with caffeine, and neural inflammation is decreased. A large observational study of caffeine intake showed a 22 percent reduction in Parkinson's disease with coffee and a 28 percent reduction with tea.

Although there are no clinical trials of caffeine in brain injury, there is much suggestion of its effectiveness. Adenosine levels, which are affected by caffeine, are elevated following TBI, and subsequent elevated caffeine levels in the cerebrospinal fluid are associated with improved outcome of TBI.

One of my favorite natural products that shows promise in reversing the effects of TBI is another flavonoid, called baicalin. This substance from the scutellaria (skullcap) plant has been studied for its effectiveness in cancer and inflammatory diseases, as well as in brain disorders.

Multiple studies of all kinds have demonstrated the positive effects of baicalin and the other components of skullcap in decreasing inflammatory messages in the brain—particularly something called NFkB, an inflammatory messenger that's implicated in much of the damage to the brain following injury.

You can bounce back

Several studies have shown vitamin E to be effective in protecting the brain from the damages of injury.

In one animal study, daily intravenous vitamin E improved function after TBI, in a six-month follow-up. In another study, vitamin E reduced the damage and loss of cognitive function of even repetitive concussions.

The high antioxidant activity of vitamin E can sometimes result in altering the vitamin E itself, leading to increased oxidation, so it's frequently given along with vitamin C, which prevents this from happening.

High-dose vitamin C therapy has also been shown to have neuroprotective effects and to enhance nerve healing after an injury.

Vitamin D is another nutrient that has been studied for its potential use following TBI. Vitamin D actually acts as a hormone—and, as such, it can be used to enhance hormone therapy.

In the case of TBI, Vitamin D seems to enhance the positive effects of the hormone progesterone. Currently, Phase III multi-center studies are underway of progesterone's use in treatment of TBI.

Finally, creatine is an amino acid that's useful in maintaining proper brain and muscle function, and there seems to be enough evidence that creatine is useful in improving recovery from brain injury if given soon after.

We know that TBI lowers the creatine level in animal brains and that giving creatine to animals lessens the amount of brain damage caused by subsequent injury. But we also think that the role of creatine in improving metabolism and energy in tissues, including brain tissue, is responsible for its role in protecting the brain from damage.

In one study, children who were given creatine within a few hours of a concussion seemed to have less cognitive problems afterwards. Other studies have shown similar results in adults.

In one study of TBI in adults, creatine therapy showed significantly better function, including cognitive function and behavior, than those who did not receive the supplement.

Turn back the clock on brain injury

We are just beginning to recognize to recognize how thoroughly a knock to the noggin can affect us in the long run—and its effects may take decades to manifest.

So as we discover even more natural substances and treatments that protect our fragile nervous systems, I'll be sure to continue sharing the latest with you.

And if you've already taken a few punches to the skull, it's not too late to start trying to repair the damage that's been done. Because while you keep taking hits, your opponent in the ring isn't tiring out anytime soon.

Chapter 4:

This toxic crud could be hiding in your home, attacking your brain and making you sick!

Have you ever had the feeling your home is making you ill? Do some of your most persistent symptoms—like fatigue, headaches, brain fog and frequent colds—seem to magically clear up when you're on vacation?

If you've ever had a suspicion that your house is causing some of your health issues… you're probably correct. And the most likely culprit for your misery is mold.

Mold is made up of living organisms, and all living organisms have the internal drive to grow and expand. They produce toxins both as protection, and as a means to weaken the environment around them making it easier for them to spread. Similar to a skunk's odor, nature has given mold a powerful tool that's necessary for its survival, but toxic to everyone around it.

I myself have been helping patients fight this formidable health-destroying opponent for the last decade now. I've even locked horns with toxic mold in my own personal battle.

In 2001 we had an addition put onto our house, with a master bedroom and bathroom on the second floor. My Parkinson's symptoms first surfaced in early 2005—and two years after that, we finally realized the bathroom shower had been installed incorrectly and had been leaking water into the walls.

When we opened the walls, to our horror we discovered that dreaded black mold had obviously been growing in them for years. I firmly believe that this insidious substance—and the toxins it produced—are responsible for triggering my illness.

And I've committed myself to helping patients better understand the risks of mold exposure and to heal them of mold-related sicknesses that may have gone undiagnosed for years.

The sickening fungus among us

Mold is the true definition of a hidden killer. It's growing unseen in walls, attics and basements. In fact an estimated 40 percent of all America households are contaminated with some form of fungus. And this is way more than just a little bit of mold in the bathtub that we're talking about here.

Mold toxins irritate your brain and central nervous system causing a myriad of seemingly unrelated symptoms including (but not limited to)…

- fatigue

- headaches

- twitching

- tremors

- brain fog

- muscle pains

- insomnia

- abdominal pain, and

- frequent illnesses or colds

While mold is not good for anyone, and some people are allergic to it, it can also cause severe symptoms in certain people with a specific genetic susceptibility. For these individuals, mold is incredibly toxic and continual mold exposure at home, work or school can cause severe neurological symptoms and even trigger devastating neurological diseases like my own Parkinson's.

Most people, many of my own patients included, believe that the mold in their homes is no big deal if it isn't the "black mold" variety. The truth is ALL mold is toxic regardless if it's green, brown or black. Some people are able to excrete the mold toxins once they're breathed in, and have little long-term consequences from their exposure. But those of us who are genetically handicapped can't rid our bodies of them, and the toxins continue to build up leading to those health shattering symptoms.

Unfortunately, most people who are genetically handicapped to be susceptible to mold toxins have no idea, and very few ever get a correct diagnosis even after their health is destroyed by the creeping crud. But the good news is that you don't have to remain in the dark. You can find out if you are genetically susceptible by having an Integrative Medicine practitioner run an HLA (human leukocyte antigen) genetic test which looks specifically at the HLA or immune response gene.

Toxic schools produce toxic kids

Most parents would be horrified to learn that their kids are in danger every day at school. Unfortunately many American schools are breeding grounds for toxic mold. School buildings are often old with water damage. Air conditioning typically gets switched off in the summer months, and the rising humidity levels in the sealed empty buildings produces the perfect environment for growing mold.

Countless kids are being exposed to these hidden molds and that exposure can have terrible consequences, including some children being misdiagnosed and treated for conditions they don't even have such as ADD and ADHD.

Simple tests for toxicity

If you're experiencing troubling symptoms and suspect mold toxicity may be to blame, there are several different blood tests that could help with a diagnosis. I routinely order these tests in my own office (as do many other toxin-literate doctors) and find that the results are consistently abnormal in patients who suffer from the persistent and disabling symptoms that are often linked with mold exposure.

Although the tests—which go by acronym-laden names including the VIP, MSH, C4a and TGFbeta 1 tests—can be ordered from major local labs such as Quest and LabCorp, many conventional medicine doctors will not be familiar with them. But if you can't find a mold literate physician in your area to order the tests for you, there's a vision test that you can take on your own computer that can help clue you in to whether mold toxins are at the root of your own health challenges.

In the genetically susceptible individual, the mold toxin irritates the central nervous system and one of the most sensitive parts of the central nervous system is a nerve that controls how your eyes distinguish between shades of grey, black and white. The VCS test (visual contrast sensitivity test), sometimes known as FACT (functional acuity contrast test), evaluates how well your eyes distinguish contrast (black vs. white and especially your night vision).

I can't tell you how many patients I've seen over the years with this condition that continuously complain to their eye doctors that their glasses or vision are "off," but are told that the vision is fine and their glasses don't need to be altered. It's these very same patients who fail horribly at the VCS test. The test (there's a small fee for the VCS), and a wealth of mold toxicity information, can be found on the website www. SurvivingMold.com. This site was set up by Dr. Ritchie Shoemaker, a pioneer in the field of mold toxicity.

And for further testing you can do yourself, Real Time Labs (www. RealTimeLab.com) and BioTrek Labs (www.BioTrekLabs.com) specialize in urinary testing for mold toxins.

Detecting mold in your home and in YOU

If you're unsure if there's mold in your home but you fail the VCS test or have other symptoms, then you should attempt some form of mold detection. The telltale sign that there's mold in your home is a musty smell, especially if the house has experienced moderate to significant flood or water damage.

The cheapest first step (but not totally 100 percent foolproof) is to get mold test kits from your local home improvement store such as Home Depot or Lowe's. Leave them for the required time in the areas of your home where you suspect there might be mold and where you spend the most time.

For a more scientific and complete examination, you might want to consider using a special mold DNA test called the ERMI (www.mycometrics.com). And it may be worth the investment to have a mold remediation specialist come to your home for an inspection, or even to hire a mold sniffing dog (I'm not kidding!) for a more thorough job.

If you're sure you have mold in your home, either from the results of testing or symptoms of mold toxicity, then you should start some form of mold remediation. I won't claim this is an easy task, but it's a necessary one and well worth the effort to get rid of the fungal intrusion. The first steps, which you can do on your own, are cleansing away of any of the obvious mold (be sure to wear a breathing mask and avoid tackling black mold on your own), stopping any water leaks and de-humidification. Try to keep the house at 50 percent humidity. If your symptoms are severe and the mold issue in your home is a more serious case, you should consider employing the help of a mold remediation specialist.

Simple 3 step mold detox plan

Now that you're getting the mold out of your home it's time to think about getting the mold out of YOU. There are both nutraceutical and lifestyle changes that can rid your body of the mold toxins. In the genetically susceptible individual these toxins need some extra prodding to be fully excreted. Without this extra help the toxins will continuously recirculate, wreaking havoc on your central nervous system.

While some of my sickest patients need much more sophisticated and intense regimens, there are three steps that anyone can do on their own to help rid their body of these toxins.

Step 1: Purge toxins with binders—The most important part of the regimen is to use something that can "bind" with the toxin—sopping it up like a sponge so it can be shuttled it out of the body. My favorite "sponge" is edible bentonite clay (taken on an empty stomach), but you could also use any good source of fiber because of fiber's wonderful natural binding properties. For example, chlorella (a green sea vegetable in capsule or powdered form) is a good binder for neurotoxins. And activated charcoal tablets, available in most drug stores, can also be helpful.

Step 2: Support your liver and detox with supplements—Milk thistle and NAC (N-acetyl cysteine) will support your liver and raise your glutathione (your body's natural detoxifier) levels. This helps your body rid itself of the toxic invaders.

Step 3: Sweat it out—Last but not least, one of the best ways to get these toxins out of your body is to simply sweat them out. If your liver is overwhelmed by the toxins and unable to process them all, then you can force some of them to exit right through your skin. Exercise and saunas can raise your body temperature and help you sweat those toxins out once and for all.

PART III

Heart

Chapter 1:

Five blood-flow secrets to slash your risk of heart attack and stroke

Is your blood like wine or ketchup? Does it flow freely through your arteries like a fine Bordeaux or creep along like a cheap bottle of sticky Heinz?

The medical term for sticky thick blood is hyperviscosity and although it might seem like a silly idea to compare your blood to alcohol and condiments, studies confirm having sticky thick blood is a huge risk factor for strokes and heart attacks. And the reason why is simple—sludgy blood is significantly harder for your heart to pump around your body, and far more likely to clot and cause heart problems.

Mainstream medicine typically turns to drugs

Conventional docs deal with the sticky blood problem by recommending daily aspirin (see my sidebar to learn more about aspirin therapy) for patients with diabetes, hypertension or high cholesterol to reduce their risk of a heart attack or stroke. And if you've already had a blood clot, atrial fibrillation or a heart attack your doctor will likely also insist on a strong blood thinning medication such as coumadin.

But what if you *haven't* already been diagnosed with a medical condition that's linked to heart attack and stroke? What can the rest of us do to keep our blood flowing like wine?

Five natural blood-thinning tricks to try

Fortunately if you want to reduce your risk of heart attack or stroke, there are five simple (and safe) natural options you can try.

1) Give blood: It turns out that regularly donating blood isn't *just* a good deed—it's also good for your blood flow. It helps thin your blood, reducing damage to your blood vessels and possibly preventing blockages.

In one study out of Finland men who donated blood had an astounding 88 percent less chance of having a heart attack then men who didn't. This is also likely the reason that menstruating women rarely have heart attacks or strokes.

2) Add more garlic to your diet: Pungent and delicious garlic isn't just for cooking. In fact, the herb has been used medicinally for thousands of years, and has been proven to make your blood less sticky. And, of course, keeping blood platelets from sticking together reduces the risk

---

Aspirin benefits from a natural source

Taking an aspirin a day can thin your blood. So it might seem to make sense for all of us to simply start popping these cheap and easy to get pills. But the truth is aspirin *can* come with a serious potential side effect. The drug can lead to gastrointestinal bleeding for some users, and for some people it may even do far more harm than good.

Many of my patients are surprised to learn that aspirin is a synthesized version of the active component of an extract from the bark of a willow tree. You can get many of the same benefits of aspirin— much more safely—by taking a white willow supplement instead.

of blood clots. The herb has even been shown to help lower blood pressure slightly in some people (probably due to that free-flowing blood).

3) Load up on vitamin E: Vitamin E may be another effective way to thin your blood naturally. One study that looked at data from 26 different countries found that people with the lowest vitamin E levels had the highest risk of heart disease and stroke. While another study showed that 100 IU of E a day could reduce your chances of suffering a heart attack by a third.

If you're going to try a vitamin E supplement just be sure to choose the natural form of the vitamin, d-alpha-tocopherol.

4) Don't forget the fish oil: The omega 3's found in fish oil can do a lot more for you than simply make your blood less sticky. They can also reduce inflammation, lower cholesterol and improve your brain health while they're at it.

One precaution—if you're on a blood thinning medication such as coumadin, talk with your doctor before taking omega 3's to make sure the combined action of both don't thin your blood *too* much.

5) Get plenty of H2O: This final blood-thinning solution is so obvious that most doctors overlook it. And that's simply drinking more water. If your blood happens to be sludgy you can make it less "ketch-up-y" by diluting it in your bloodstream with simple H20. Especially if you have a history (or a family history) of heart attack or stroke, staying hydrated is essential.

Chapter 2:

Beware of the statin drug trap. Lower cholesterol is making us OLD and SICK!

What if I told you everything you've ever been told about cholesterol is a lie? That the need to aggressively lower cholesterol levels by any means necessary is nothing but a dangerous fraud foisted on us by the greedy pharmaceuticals industry designed simply to sell us statin drugs?

And what if I said that I can prove it with a basic lesson in chemistry?

You'd probably call me crazy; And that's exactly what the drug companies want you to think about anyone who dares to challenge their carefully constructed cholesterol myth. But the truth is your body NEEDS cholesterol to function.

Not only is a significant portion of your brain literally constructed of cholesterol, if you remember your high school chemistry you might also recall that many of the major hormones in our bodies come from cholesterol. In fact, if you look at testosterone or estrogen under the microscope, the very backbone of these critical-to-life sex hormones IS a cholesterol molecule.

Statins rob your body of hormone building blocks

That means that when we aggressively try to lower our cholesterol levels we're actually in direct conflict with what our body is trying to accomplish. As our body struggles to increase its hormone levels we're robbing it of the very building blocks it needs to do it.

While it's true that around 25 percent of the cholesterol in your body comes from the foods that you eat, a whopping 75 of your cholesterol profile comes from your own liver! And your liver is making those cholesterol molecules in order for your body to perform major and crucial life functions.

To make the sex hormones testosterone, progesterone and estrogen as well as the stress hormone cortisol your body takes cholesterol from your liver and turns it in to a hormone called pregnenolone. Pregnenolone is then converted into progesterone which, eventually, becomes cortisol, testosterone and estrogen.

This process is known as the "steroid pathway," and you may even remember it from a high school biology or chemistry class. And doctors should CERTAINLY remember it from their basic med school training, yet most seem to have forgotten it.

Both LDL and total cholesterol levels naturally rise in women as they enter menopause. A study in 2009 followed about 1,000 women for 10 years and found that their total and LDL cholesterol dramatically rose starting a year before stopping menstruation. This sudden spike happens for a reason, and it's one that should seem as obvious to any doctor out there as the nose on his own face. And it probably would if his vision weren't so obscured by the statin snow screen Big Pharma has produced.

Cholesterol drugs cause us to age faster!

There's really no mystery here. A woman's cholesterol spikes so dramatically at menopause because as her ovaries start to slow down on sex-hormone production her body begins to crave more of the hormones. As her levels of estrogen and testosterone drop her body starts to churn out more of the cholesterol it needs to make more of them so it can help stave off aging.

When we introduce heavy-duty statin drugs we kick off a demented game of tug-of-war with the master of our hormones, the pituitary gland. As the gland attempts to orchestrate the production of more cholesterol to make more hormones, the statins put the brakes on cholesterol production in our liver.

It's really no wonder that we see so many side effects from statins when the body is being subjected to this constant push and pull. And we are, no doubt, fast-forwarding the aging process in countless women as a result.

Men don't experience as sharp of a decline in their hormone production and as a result their cholesterol levels don't rise quite so dramatically. However statins do cause testosterone levels to drop, according to a brand new study out of Europe. And as their testosterone levels fall men are being set up for the same sort of statin drug and pituitary gland tug-of-war as the ladies.

Low T levels could lead to heart troubles

Even worse, low testosterone has been linked to heart problems, which means that by artificially lowering men's cholesterol to bargain basement lows we're likely threatening their heart health along with accelerating their aging process overall.

It's pretty obvious that statins are robbing us of the precious resources our bodies need to create the hormones that help keep us young. As a result countless men and women are being left hormone deficient with weak muscles, mushy memories and feeling old before their time.

And it's not just me that's making this critical connection. In one clinical study 41 patients with high cholesterol were given bio-identical steroidal hormones to replace those they had lost during normal aging.

Astoundingly, cholesterol levels plummeted in 100 percent of the participants. Their LDL (bad) cholesterol levels dove a whopping 24 percent on average, and their total cholesterol levels plunged 25.6 percent. And equally as exciting, 100 percent of the volunteers also reported a significant improvement in their quality of life.

You DESERVE individualized healthcare

If a new drug hit the market with similar numbers it would be FLYING off the shelves. But the researchers in this groundbreaking study didn't simply dump a one-size-fits-all drug on these folks. Instead they individualized the dosages of the bio-identical hormones including DHEA, pregnenolone, testosterone, estrogen and progesterone. In other words, every single participant got exactly what they needed to restore their hormones to youthful levels.

While the drug companies have made most people accustomed to the exact opposite of this customized approach to medicine, for anti-aging doctors (like myself) it's simply business as usual. The truth is you can, and SHOULD expect, individualized healthcare. If your current doctor doesn't fit the bill I suggest you look for one that does. Check the Alternative Health Resources section on page 449 for the contact information of some organizations that may be able to help.

Chapter 3:

Two signs on your body that may point to heart trouble

There are some physical signs to look for on your body that can be used as a basis for further investigation or treatment. Of course, this method isn't 100 percent accurate—and you must keep in mind that self-diagnosis can be tricky and deceptive. Any serious symptoms deserve medical attention. With that said, these physical signs can be a great starting point on your way to good health.

A message to your heart written on your earlobes

If you have diagonal creases across your earlobes, it may be a sign of increased susceptibility to cardiovascular disease. If you're eating right, getting regular exercise, and taking vitamin E, it's probably not anything to worry about. But just to be on the safe side, you may want to have your cholesterol, triglyceride, homocysteine, and C-reactive protein levels checked.

Beware of a pink nose and rosy cheeks

If you have dilated capillaries in your cheeks and nose (a red nose or rosy cheeks), it could be a sign of low stomach acidity. This means that you may not be properly digesting and absorbing important nutrients, supplements, or medications.

Also, low production of hydrochloric acid and pepsin in the stomach is associated with hardened arteries, high cholesterol, high triglycerides, high blood pressure, and even obesity—all of which can spell trouble for your heart.

Chapter 4:

OPCs—what are they and how do they help your heart?

Contributor: Jenny Thompson, Health Sciences Institute

Scientists are still baffled by the French paradox: Although the French have a similar intake of saturated fat to the British, their incidence of heart disease is substantially lower. Various causes have been attributed to this phenomenon, but much attention has focused on the high French intake of red wine. Red wine is rich in OPCs. OPC stands for oligomeric procyanidins, compounds that have been found to be useful in the prevention and treatment of a wide variety of heart problems.

OPCs are also a key chemical component in hawthorn, a popular herbal cardiac treatment. Some people will obviously prefer to take their OPCs in the form of wine. The quality of the wine does make a difference to its potential health benefits. If the wine contains any sort of preservative, like sulfites, it's just as likely—if not more so—to do harm as it is to do any good. Vineyards are required to state the presence of sulfite on the label of any wine containing it, so this is another instance where it's important to read labels. The key word in terms of wine's health benefits is moderation. Of course, there's no final word about how much wine is "optimum" for your health. But it's pretty safe to say that the negatives associated from drinking too much would undoubtedly outweigh any positives. Stick with a glass or two a day, at the most.

If you prefer not to drink wine, there are various OPC herbal products, including hawthorn that have strong clinical support. And they are available in most natural food stores. Just take a look at the evidence in the following studies...

Studies Confirm Hawthorn Extract is Beneficial for Heart Disease Patients

In 2003, researchers conducted a study in which more than 200 patients with chronic congestive heart failure (CHF) were divided into three groups to receive either 900 mg or 1,800 mg of hawthorn extract daily or placebo. After 16 weeks, maximum exercise tolerance increased significantly in the high-dose group compared to the other two groups, and heart failure symptoms improved in both of the extract groups, but not the placebo group.

That study was included in an Exeter University meta-analysis of clinical trials in which hawthorn was tested on hundreds of patients.

Here's how the analysis was conducted:

- Researchers combed through five medical databases looking for randomized, double-blind, placebo controlled trials in which extracts of hawthorn leaf and flower were tested on CHF patients

- Fourteen trials, which included more than 1,100 subjects, met the criteria for inclusion

- In most of the trials hawthorn was used as a complementary treatment along with conventional drug treatments for CHF

- As in the trial mentioned above, exercise tolerance was significantly improved by hawthorn intervention, as was maximal workload and pressure-heart rate product (an index of cardiac oxygen consumption)

- Analysis showed that CHF symptoms such as shortness of breath and fatigue also improved

In the most recent issue of the Cochrane Database of Systematic Reviews, the Exeter team writes: "These results suggest that there is a significant benefit in symptom control and physiologic outcomes from hawthorn extract as an adjunctive treatment for chronic heart failure."

Adverse side effects were described as "infrequent, mild, and transient."

The Exeter study shows that hawthorn extract may improve quality of life measures for CHF patients. Granted, hawthorn may not actually save the lives of gravely ill patients, but many CHF patients will likely find the extract to be "particularly helpful" in coping with the day-to-day challenges of their disease.

It should also be noted that at the 18-month follow up assessment in the 2007 study, patients who were taking the extract had a 20 percent reduced risk of CHF-related death compared to placebo – a difference that equaled four additional months of survival time.

Talk to your doctor before adding hawthorn to your daily regimen. CHF patients might want to consult with an experienced herbalist to make sure they receive a potent, high-quality hawthorn extract.

Chapter 5:

How to drop your cholesterol level by as much as 134 points without drugs or deprivation

Until recently, the general consensus among mainstream health "authorities" was that saturated fats are bad and unsaturated fats are good. But as some research supporting high-fat, high-protein diets (like the Atkins diet) suggests, it's not quite that simple.

There's only one general type of fat that you should always avoid, and that's the artificial, man-made type of fats—especially hydrogenated and partially hydrogenated vegetable oils.

You've probably noticed that these oils have been inserted into a myriad of products in the supermarket. Snack foods are the worst offenders: Try to find a potato or corn chip without it and you'll see what I mean. Even natural food stores carry a lot of products that contain partially hydrogenated oils. Make sure to read the labels of the packaged foods you buy. If it contains hydrogenated or partially hydrogenated oil, don't buy it.

So these man-made fats are definitely the ones you should stay away from. But you can't go without any fat at all. Essential fatty acids are definitely a must. The best way to make sure you are getting enough essential fatty acids is to eat whole foods containing them. The best food sources are fish and unroasted nuts and seeds.

Other naturally occurring fats (polyunsaturated, monounsaturated, and even saturated) are also safe as long as you eat them as part of a whole, unprocessed, unrefined diet.

Even though milk, ice cream, and cheese aren't on that list of man-made fats to avoid at all costs, it's still a good idea to eliminate as much dairy from your diet as possible. Dairy is one of the most common food allergens and just generally does more harm than good. It's like I always say: Milk is for baby cows—not people!

On the other hand, you should eat eggs. They've gotten a bad reputation because of their cholesterol content. But they contain phospholipids, which offset any possible adverse effects of egg cholesterol. Plus, phospholipids have a unique function in keeping brain cell membranes healthy. Eggs and soy are the only dietary sources of phospholipids. Soy is still rather controversial, and while I don't think it's necessary to give it up entirely, I do think it's a good idea to limit how much you eat to just a couple of servings a week at the most. So eggs are your only other food option for getting those nutrients that are crucial to brain cells.

Also try to include plenty of the following in your diet as good cholesterol-lowering foods: Garlic, onions, oat bran, carrots, and alfalfa sprouts.

Supplement, supplement, supplement!

There are so many vitamins, minerals, and botanicals known to lower serum cholesterol that drugs are almost never necessary. There's inositol hexaniacinate, lecithin, pantethine, L-carnitine, beta-sitosterol, fish oil and fish-oil concentrates, phosphatidyl choline, choline itself (usually with inositol and methionone), vitamin C, calcium, vanadium, magnesium, chromium, and vitamin E, which have all been found to raise levels of HDL cholesterol, the "good" cholesterol. Then there are the botanicals, including guggulipid, garlic oil, "red yeast rice," ginger, pectin, curcumin, fenugreek powder, reishi mushrooms, silymarin, turmeric, garcinia, and artichokes.

But perhaps the most effective way to lower cholesterol naturally is with something called policosanol, a natural supplement derived from sugar cane. In numerous studies comparing it directly with patent cholesterol-lowering medicines, policosanol was more effective at lowering levels of LDL (bad) cholesterol. But that's not all.

Unlike the patent medicine products, policosanol also lowered triglyceride levels and elevated HDL (good) cholesterol levels. In two studies, it also significantly lowered blood pressure as well. The good news is that it does not require a prescription and is available at most natural food stores, compounding pharmacies, and even online. And it doesn't come with the negative side effects associated with statin drugs.

You don't need to take ALL of these different supplements, of course; the point is, there are so many to try that chances are good you won't ever need to take cholesterol-lowering drugs.

Cholesterol: How low should you go?

Let's face it: Much more attention is given to high cholesterol than low cholesterol. But like any other biologic marker, there's always a range that's "too high," "too low," or "just right."

I'm not denying that having high serum cholesterol carries a risk for heart disease. I'm just saying that many people probably don't know that low serum cholesterol may also carry risks—namely cancer, stroke, and depression.

All naturally occurring steroid hormones such as DHEA, estrogens, progesterone, testosterone, and pregnenolone are made in our bodies from a single starting material: Cholesterol. And cholesterol is a key component in every cell membrane in our bodies. That's why it's important not just to make sure cholesterol isn't too high or too low, but that it's just right.

High serum cholesterol is usually considered at or above 200 mg/dl (milligrams per 100 cc's of blood). Low cholesterol is defined by many researchers as being at or below 160 mg/dl.

I pay particular attention to low cholesterol levels when they get to be around 140 mg/dl and advise them to take manganese. Manganese is a key co-factor in the transformation of cholesterol to steroid hormones. Although manganese doesn't raise serum cholesterol to the normal range 100 percent of the time, it is partially or completely effective in more than 50 percent of the cases. I usually recommend 50 milligrams of manganese citrate, once or twice daily. Once your level returns to normal, you can cut your dose to 10 to 15 milligrams a day.

There is one caution in regards to manganese supplementation: Very high levels of manganese intake have been found to cause Parkinson's disease in manganese miners and other industrial workers. However, case reports of manganese poisoning from oral intake are extremely rare (only one case report exists of toxicity from supplementation; others have been from well water with excess manganese).

But in my experience, I've never observed problems from the doses necessary to raise low serum cholesterol.

The high-fat/low-fat debate: Choosing which diet is best for you

There are two basic approaches to a cholesterol-lowering diet: The first is the politically correct, low-fat, high-complex-carbohydrate plan, which was the mainstay of nutritional "experts" for years. And there's also the high-protein, low-carbohydrate approach. It seems strange that such opposite plans can both work, but remember that no one diet is best for every person. Before choosing what's best for you, you will need to find out a bit more about your insulin response to sugar and carbohydrates (yes, sugar and carbohydrates, even though the subject is cholesterol regulation).

High-protein diets work well for many people struggling with cholesterol problems because these individuals' bodies generally manufacture much more insulin than others in response to sugar, refined carbohydrates, and excess carbs in general. This overproduction of insulin causes the liver to produce too much total cholesterol and triglycerides, and not enough HDL cholesterol.

Insulin is one of the hormones that regulates blood sugar. Some people (especially if they have type 2 diabetes or even have a genetic family tendency toward type 2 diabetes) have high insulin levels that go up much more rapidly in response to sugar and carbohydrate intake. In this case, the insulin is not used properly by the cell membranes, so the insulin can't take the sugar from the blood into the cells as it's supposed to. Then, their bodies keep making more and more insulin to try to force the sugar from the blood into the cells. The excess insulin causes other problems, including high blood pressure and cholesterol abnormalities.

Just recently, more and more evidence has been coming out in favor of the high-protein, low-carb approach to lowering cholesterol and triglyceride levels. In fact, according to a study published in the May 22, 2003 edition of the *New England Journal of Medicine*, people following a high-protein diet for six months had higher levels of HDL (good) cholesterol and bigger decreases in triglyceride levels than those people following a low-fat diet. There was no difference between the groups' LDL (bad) cholesterol levels, which shows that restricting protein and fat intake doesn't do as much to help cholesterol levels as the "experts" once thought.

It's possible that many people with weight problems have them due to this excess insulin response to sugar and carbohydrates. If your cholesterol levels are high, ask your doctor to administer a glucose-insulin tolerance test, which can tell you how much insulin your body makes in response to a standard amount of sugar. Then you can make an informed choice about your diet.

The hidden high cholesterol culprit you might not be looking for

Saturated fat gets a lot of blame when it comes to high cholesterol. Carbohydrates come in a close second. While they're both important factors, they aren't the only ones to consider. Diets high in saturated fat are responsible for approximately one in five cases of high serum cholesterol, and high carbohydrate intake is responsible for approximately one in three. That still leaves a little less than half of all high serum cholesterol cases unaccounted for.

The fact is, if you have high cholesterol, you may need to look further than your diet to find the real culprit.

Researchers from the Japanese National Institute of Agrobiological Sciences think they may have found a missing piece of the cholesterol puzzle. They discovered that small quantities of lead caused elevated serum cholesterol in experimental animals. In their experiments they found that lead induces the genes responsible for creating the liver enzymes that produce cholesterol.

To compound the problem, lead also suppresses a gene responsible for the production of a liver enzyme that breaks down and destroys cholesterol. With cholesterol production "turned on" and cholesterol breakdown "turned off" by lead, the animals' serum cholesterol increased significantly.

Although the lead/cholesterol connection hasn't been proven by research on humans yet, it still helps to explain some observations that holistic doctors have made over the years. Holistic doctors who do chelation therapy (a process that removes lead and other toxic metals from the body) have noted that cholesterol levels often drop after chelation.

If you've tried following a strict diet and your serum cholesterol is still high, have a physician skilled and knowledgeable in nutritional and natural medicine check your lead levels. The most accurate way to test for lead is to get an intravenous drip of a chelating agent (EDTA is typically used for lead chelation) followed by a six- to eight-hour urine collection, which is then tested for lead and other toxic metals.

If a chelation test shows you have too much lead (or other toxic heavy metal) in your system, work with your physician to get the lead out. Not only will it help your serum cholesterol levels, but it will also help lots of other natural biochemical processes in your body operate better.

Chapter 6:

Red yeast rice drops LDL cholesterol 35 points

Mainstream admits power of red yeast rice

Just as the mainstream is pushing statins for even healthy people, good news comes from an unlikely source. Red yeast rice continues to show its power, and it's getting harder to ignore.

Sometimes, good news comes from surprising places. This time, it's a small beam of support for alternative medicine from a very mainstream source.

In a video from Medscape (a very conventional online news source for doctors), Dr. Sandra Fryhofer pays the mildest of lip service to the dangers of statins before giving a reluctant report of an alternative.

She calls it statin-associated myalgia, or SAM–because what mainstream news outlet wants to come right out and admit to the debilitating muscle pain and weakness that statins can cause?

The report also becomes a test in how many times one person can say the phrase "some patients."

"Some patients" are "bothered" by statin side effects. "Some patients" experience statin-associated myalgias. "Some patients" are seeking an alternative. Say it enough, and "some patients" starts to sound like some foreign group, completely outside all of the normal, statin-loving people.

But we know better than that.

The study–published in the Annals of Internal Medicine– had 62 patients who'd quit taking statins because of terrible pain on 3 600 mg capsules of red yeast rice or placebo 2 times a day for 26 weeks. Both groups also made lifestyle changes, incorporating diet and exercise plans, yoga, and massage. (Sounds pretty nice to me!)

You can tell she doesn't want to admit it–in fact, she offers a slew of caveats you just don't see when the media fawns over the latest Big Pharma poison–but she has to.

The red yeast rice worked, bringing on a 35-point drop in LDL cholesterol. The group on placebo (but who still made lifestyle changes) saw a 15-point drop.

The doctor is critical, calling the study small and saying red yeast rice "seemed to help." She even speculates that, because red yeast rice has the same basic action as statins, maybe the dose of red yeast rice is just too small to cause unwanted side effects.

No unwanted side effects, and it still works? Sold!

This news couldn't come at a better time, with the FDA showing its support for statin use to prevent heart attacks in healthy people. That's right–the very thing we have been cautioning against is coming true: Statins for everyone!

One doctor called the FDA advisory panel's recommendation for Crestor use in healthy people "courageous." I call it something else…but I can't write that word here.

Chapter 7:

The ONE number that can really predict your heart attack risk

This wasn't supposed to happen to you.

Your cholesterol numbers are perfect. Maybe you even use a statin drug to keep them low.

But there you are, stretched out on a hospital bed, listening to some doctor tell you that you've had a heart attack.

It happens more often than you'd think. And that's because millions of Americans—and their doctors—have fallen for the "cholesterol myth."

It goes something like this—keep your cholesterol low (preferably by taking statin drugs) and you'll never have to worry about a heart attack. But studies have shown that lowering your cholesterol using statins doesn't do a thing to prevent heart attacks or strokes.

There's a lot more to predicting a heart attack than your cholesterol count. In fact, there's an important missing link in the whole cholesterol discussion that many mainstream doctors have never figured out.

But once you understand it (and how to test for it) you'll see how it just may be possible to stop heart disease—or even a deadly heart attack—before they strike.

The cholesterol secret that could save your life

For years in my own medical practice, I've seen evidence that the root cause of stroke and heart attack is not JUST elevated cholesterol.

In fact, one of my patients has a life-long total cholesterol ranging near 1,000 and a LDL (bad cholesterol) near 600. If high cholesterol was the only cause of cardiovascular disease, she would have been dead a long time ago!

Thankfully, she's still healthy and vibrant—at the ripe old age of 90.

And, there's already plenty of research to back up my own findings. A landmark study published in 2009 in the *American Heart Journal*[1] showed that 75 percent of 135,000 patients that were hospitalized for a heart attack showed cholesterol values that were not high, per the current guidelines at that time.

Half of them even had cholesterol levels that were considered IDEAL, to boot![2]

That surprised a lot of folks in the mainstream—but it shouldn't have. As far back as 1979, scientists knew that just having high LDL cholesterol was not the ONLY factor involved in cardiovascular disease.

Clearly, the LDL cholesterol needed to be MODIFIED in some way to be rendered "dangerous"—that is, to spark off the chemical process of clogging an artery.

Oxidation puts you on the fast track to Heart Attack City

You see, LDL cholesterol isn't bad on its own. It's when it becomes "oxidized" through inflammation that it sticks to and clogs your arteries.

So how much LDL cholesterol you have isn't all that important. It's how much of it is oxidized that counts.

Fortunately, there's an oxidized LDL—or "OxLDL"—blood test that doesn't measure the AMOUNT of LDL in your body, but how much damage has actually been done to your arteries once the LDL became oxidized.

Since oxidized LDL testing was first developed in 1986, there have been over 5,000 published articles that support using oxidized LDL as a marker and predictor of heart attacks.

And it's WAY more accurate than a standard cholesterol test. One of the larger studies showed that patients with an elevated oxidized LDL were over *four times more likely* to have a heart attack than if their LDL wasn't oxidized.[3]

Unfortunately, for years oxidized LDL testing wasn't reliable and affordable enough to provide to the masses, so it went largely ignored.

The great news is that's all changed, and oxidized LDL testing has become more widely available and economical. There are labs all across the country that can do the test, and I regularly use it as a screening tool for my high-risk patients.

If you're like most patients, you've never had an oxidized LDL test. But you should get one, as it will give you a much more complete picture of your heart attack risk.

Ask your doctor to order the test. If he's not familiar with it, or doesn't know how to interpret it, there are a number of blood labs that can refer you to a doctor who does.

Powerful supplements fight oxidation... *naturally!*

So what can you do if your oxidized LDL is high—or you're just interested in preventing oxidation in your body?

Common sense tells us that if oxidation is the problem, antioxidants are the solution.

Unfortunately, a lot of patients and doctors are steered away from this course of action because of studies about a decade ago that claimed antioxidants didn't work in fighting heart disease.[4]

Well, those studies only tested two antioxidants: vitamin E and beta carotene. And the doses used were much too small to be of any clinical benefit.

Believe it or not, some old studies actually DID show the amazing powers of vitamin E in select groups of patients, but were swept under the rug. In fact, in one study of patients with known excessive oxidation, 800 IU of vitamin E a day provided an amazing 75 percent reduction in heart attack risk![5]

To top that, the results were SO good in another study that it was deemed unethical to keep giving anyone a placebo dummy pill when the vitamin E worked so well.[6]

I have tested oxidized LDL for many patients in my own clinic, and there are strong indications that supplementing with a good quality antioxidant is ESSENTIAL to stop some of the "rust" that is building up in your arteries.

As we test and learn more, I'll continue to update you about which supplements are proving to lower the oxidized LDL values the most.

Chapter 8:

How to drop your blood pressure by 20, 30, or even 40 points—naturally

The mainstream medical industry certainly seems determined to get us all on patent hypertension (blood pressure) medications. With the new guidelines issued by the National Heart, Lung and Blood Institute, people whose blood pressure levels were once considered well below normal (a 120 over 80 reading) suddenly became "pre-hypertensive"—essentially overnight. And, of course, one of the first recommendations out of all the so-called "experts'" mouths was more widespread use of patent hypertension medications.

But you can beat high blood pressure—most of the time without drugs. And even if you can't completely avoid patent medicines, taking the right natural measures may be able to help you use substantially less.

What works for someone else may not work for you

In many cases, the old saying "you are what you eat" holds true. It might do some good in some cases to cut out a few of the cream sauces and slices of pizza. In some cases, a diet containing more fruits, vegetables, and whole, natural starches rather than a lot of protein could be your best bet. However, the key words here are "in some cases" and "could."

Decades ago, public health researchers observed that women and men who had been strictly vegetarian all their lives had lower blood pressure readings in their 60s and 70s than did men and women who ate considerable animal protein. A vegetarian diet provides a better potassium-to-sodium ratio. Having more potassium and less sodium helps regulate blood pressure. But a vegetarian diet isn't the best choice for everyone and, in fact, could cause more harm than good for some.

People with high blood pressure who have personal or family histories of type 2 (adult onset) diabetes usually have insulin resistance/hyperinsulinemia. The term insulin resistance refers to the impaired use of insulin by cell membranes. Hyperinsulinemia occurs when the pancreas overproduces insulin in an attempt to overcome insulin resistance. (Insulin resistance/hyperinsulinemia is easily diagnosed via a glucose-insulin tolerance test.)

Hyperinsulinemia is a known cause of high blood pressure. To bring insulin overproduction under control, the most necessary dietary changes are total elimination of sugar and refined carbohydrates and a sharp reduction in overall carbohydrate intake. It's especially important to eliminate such starches as potatoes, beans, pasta, and grains. Obviously, this diet pattern is not vegetarian, but, as it helps bring hyperinsulinism under control, blood pressure is also better regulated.

You can also take natural supplements to help regulate your insulin. There are so many nutrients shown to be helpful in type 2 diabetes that taking them all individually would be a real chore. You'll find several "multiple" formulas designed specifically to aid in blood sugar control in natural food stores. One of the most common ingredients in these formulas is chromium, which restores the cell membrane response to insulin.

There are also two more ingredients you should take in addition to your blood sugar controlling multiple supplement. The first is niacin. With chromium, niacin forms part of a molecule called the glucose-tolerance factor, which helps insulin do its job. Both chromium and niacin will get your cells to pay attention to the insulin again, so your insulin and blood sugar levels should go down. It's important to do initial and follow-up testing with your doctor to monitor your progress. Finally, you should also consider taking flaxseed or flaxseed oil capsules. Flaxseed also helps your cells use insulin.

However, there has been a shadow cast over it recently because it contains the essential fatty acid alpha-linolenic acid (ALA), which several studies have linked to a higher risk of prostate cancer and cataracts. While not all the research agreed, there's definitely enough to be cause for concern.

However, these studies definitely aren't the "last word" on ALA. It's important to remember that ALA is an essential-to-life fatty acid, and it's highly unlikely that Nature would require us to have it in order to survive if there was no way around these potential negative effects. It's very possible that another nutrient or several nutrients are involved in the ALA-prostate cancer and ALA-cataract connection, and that using more (or less) of these would "erase" any possible harm from higher levels of ALA. Unfortunately, researchers rarely consider nutrients in more complex interactions. So it'll likely be a long time until this aspect of the "ALA question" is considered.

In the meantime, this does not mean that you need to eliminate flaxseed and flaxseed oil from your diet! In addition to ALA there are many other healthful nutrients present, especially in whole flaxseed. However, it's probably wisest to consult your nutritionally knowledgeable physician about what quantity of flaxseed or flaxseed oil might be best for you. And since too much ALA can suppress "5-alpha-reductase," if you're a man, you might want to have your "5-alpha reductase" enzyme activity measured. This is easily done from a 24-hour urinary steroid test. Some physicians may also recommend a red blood cell membrane essential fatty acid test to make sure your ALA levels aren't out of balance with other fatty acids.

Food allergy may be the culprit

For some people with hypertension, food allergies can play a big part in the problem. Eliminating the allergens or desensitizing to them can help lower blood pressure levels, though no one has been able to successfully explain the connection. If you have a personal or family history of allergies, it's worth investigating. Contact a member of the American Academy of Environmental Medicine (316-684-5500; www.aaemonline.org) for a list of doctors near you who can help with thorough allergy screening.

The most notable individual case of allergy aggravated hypertension involved a gentleman who was undergoing maximum antihypertensive drug therapy but still had blood pressure readings ranging from a minimum 180/120 to a maximum 220/150. Once he discovered and eliminated all food allergies, his blood pressure dropped to a level ranging from 160/100 minimum to 180/120 maximum.

Biofeedback and exercise—old news, but underrated and underused

Biofeedback is another valuable and frequently effective "non-drug" tool for lowering blood pressure. It's not so much a "treatment" as it is a training program. Using external instruments, a reading is obtained of your body's reactions to stress. Through practice, you learn to recognize the physiological responses you have that might be causing unhealthy reactions and teach yourself how to control those responses. Biofeedback centers are found in all major and most midsize cities. Check your local Yellow Pages for listings.

Exercise also can significantly lower high blood pressure. Even light exercise can make a big difference. The amount that's healthy varies from person to person. Of course, it's best to check with a doctor or other knowledgeable individual before starting a strenuous exercise program.

If you're concerned about blood pressure and wonder what your level might be, there are many places to have it measured for free, including drugstores, fire stations (when the firemen aren't fighting fires), health fairs, and "senior centers." Home blood pressure monitoring equipment is quite accurate, and most places that sell it will teach you how to use it as well.

Nutrients: Which to cut back on and which to increase

Sodium. You've probably heard that cutting WAY back on salt intake is an important step in lowering high blood pressure. However, researchers are finding more and more evidence that sodium restriction might not be best for everyone after all. If you have high blood pressure you might want to determine through trial and error whether or not salt restriction makes a difference for you.

Potassium. Sometimes it reduces blood pressure, sometimes it doesn't. Since a higher potassium level does reduce the risk of stroke, it's always wisest to take extra potassium if you have high blood pressure, even if it doesn't lower your actual blood pressure numbers.

Calcium and magnesium. For some individuals, about 1 gram (1,000 milligrams) of calcium daily can greatly reduce blood pressure by five to 10 points. For others, calcium makes very little difference. It appears to work more often for those with insulin resistance/hyperinsulinemia. If you do supplement with calcium, it's important to balance it with magnesium. Magnesium by itself can lower your blood pressure level, since it helps relax muscles, including those of the smaller blood vessels, thus helping to dilate them and improve blood flow. Supplementing with 300 to 400 milligrams daily is usually sufficient.

Vitamin C. A recent research letter sent to the medical journal *Lancet* reconfirmed that vitamin C lowers elevated blood pressure. Although this study used less, you should take a minimum of 1 gram twice daily.

Vitamin D. Vitamin D achieves its blood pressure lowering effect by addressing one of the major causes of high blood pressure—a substance called angiotensin II.

Without adequate vitamin D, one of your genes (a tiny part of your DNA) initiates the formation of excess quantities of a molecule called renin. Renin breaks down another molecule, called angiotensinogen, into angiotensin I. Angiotensin I is converted into angiotensin II by a substance known as angiotensin converting enzyme (ACE). That's why most popular patented "space alien" antihypertensives are ACE inhibitors and angiotensin II receptor blockers (ARBs).

But vitamin D helps prevent high blood pressure by targeting the very first step in the process: It persuades the gene that controls the production of renin to become less active. When less renin is produced, less angiotensin is produced.

While vitamin D is very effective at lowering blood pressure, don't expect overnight miracles: It frequently takes two to three months for significant changes to start taking place and six to eight months for the vitamin D to take full effect.

How much do you need? Well, recent research has reevaluated the safe upper limit for this vitamin, and many experts now agree that it's 10,000 IU daily (though some say it's as low as 4,000 IU daily). But my target for optimal vitamin D intake is whatever it takes to achieve a serum level of approximately 60 ng/ml. Since achieving this level will mean a different dose for everyone, it's always best to work with your doctor to monitor your blood level of vitamin D.

The building blocks of healthy blood pressure

Amino acids are the "building blocks" from which all proteins are made. In certain cases, supplementing with them has led to lower blood pressure.

At least one study devoted to each demonstrated that L-tryptophan and taurine can lower blood pressure in essential hypertension (high blood pressure with no known cause). The amount of L-tryptophan used was 3 grams daily. L-tryptophan has been available by prescription for two to three years now, but it also very recently became available over the counter once again (as it used to be until about 1989). At present, over-the-counter L-tryptophan can be found in a few natural food stores, and compounding pharmacies.

Quantities of taurine used in the study were relatively large (but safe)—6 grams daily. However, when taurine is used in combination with other nutrients and botanicals, you need only 1 to 2 grams daily.

L-arginine has gained considerable "notoriety" lately as the precursor to nitric oxide (NO), the blood vessel-dilating metabolite essential to male sexual function. However, that same blood vessel-dilating ability has been found to improve heart function in cases of congestive heart failure, and there are many cases in which this same blood vessel-dilating effect has lowered blood pressure.

The benefits of metabolites: Coenzyme Q10 and DHA

Metabolites are molecules made in our bodies from other (precursor) materials. Sometimes, directly supplying the body with extra quantities of certain metabolites can be much more effective than supplying the precursor materials. This is definitely the case with coenzyme Q10, as our bodies make less and less of this metabolite as we grow older.

Coenzyme Q10 aids in metabolism in every cell in the body. It's found in greatest concentration in the mitochondria, the "energy engines" of the cells. It's such an important metabolite that, even though it can be fairly expensive, I recommend a small amount (30 milligrams) for everyone over 60 and more (50 to 150 milligrams daily) for everyone with high blood pressure.

Another important metabolite that helps lower blood pressure levels is docosahexaenoic acid, or DHA (not to be confused with DHEA). This is an omega-3 fatty acid, a metabolite of the essential fatty acid called alpha-linolenic acid. A recent study reported that 4 grams daily of DHA lowered blood pressure in hypertensive patients by a small but significant degree.

The garlic and herb recipe for blood pressure success

Although you'll encounter a few foods that your doctor will tell you to stay away from if you have high blood pressure, there are certain foods and herbs that can help. Garlic may not make for the freshest breath, but it does usually help to lower blood pressure readings.

A lesser-known (but still important) blood pressure-lowering botanical is olive leaf. Only powdered olive leaf in capsule form is presently available in the United States, and you should take 500 milligrams four times daily. Like many of the items noted above, olive leaf can take three to four months to show an effect.

Sarpagandha (better known in Western medicine as rauwolfia) has been used in India for centuries to treat ailments like fevers and snakebites. Early 20th century pharmaceutical chemists searching for a "magic bullet," single-ingredient, patentable, FDA-"approvable" drug treatment managed to isolate one of the active ingredients in sarpagandha—reserpine.

Herbalists have been telling us for most of the 20th century that it's really better to use the whole herb containing the active ingredient(s), for at least two reasons. First, a smaller quantity of an active ingredient is usually effective because of synergistic effects of other parts of the herb—and the whole herb usually holds less potential danger than the isolated active ingredients. Second, herbalists have told us that combining the whole herb with other selected herbs can further lessen the quantity of each active ingredient necessary to achieve significant results and further lessen potential danger.

But western physicians still went ahead using reserpine instead of whole natural sarpagandha to combat high blood pressure. Unfortunately, many of them prescribed excess dosages of reserpine. These excess dosages caused various ailments, including depression and occasional suicide, so reserpine fell out of common use.

Unfortunately, since there's not as much money to be made with the whole, natural herb itself, the medical world basically forgot about sarpagandha after the problems with reserpine: Only a few practitioners outside of Ayurvedic medicine are even aware of its existence. Most of the sarpaganda products available these days combine this herb with others also useful for the heart. Although side effects are rare and sarpagandha is definitely a very effective "big gun" in hypertension treatment, products containing sarpagandha are usually only available through health care practitioners.

I usually recommend sarpagandha as a part of the Ayurvedic combination, Cardiotone, which contains 50 milligrams of sarpagandha per capsule; take one capsule three to four times daily.

An underactive thyroid: An often overlooked culprit

Incidence of hypothyroidism (an underactive thyroid) is higher in individuals with high blood pressure than in those with normal blood pressure. Even the most up-to-date thyroid blood tests can miss instances of "subclinical" hypothyroidism. Some signs of an underactive thyroid are low body temperature, dry skin, and a slow ankle reflex. It's best to talk to your doctor if you think there's a problem.

Make sure you know how much metal you're really carrying around

Heavy metal toxicity is another often-overlooked cause of high blood pressure. But even if your doctor does test you for heavy metal toxicity, chances are the results won't be accurate. That's because blood tests for heavy metals are virtually useless.

Since these toxic substances are damaging to so many different cell structures, your body clears them from your bloodstream as rapidly as possible. If there's too much toxic metal to be immediately excreted through your liver and kidneys (and there usually is), it gets tucked away in your bones or other less metabolically active tissue where it causes less immediate damage. So a blood test won't necessarily pick up any toxicity—even if there's a ton of it stored in your body.

Unfortunately, wherever the unexcreted toxic metal is stored, it still does some damage, and if and when it's finally released from storage, it can do further damage.

Hair testing for toxic minerals isn't much better than blood tests. If one or more metals are found to be high based on a hair test, there's definitely a toxic mineral problem. But if the hair test comes back negative, it doesn't necessarily mean that you're free from heavy metal toxicity.

The best test for the presence of heavy metals is a chelation test. In my experience, more than 50 percent of individuals with blood pressure higher than 140/90 have significant excretion of toxic metals found by a chelation test.

And if you do have heavy metal toxicity, chelation therapy will usually help lower your blood pressure. Chelation therapy is an intravenous process that binds to the heavy metals and removes them from the body. Oral chelation can also be effective, but it takes considerably longer and doesn't necessarily remove as much toxic metal.

For more information or advice about both chelation testing and treatment for toxic metals, consult a physician from any of the groups listed below:

- The American College of Advancement in Medicine: (800)532-3688; www.acam.org

- The International College of Integrative Medicine: (419)358-0273; www.icimed.com

- The American Academy of Environmental Medicine: (316)684-5500; www.aaemonline.org

- The American Association of Naturopathic Physicians: (866)538-2267; www.naturopathic.org

If you have high blood pressure, nearly all the diet and supplementation ideas discussed are safe to try. If you don't have high blood pressure but it runs in your family, it can't hurt and may help in prevention to follow a few of the basic suggestions outlined in this section.

Chapter 9:

Can this one "hero mineral" keep you from EVER having a heart attack?

Forget those prescription drugs or the latest exercise fads—it turns out Dr. Mom has had the key to preventing heart disease all along!

Moms and grandmoms have known forever about the importance of magnesium. It's been used to heal wounds since the 1600s, and I bet at some point your mother threw you into an epsom salt (a.k.a. magnesium salt) bath to help relieve sore muscles or even a stubborn cold.

But when it comes to preventing serious and chronic health conditions, magnesium is like the Rodney Dangerfield of minerals. It just can't seem to get any respect!

Magnesium helps promote everything from strong bones to a good night's sleep—but other supplements like calcium and melatonin seem to grab all the headlines.

But now it looks like magnesium is about to be recognized as the hero mineral it is. Because a growing body of research is proving that it can hold the key to protecting your heart—and even stopping a deadly heart attack before it ever strikes.

The heart's silent savior

Magnesium's ability to fight inflammation has long been tremendously underappreciated. But it's so important, because we're learning that inflammation is the hidden culprit that starts to break down your body's organs, including your cardiovascular system.

It begins when the cells that line your arteries (a.k.a. the "endothelium") become inflamed. In response, your body produces inflammatory messengers (like C-reactive protein, nuclear factor kappa B, and cytokines) and puts platelets on the injured cells in a process called thrombosis. Your body further attempts to heal the area by using cholesterol and other substances to "patch" the wound.

But the patch, called an atheroma, later collects calcium and fibrous tissue, which eventually harden into plaque and obstruct the artery. That's when you develop a serious condition like atherosclerosis.

And hardened arteries can lead to high blood pressure, heart attacks, strokes, or other problems that collectively are called ASCVD (atherosclerotic cardio-vascular disease).

Stop cardiovascular disease
before it starts

Research shows that if you're getting enough magnesium, your body is less likely to go through that inflammatory response in the first place.

In one of the studies that supports the use of magnesium in atherosclerosis, rabbits with varying levels of cholesterol (from low to high) were fed a diet either low or high in magnesium. As expected, the most aortic plaque formation occurred in the group with high cholesterol and low magnesium.[1]

But here's the really interesting part: The ones with both high cholesterol AND high magnesium were almost plaque-free!

Since then, several other animal studies have supported the same conclusion: Dietary magnesium can prevent arterial clot formation and therefore prevent ASCVD.

But it's not *just* about inflammation. Magnesium can also prevent you from having a heart attack, keep your blood pressure from getting too high, and make sure you've got enough good cholesterol and not too much of the bad stuff.

Blocking calcium: Magnesium is the body's natural calcium-channel blocker. That's a good thing because too much calcium in the cells can result in too much muscle contraction—and since your heart is a muscle, you'll want to keep it nice and relaxed if you want to avoid a heart attack.

Here's how it works: when magnesium moves from its regular place inside your body's cells, through the cell membrane to outside the cell, it blocks calcium from entering the cells. This leads to less production of the two main hormones that contribute to high blood pressure—angiotensin and aldosterone—and the result is lowered blood pressure.

Balanced cholesterol: Additionally, magnesium can help keep your cholesterol balance in check. Its presence is necessary for many of your body's enzymes to work properly—including "lipoprotein lipase," the enzyme that increases your production of "good" cholesterol (HDL) and keeps your triglycerides from getting too high.

On the other side of the coin, magnesium also lowers the "bad" cholesterol LDL by a mechanism related to its role in metabolizing lecithin, a nutrient mixture critical in balancing lipids in the body.

Finally, magnesium can also work in the same way that statins do: by inhibiting HMG-CoA, the enzyme that makes cholesterol in your body in the first place. Only, with magnesium, you don't get all those scary side effects and risks.

Without magnesium, your heart disease gets worse fast

Even if you've already got ASCVD, studies show that magnesium can prevent it from getting any worse—and can even improve your condition!

A common way doctors evaluate the severity of your atherosclerosis is by measuring a biomarker called Carotid Artery Intima Medial Thickness, or CIMT. The thicker the artery, the more severe the condition.

One study showed that supplementing hemodialysis patients with just 100 mg of magnesium a day for two months actually lowered their CIMT—that is, the magnesium REDUCED the thickness of their arteries![2]

The reverse is also true. The Atherosclerosis Risk in Communities (ARIC) study[3] showed that lower levels of magnesium intake resulted in thicker arteries (and therefore a higher CIMT). This was more significant in women than in men in this study, and it appears from other studies as well that women are particularly susceptible to the cardiovascular damage associated with low magnesium.

Magnesium also seems to protect against some of the potentially disastrous consequences of ASCVD, including getting hit with a stroke.

In 2012, several studies on the link between magnesium and stroke were compared for common effects and combined, so that the researchers can see possibly significant findings that weren't obvious in the individual studies. Among the 240,000 some-odd participants who were included, 100 mg of magnesium daily was associated with an 8 percent reduction in the type of stroke caused by a blockage of an artery that brings blood to the brain (called "ischemic stroke").[4]

Your risk of stroke can also be increased by atrial fibrillation, a dangerous complication of cardiovascular surgery that can also be lessened by magnesium before you go under the knife. In one study, only 2 percent of patients treated with IV magnesium sulfate before cardiac bypass surgery experienced the irregular heart rate associated with atrial fibrillation—far less than 21 percent of the untreated group.

I always wonder how many lives could be saved by loading a patient with magnesium before performing the thousands of potentially dangerous cardiovascular surgeries that are the bread-and-butter of many modern hospitals.

And that's just the beginning...

I've got lots more to talk about regarding magnesium, so stay tuned for a continuation on the topic in next month's newsletter. I'll talk more about intravenous magnesium therapy, which can be beneficial for lots of other conditions. In my office, we use it for everything from chronic fatigue and fibromyalgia to hypertension, angina, asthma, and even panic disorder. In next month's issue, I'll also take you through the various forms of oral magnesium supplements and ways to get your magnesium levels checked.

In the meantime, it can't hurt to load up on a magnesium-rich diet, like spinach and other dark leafy greens, bananas, nuts and seeds, fish, avocado, and even...wait for it...dark chocolate! Magnesium is hiding in all of these delicious foods, just waiting to work its wonders on your heart health.

Chapter 10:

Don't TOUCH that next dose of aspirin until you've had this important test

If I had a dime for every time a patient asked me whether they should be taking a daily aspirin for their heart, I'd be sipping margaritas on a tropical island by now.

And I don't blame them (or you) for being confused. Because when it comes to aspirin guidelines, most doctors have been flying blind for years!

Say what you will about the dangerous cholesterol and blood pressure medications on the market today (and I have plenty to say about them). But at least doctors will actually *test* you before prescribing them.

But aspirin may be the one drug that docs will tell you to take without performing *any* diagnostics—and without barely giving you a once-over.

And that's a serious mistake. Because there actually *is* a test that doctors like me have been using for years to make smart aspirin recommendations to our patients.

It could keep you from starting an aspirin regimen you don't need—and prevent you from taking a dose that could be downright dangerous.

Your blood may be thicker than it should be

First, it's helpful to understand why some doctors recommend aspirin for preventing a heart attack or stroke (especially if you've already had one).

You see, a heart attack, stroke, or pulmonary embolism will occur due to the formation of a blood clot (a thrombosis). While not all blood clots are fatal, anytime one of these events does take a life, you can blame the blood clot. Blood clots can stop your heart, brain, and lungs dead in their tracks.

I'm a big believer in keeping your blood relatively thin to prevent those clots from forming. The thinner your blood is, the less likely you are to develop a life-threatening clot. I like to say that your blood should flow more like wine than ketchup.

And while there are many natural and non-natural ways to thin your blood, the cheapest and most reliable way is...you guessed it, aspirin. That's the reason so many doctors have been pushing it for years.

Get an answer that's as simple as "yes" or "no"

So to determine whether you need to (or even should) take aspirin, there's a test called "AspirinWorks."

It actually measures the chemical biomarker of thromboxane (specifically, 11-Dehydro Thromboxane B2), the chemical that makes your blood platelets sticky and therefore more likely to form a clot.[1]

So, elevated thromboxane levels in the urine—and the indication that your blood may be too "sticky"—can reveal a higher risk of stroke and heart attack. In fact, one large study showed that an elevated urinary thromboxane level in an AspirinWorks test result could increase your risk of one of these life-threatening cardiovascular events *four times over*.[2]

And you know how aspirin thins your blood? By reducing your levels of thromboxane.

Therefore, if the AspirinWorks test detects that you have elevated urinary thromboxane levels, then it's relatively conclusive that your blood could use some thinning, and taking aspirin as a preventative measure may be the way to go. That's a pretty reliable recommendation based on your own body chemistry.

And the feds just keep muddying things up

I'm excited to tell you about this test because without it, your conventional primary care doctor and cardiologist are about to get even more befuddled than before.

That's because the new draft recommendations released by the US Preventive Services Task Force[3] regarding daily aspirin use are so elaborate, it's hard to figure out whether or not you fit the profile they're describing!

The USPSTF recommends taking low-dose aspirin daily to prevent cardiovascular disease if you...

☒ are an adult, 50 to 59 years old AND

☒ have a 10-year risk of developing cardiovascular disease that's 10 percent or higher AND

☒ are not at increased risk for bleeding AND

☒ have a life expectancy of at least 10 years AND

☒ are willing to take low-dose aspirin daily for at least 10 years.

So...should you take aspirin to prevent a heart attack or stroke? Without the AspirinWorks test, the best answer you could probably get is a big ol' shrug.

Get the download on your ideal dose

Since introducing it into my practice, I have found the AspirinWorks test to be reliable, easy, and incredibly informative. I feel so relieved to have the confidence to help patients make this important decision. It's also been eye-opening to see that a good number of my patients actually do have elevated urinary thromboxane levels.

This test is also incredibly useful because it can even direct HOW MUCH aspirin you should take so that you can stay at the lowest possible dose.

This is such an important aspect of the test because the side effects of ANY drug—prescription or over-the-counter—accrue and become compounded as the dosage increases. In the case of aspirin, you run the risk of bleeding in the gastrointestinal system and brain when you take it—so it's best if you take as little as possible of it, if you take it at all.

On the other side of the coin, the test also can tell you if you're one of the 25 percent of Americans who are resistant to the effects of aspirin—which may mean you'll need a higher dosage than normal, or you shouldn't bother taking it at all.

So now what?

If you do decide to start taking aspirin, there is yet another debate you should be aware of: coated versus uncoated. The "safety" coating has been added to some versions to make them easier to swallow, but it doesn't really make them any safer once they're in your system (especially as it relates to stomach bleeding), and the coating may actually inhibit aspirin's ability to prevent blood clotting.

Typically, the consensus is to start with "baby" aspirin, which you can chew, crush, or swallow whole. You should take it with food keep your stomach from getting irritated.

Of course, you don't have to take aspirin to thin your blood. While there aren't many supplements that naturally lower thromboxane levels, aspirin's natural alternative, white willow bark, is available.

This supplement isn't as powerful as taking an aspirin (which, if you're sensitive to aspirin, can be a good thing), but it can still do the trick. White willow bark, which has been dubbed "Mother Nature's rival to aspirin," is available in both capsule form and as an extract at your local health food store. Talk to your doctor about any interactions with other medications you may be taking, and what dosage may be right for you as an alternative to a daily aspirin.

But first: start with the AspirinWorks test. You'll be happy to know that this very useful, potentially life-saving test is widely available and offered by large laboratories such as Labcorp and Quest. Your doctor should be willing to order one for you.

Chapter 11:

Could this "blacklisted" treatment end up saving your life?

A treatment the mainstream has been trying to kill for decades just may hold the secret to adding years to your life. And the proof is now so rock solid, even conventional doctors are going to have to take a second look.

I'm talking about intravenous chelation therapy, which can attract, capture, and sweep toxins out of your body, especially heavy metals that can attack everything from your heart to your brain.

The American College for Advancement in Medicine (ACAM, a non-profit organization of which I'm a member) has been teaching physicians how to perform chelation therapy for over 30 years.[1] Still, many mainstream docs—and even groups like the American Heart Association—have done everything they can to blacklist chelation.

But a major study has definitively proven that chelation can help you ranging from heart disease to diabetes. And this treatment that has spent too long in the shadows may now be ready for prime-time.

One small step for chelation therapy... one giant leap for cardiovascular disease

ACAM first partnered with the National Institutes of Health (NIH) in 2003 to produce even MORE proof of how chelation can be used to successfully treat cardiovascular disease.

Their joint, large-scale study called the Trial to Assess Chelation Therapy (TACT) involved a course of 40 ethylene diamine tetraacetic acid (EDTA) chelation infusions—just like the ones we've all been giving for years. Over 1,700 patients across 134 sites in both the U.S. and Canada received a total of 55,222 infusions. They were randomized to receive either (a) intravenous chelation and oral vitamins or (b) placebo chelation and placebo vitamins.

In the end, the EDTA-based chelation therapy reduced overall cardiovascular events (heart attacks, strokes, etc.) in patients who had some history of prior heart attacks and were being treated medically. Not only that, but IV EDTA chelation therapy and high-dose oral vitamin therapy significantly reduced cardiovascular events when combined with standard medical therapy as compared to standard medical therapy combined only with a placebo.[2]

And that's not the only good news that came out of TACT. Chelation therapy actually outperformed statins in terms of preventing cardiovascular events, especially among diabetics.[3] Adding oral high-dose vitamins seems to have made the EDTA effects for diabetics even greater.

And the best news of all? EDTA chelation has a remarkable safety history, while statin therapy causes all sorts of side effects, some quite dangerous.

Toss out the one bad apple that's spoiling the bunch... in your body

To be honest, we don't yet know exactly why chelation might work for cardiovascular disease—which is why studies like TACT are so important. Right now the resounding theory is that it removes the metals in your body that can cause the abnormal proteins and oxidative stress that can lead to circulatory damage and diabetes.

Lead and cadmium in particular seem to enhance oxidative stress and cell damage, and chelators like EDTA act as a powerful antioxidant when introduced to a toxic environment like that.

These processes of oxidation are sometimes called "browning reactions," because they're the same thing that toasts your bread, caramelizes your onions, and turns your apples brown. And, like food, once the walls of our vessels are "browned," they can't ever go back.

EDTA has been known to block the browning reaction—at least, in chemical studies on food. And it may have the same reaction in the human body—but to find out for sure, human clinical trials are needed.

It's going to take a little more convincing

You would THINK that the prospect of a safe and effective therapy would excite mainstream cardiologists, but the TACT results don't seem to have impressed the American Heart Association very much. Their latest recommendations state that "the usefulness of chelation therapy in cardiac disease is highly questionable."[4]

Well, any good researcher would tell you that one study by itself shouldn't be considered proof positive—no matter how good the design—so the principal investigators from TACT have submitted an application and are seeking funding for a follow-up study to see if they can get the same positive results a second time. The design of the so-called "TACT2" will be the same as TACT1, involving 1,200 diabetic patients age 50 or older who have had heart attacks prior to the study.[5]

Hopefully, the results will be positive enough to finally convince those bubble-bursting naysayers that there IS a safe and effective alternative to statins and surgery, and that there's PROOF of it.

In the meantime, physicians like myself are continuing to seeing the positive effects of this remarkable therapy first-hand in patients like you, in hundreds of offices globally.

I'm keeping my eyes on this story, and will be sure you update you on any new developments as they happen.

Chapter 12:

The "broken heart syndrome" that could kill you—and that lots of doctors miss

They say that time heals all wounds—but when it comes to the heart, that may not always be the case.

We talk a lot about our hearts breaking when a relationship ends or someone close to us dies.

But did you know that when your heart breaks *figuratively,* it also can be breaking *literally?* And you can feel just like you're having a heart attack, without having ANY blockages in any of the arteries of your heart.

A stressful, sad, or emotionally taxing event can cause the muscular part of your heart to swell for a period of time and, as they say, "break."

It's a medical condition called Takotsubo Cardiomyopathy, nicknamed "broken heart syndrome." The heart muscle is stunned by some tragic event and is not able to beat properly and effectively.

Takotsubo is the Japanese term for a fishing pot used for trapping an octopus—which is exactly what the heart looks like when the top part of the heart's left side contracts differently than the bottom part.

Broken heart cases skyrocketing

Takotsubo Cardiomyopathy initially feels identical to a heart attack. The symptoms include chest pain, shortness of breath, sweating, irregular heartbeat, nausea, and vomiting, as well as fatigue.

A few years ago, people used to be told that it was "all in their head" and were sent home—when, in fact, they'd had a serious, life-threatening health event.

However, this syndrome is becoming much more recognized and diagnosed. A July 2015 study showed that the number of reported cases grew from 315 in 2006 to 6,230 in 20121— probably because technology and testing at the time of hospital admission is more sensitive now than it used to be.

The good news is that the basic blood tests and EKG that all respectable emergency rooms will conduct will usually pick up the seriousness of this event.

When stress can be a real heartbreaker

The bad news is that there's not much that modern medicine can do to prevent an occurrence of Takotsubo Cardiomyopathy or a repeat episode of it.

Interestingly, most of the patients that are diagnosed with it have less of the common risk factors for heart disease, such as obesity, smoking, high blood pressure, diabetes, or high cholesterol. And interestingly, about 90 percent of patients who suffer from Takotsubo Cardiomyopathy are postmenopausal women.

And the common factor among them? They're usually anxious, and have high levels of adrenaline in their blood.

Therefore, reducing stress and anxiety is important—especially since a recent *New England Journal of Medicine* article showed that blood pressure medications don't do a thing to prevent a reoccurrence of Takotsubo Cardiomyopathy.

But the good news is that there are natural ways to heal your heart from Takotsubo Cardiomyopathy and to keep it from striking again.

This is how you mend a broken heart

A few years ago, a patient came to me for this exact purpose. She wanted to recover from her recent Takotsubo Cardiomyopathy "heart attack," which occurred after a sudden and horrific car accident. Within minutes after the accident, she'd started having severe chest pain and was rushed to the hospital.

The blood tests and an EKG confirmed that she'd had a heart "attack," but the angiogram (putting dye through the arteries of the heart) showed that her arteries were crystal clear. So, she was diagnosed with this condition.

The cardiologist prescribed some basic medications, but he told her that the only way to help her and to help prevent another attack was to reduce her stress and anxiety levels. Of course, he didn't tell her how to do that, and he sent her to a "shrink."

In fact, the main reason that she came to me was that she couldn't tolerate any of the normal antidepressants or anxiety medications—and they didn't work for her, anyway.

So in my office, we began by trying to improve her heart function. The heart is a muscle, and so I treat Takotsubo Cardiomyopathy as I would any other muscular problem. I had her start exercising slowly because I wanted the heart muscle to regain strength.

I also asked her to take magnesium and CoQ10 as well as ribose because I wanted to make sure the mitochondria of her heart were as strong as possible. That way, they'd be able to not only repair from the event (that is, "fix" her broken heart) but also strengthen her heart so that an event like this wouldn't reoccur.

We also used amino acids and herbs to bolster her brain chemistry and help her deal with her excessive stress levels, as well as weekly acupuncture sessions to reduce her nervous system overdrive.

Finally, I sent her to a practitioner who taught her how to do some basic meditation.

And you know what? She is like a "new person," as she says, with a much better understanding of how stress affects her heart and health. She has the power over her mind and body to be able to deal with any big or small stressors that come her way.

Your heart is talking to you...so be sure to listen to it!

You need to take a proactive stance with your heart health—but even if you're at a normal weight, eating healthily, and not showing any signs of cardiovascular disease, you could still be at risk for Takotsubo Cardiomyopathy.

You should always take chest pain seriously. Even if your doctor says that your heart is fine, if you have serious chest pain or pressure, please go to the local emergency room. They should be able to determine what's really going on.

You can't avoid getting bad news...or dealing with life's (sometimes extreme) ups and downs...but there are many holistic ways to help you deal with severe stress before it affects your heart.

One of the best ways is to receive acupuncture therapy, and if you're in the Boston area, you can come see me at my clinic (as I am also a licensed acupuncturist). Or, I suggest finding a qualified physician acupuncturist near you through the American Academy of Medical Acupuncture (AAMA) www.medicalacupuncture.org.

Chapter 13:

A contaminant in your water may be clogging your arteries

There are a few, if any, communities around the world that have both chlorinated drinking water and a low incidence of atherosclerosis. Chlorine is a powerful oxidizing agent (that's why it is used for bleaching) that is capable of causing severe damage to blood vessels. American servicemen fighting in Korea and Vietnam who were killed in battle were found to have atherosclerosis in more than 75 percent of all cases. The water given to these men was so heavily chlorinated that it was virtually undrinkable. In animal studies, chlorine has been found to promote the development of atherosclerosis. The good news is that it's fairly simple to remove the chlorine from your drinking water. Just boil the water for five to 10 minutes or add a pinch of vitamin C crystals to the water.

It can also be removed by charcoal filtration, as well as through "reverse osmosis." Check with the filter manufacturer of whatever brand you choose to be certain.

Chapter 14:

The No.1 heart-protecting mineral

Among its many other heart health functions, magnesium reduces the risk of abnormal heart rhythm, helps blood vessels to relax and dilate, and raises levels of HDL ("good") cholesterol. So it makes sense that low levels of magnesium can contribute to heart problems.

The most accurate way to measure your magnesium level is by having a white blood cell magnesium (WBC-Mg) test.

The remedy for low levels of magnesium is simple: Eat more magnesium-containing food and take magnesium supplements. A general rule of thumb for finding magnesium-rich foods: Anything that's green—naturally green, that is (lime Jell-O doesn't count!)—contains magnesium. And one word of caution about supplements: Don't take more than 400 milligrams of supplemental magnesium without measuring your own "intestinal transit time." Intestinal transit time describes the length of time food takes to transit from the entrance to the exit of the gastrointestinal tract. Higher doses of magnesium can sometimes "speed things up," which means you may not be absorbing it or the other nutrients your body needs.

Although estimates vary, a reasonable range for "normal" transit time appears to vary from 12-24 hours. You can measure your own transit time by eating beets or corn or swallowing charcoal tablets and observing how long it takes them to emerge. If magnesium appears to speed up your own normal transit time, cut back on your dosage until you reach the amount that brings things back to normal.

PART IV

Chronic Pain
and Arthritis

Chapter 1:

Drive down your inflammation and relieve arthritis with these natural pain busters!

When I climb out of bed each morning, that growing twinge of stiffness reminds me that I'm no longer a spring chicken. And I'm not alone. More than 70 percent of us over 50 have some evidence of osteoarthritis (OA) in at least one of our joints. With another 1 percent of the population suffering from rheumatoid arthritis (RA), it all adds up a whole lot of sore, creaky joints.

In medical school we were taught that RA was inflammatory—due to an auto-immune illness—but that OA was merely the result of wear and tear on the joints. We were led to believe that there was just one solution to the joint damage seen with OA... or Degenerative Joint Disease as it's sometimes called... and that, of course, is joint replacement.

MILLIONS risk joint replacement every year

And judging by the rising tide of joint replacements, most of my colleagues have bought into that thinking. Over 51 million people every year in the US alone are facing the dangers of surgery and post-surgical complications like blood clots from joint replacements. And they're left with the long-term risks of having foreign metals in their bodies.

If joints aren't replaced, OA pain is usually treated with aspirin or nonsteroidal anti-inflammatory drugs (NSAIDs) such as Advil and Aleve. The reason they provide some relief is that—despite OA being labeled the wear-and-tear form of arthritis—inflammation does, in fact, play a role.

But when you understand just how these drugs work—and how they're practically guaranteed to lead to damage to your gut—you'll be clamoring for the same safe, natural alternatives I use with my own patients.

Inflammation's vicious cycle

To understand what's wrong with prescription and OTC anti-inflammatory meds like aspirin and ibuprofen, it's important to first take a look at how inflammation occurs in our bodies.

A variety of factors including diet, injuries, infections, allergies, and toxins can set off warning signals in the body. We end up producing pro-inflammatory messenger proteins (called cytokines) and enzymes (particularly cyclooxygenase or COX) that actually eat away at the collagen in our joints.

It's a vicious cycle that leads to even more inflammation and destruction of cellular tissue until, eventually, the joint space is largely obliterated.

In fact, this is the way that nearly all diseases progress; immune messengers are triggered by a variety of internal and external factors, which leads to inflammation and, eventually destruction of cells.

How common pain relievers attack your gut

Managing your levels of pro-inflammatory cytokines and enzymes is the key to reducing inflammation and controlling your arthritis pain.

In the case of OA, the cytokines that seem to do the most damage are called tumor necrosis factor alpha (TNF alpha) and interleukin one beta (IL-1b). Studies of the joint spaces of OA patients show elevated levels of both TNF alpha and IL-1b. It's also been shown that reducing TNF alpha lowers inflammation, and lowering IL-1b reduces damage to cartilage.

Aspirin and NSAIDs work by tackling pro-inflammatory enzymes. They block the pathway by which COX enzymes (both COX-1 and COX-2) work—and since COX-2 causes inflammation, this can provide some relief.

But that reduced inflammation comes at a major price, because COX-1, which is also blocked by the majority of these medicines, is needed to protect your stomach lining. And so these medications can erode the stomach and cause ulcers and gastritis, even as they have a calming effect on the joints.

In an attempt to bypass the COX-1 issue, drug companies have produced a number of selective COX-2 inhibitor drugs over the years with some disastrous results. A number of these drugs have led to serious heart issues in users, and as a result most of them—including the well-known drugs Vioxx and Bextra—have been banned. But Celebrex, another COX-2 inhibitor, is still on the market.

But while the drug companies continue to toil away trying to create a drug that effectively inhibits COX-2 and the cytokines involved in inflammation (Il-1b and TNF alpha)—while not suppressing COX-1—nature has *already* solved the problem. Certain plants are naturally anti-inflammatory, which means they can help relieve your pain without stomach damage or other side effects you get from prescription and OTC pain meds.

A recent article published in the journal *Current Opinion in Pharmacology* reviewed a number of natural substances and herbal extracts that have been proven to decrease the signals in the body that trigger and sustain painful inflammation.

The researchers listed 18 natural products that demonstrated impressive anti-arthritic activity. All of them (except the soy-derived protein Genistein) blocked COX-2.

All 18 blocked a substance called nuclear factor kappa-B (NF-kB) the signaling molecule that regulates the inflammatory process. And half of them blocked Il-1B as well. And, of course, these plant solutions manage to tamp down the inflammation *without* carrying the same harsh side effects that have been seen with drugs.

Top Four Arthritis Inflammation Busters

Of all the plant-based anti-inflammatories out there, there are four that I've seen work consistently well for arthritis symptoms. If you're suffering from the aches and pains of arthritis these Top Four Arthritis Inflammation Busters could be the answer...

1. Curcumin, which is extracted from the common kitchen herb turmeric, is a powerful natural anti-inflammatory. The herbal extract has literally hundreds of studies backing up its use for managing—and in some cases even helping to *prevent*—the symptoms of OA and RA.

There are even some studies showing that curcumin improves the function of the COX-2 inhibitor drug Celebrex, so that lower doses of the potentially dangerous drug can be used.

2. Resveratrol, another powerful anti-inflammatory herbal extract, is readily found in grapes (including wine), berries and peanuts. Resveratrol has been proven to inhibit NF-kB, IL-1B, COX-2, and another inflammatory cytokine, Interleukin 6 (IL-6). By blocking these harmful substances resveratrol slows down the destruction of joint cartilage and can even help prevent OA before it ever begins.

In a recent study researchers combined curcumin and resveratrol into special nanocapsules. The combo was able to lower both joint inflammation and tissue destruction in an animal model, without the liver irritation that occurs with drugs.

3. Boswellic acid, extracted from the Indian herb boswellia, has been used to treat OA and RA for over 30 years, and has accumulated an extensive amount of positive research over that time. It's been shown to block NF-kB, COX-2 and another inflammatory enzyme 5-LOX.

In one randomized double-blind placebo-controlled study, 30 patients with OA of the knee were given boswellia extract or placebo for eight weeks, and then (after a period of time known as a "wash-out") they were switched. The group receiving the active herbal medicine had a significant reduction in pain, they were able to walk greater distances and they had improved flexibility.

4. Avocado-soybean unsaponifiables (ASU) is a remarkable substance created by combining extracts from both avocado and soybean oils. ASU is sold as a prescription product in Europe, under the name of Piascledine, and this is the form that has been used in most studies.

ASU has repeatedly been shown to suppress pro-inflammatory cytokines, and several clinical studies have found that it has a positive effect on OA. In one study, published in the journal *Annals of the Rheumatic Diseases*, 399 patients with hip OA were treated with 300 mg ASU or a placebo, and followed for three years.

X-rays showed a significantly better joint space width in the treated group than the placebo group. In other words the ASU had stopped the progression of the OA in its tracks, and with negligible side effects.

These four natural substances, and many others, have been proven safe and effective alternatives to the dangers of NSAIDs and other arthritis drugs. And just as importantly, they suggest that taking natural medicines can be a powerful way to prevent the aches and pains of arthritis from occurring in the first place, and that they may even be able to help prevent or delay a painful and risky joint replacement.

Chapter 2:

Natural substance stops crippling arthritis pain—without the risks!

When you're struggling with the pain of osteoarthritis... when even the simplest tasks like climbing the stairs or opening a jar of mayonnaise can feel like torture... you'll do anything for relief.

And that's why so many patients I meet spend their days popping NSAID (nonsteroidal anti-inflammatory) drugs like aspirin, ibuprofen, ketoprofen, and naproxen.

Believe me, I get it. They work for a while, which is probably why one study found that 43 percent of adults had taken an NSAID in the previous two weeks.[1]

But that temporary pain relief comes with a much higher price than you may have ever imagined.

There are more than 100,000 NSAID-related hospitalizations each year in the United States and over 16,000 NSAID-related deaths. Most of the problems come from serious gastrointestinal bleeding, followed by permanent damage to your kidneys.[2]

Nobody should have to endure those risks for a little pain relief. That's why I've worked to find new, alternative therapies that won't just turn the dial down on your pain, but will also save you from harmful side effects and keep you out of the hospital.

A natural remedy that measures up to powerful anti-inflammatory meds

I've recently discovered a remedy that works just as well as NSAIDs— with a small fraction (if any) of the scary side effects.

I've been having such success with this product...and the science behind it is so good...that I'm surprised that I had to do so much digging to uncover it myself.

The product is called Limbrel, a "medical food" that's used to treat osteoarthritis. Also known as "flavocoxid," it's a proprietary blend of the extracts of powerful compounds from two different natural plants. The inventors of this medical food figured out how to isolate those molecules and put them into a supplement that can pack the same punch as a prescription drug.

The compounds in Limbrel are called "flavonoids"—and they're basically the "good stuff" that make colored fruits and vegetables, green tea, and red wine classify as "superfoods."

For this blend, however, scientists used portions of the Chinese skullcap (*Scutellaria baicalensis*) and the Acacia catechu tree (also known as the Cutch Tree, *Senegalia catechu*).

The studies of Limbrel are staggering—because they show this medical food to be equally as effective as an NSAID and just as safe as a placebo.[3]

There's a very well-done study out of Russia that showed that Limbrel relieved pain just as well as a naproxen (Aleve).[4,5]

Limbrel was able to reduce pain by an average of 85 percent[6]—with significantly fewer adverse effects to the patients' stomach and kidneys.

That's a big feat...and very impressive for a natural remedy.

These plant extracts do more than just mask your OA pain

Instead of just treating your symptoms, or covering up the pain, Limbrel also uses natural ways of reducing your body's ability to trigger inflammation.

Now this gets a little technical, but common NSAIDs work by drastically reducing the amount of inflammation being produced by two of the body's three pathways (COX 1 and COX 2).

But your body isn't dumb. It knows that it needs to main a supply of some of these inflammation-causing chemicals for jobs that aren't necessarily related to inflammation. So it just sends them through the third, remaining pathway (LOX) in order to meet the needs.[7] And, believe it or not, that's what causes a lot of the side effects with NSAIDs.

Limbrel, on the other hand, "spreads its wealth" by slowing down each of the three arms of the inflammation cascade (COX1, COX2, and LOX)—and thus the body does not panic and divert the chemicals to the unblocked pathway.

Limbrel is one of the first remedies to be shown to reduce COX1, COX2, and LOX at the same time, which manages the UNDERLYING processes that lead to inflammation and arthritis.

And that's precisely what we holistic doctors are always trying to get to—the root cause of the condition.

Now, all of this is pretty encouraging; but the most amazing thing is that there's yet ANOTHER huge bang for your buck with Limbrel.

As you know, flavonoids act as a powerful antioxidant in the body. This means that the natural substances in this medical food will go around your body and clear out free radicals—the molecules that are actually causing the joint damage in the first place.

Your gut will thank you for making the switch

The really good news about Limbrel is that it has almost ZERO risk to the stomach. Little to no gastrointestinal side effects have been found in studies, and I haven't seen any problems with my patients.

In one study, Limbrel was better-tolerated than NSAIDs in 90 percent of patients who had to stop NSAIDs due to gastrointestinal side effects.[8] In fact, there were no reports of anyone experiencing gastrointestinal difficulties in a 90-day human clinical trial.[9]

On top of that, another study gave rats normal dosages of Limbrel, and after two months, the scientists found zero damage in their stomach linings when examined under a microscope.[10] In comparison, when rats are given NSAIDs, they almost always develop some damage that can be seen under the microscope at the two-month mark.[11]

In fact, scientists have not been able to find a dose high enough to kill even ONE of their experimental animals![12]

Since you're a human and not a rat, you can rest assured that there are very few interactions with other drugs[13]—but you should always make sure your healthcare provider knows everything you're taking just to be sure.

A prescription-strength alternative you can trust

There is one slight wrinkle to this powerful remedy: medical foods are natural remedies that are so strong that the FDA requires you to get a prescription for them.

But if you are (or have been) on a NSAID and have not found a natural remedy that can help manage your pain, consider talking to your primary care doctor about Limbrel.

Due to the science behind it—and the known dangers of the only mainstream alternative—I don't see why your doctor wouldn't be willing to write a prescription for you. After all, it's been around since 2004 and in the *Physicians' Desk Reference* since 2009.

If you need to educate your doctor, you can go to www.limbrel.com and print out some information.

Make sure you tell him that both of the main components of Limbrel have been approved for use in prescription products in Japan for over 20 years and often qualify for reimbursement by their national health insurance.

There are other exciting studies in progress with this medical food for use in treating other inflammatory conditions, so I'll be sure to update you as the findings are reviewed and released.

But with any joint-care product, no matter what you use, the key is to start early—the longer you wait, the more pain, joint inflammation and damage you'll be dealing with.

Chapter 3:

Catch the culprit behind your arthritis pain

The first thing to determine is which type of arthritis you have. There are two major forms of arthritis: Degenerative arthritis (also known as osteoarthritis) and rheumatoid arthritis.

Osteoarthritis is the most common form of the disease and occurs when the cartilage between the joints begins to break down and wear away, causing pain and stiffness. This cartilage damage is one of the hallmarks of osteoarthritis, but oddly enough, heavy use of the joints isn't necessarily what causes this problem. In fact, many former long-distance runners have perfectly normal hips and knees, while their more sedentary friends become plagued with degenerating joints. No one knows for sure exactly why the cartilage wears away, but those of us who practice natural medicine do know that there are plenty of ways to alleviate the pain it causes. More on that in a minute.

Rheumatoid arthritis involves inflammation, pain, and stiffness of the lining of joints in your body and also causes redness and swelling in most cases. If you aren't sure which form of arthritis you have, your doctor can help determine that. Although both types have very different causes, some of the natural treatments for each type overlap.

And no matter which type of arthritis pain you're battling, you'll need a good starting point for all of the nutrients that can help. So the first thing I recommend is a basic, healthy diet. This includes whole, unprocessed foods, with no added sugar, no so-called "soft drinks," no chemical additives, and no flavorings, coloring, or preservatives. I suggest only whole grains (if you're not allergic or sensitive to them), no artificial sweeteners, and only small amounts of alcohol. And I know it's easier said than done, but it really is best to eliminate caffeine altogether.

Now, let's start with osteoarthritis.

The arthritis triggers that could be growing in your garden

The first thing I recommend for osteoarthritis is changing certain aspects of your diet. In the 1950s, Norman Childers, Ph.D., found that eliminating certain vegetables (known as nightshade vegetables) from the diet could completely eliminate arthritis symptoms in many cases. Nightshade vegetables include tomatoes, potatoes, peppers (including paprika, but not black pepper), eggplants, and tobacco. According to Dr. Childers, nightshade sensitivity isn't an allergy but actually a progressive loss of the ability to metabolize substances known as "solanine alkaloids," which are found in all nightshade vegetables. Unfortunately, there's no test that can tell you if your arthritis will respond to a nightshade-free diet. It's strictly a "try it and see" situation.

It's harder than it might seem to completely eliminate nightshades. Tomato and potato make their way into a wide variety of food products, and pepper gets around a lot too. Check your local library for a copy of Dr. Childers' book, variously titled (depending on the edition) *Childers' Diet; Arthritis—Childers' Diet to Stop It*; and similar titles. The information he includes can be a big help in searching out all sources of nightshades. But even eliminating the most common nightshades (the ones listed above) is definitely worth trying. Eliminate them for at least three to four months and see if it makes a difference in your symptoms. If you're not sure after three or four months, you can do a "nightshade chal-

Add some oil to those rusty joints

Fish oil is one of my favorite recommendations. There's a good reason: Omega-3 fatty acids may have replaced folic acid as America's No.1 dietary deficiency/ insufficiency. And fish oil is the best source for your body to get the omega-3s it needs.

Make sure the brand you use is "certified heavy metal free," but aside from that, fish oil— always taken with vitamin E—has practically no hazards. (That infamous "cod liver oil burp" can almost always be eliminated by "burying" the oil in the middle of a meal, by blending the oil with rice, almond, or soy milk, and a banana, or by taking it with a "high-lipase" digestive enzyme.)

For osteoarthritis, take 1 tablespoon of cod liver oil (with 400 I.U. vitamin E) once daily— twice daily if you have a particularly bad case. You can take it right along with glucosamine and niacinamide, as they all work in different ways for different aspects of the problem.

lenge" by eating lots of tomato, potato, and peppers. If the pain comes back after the challenge, you'll know that you are nightshade-sensitive and you should eliminate those foods from your diet permanently.

Sometimes, osteoarthritis is aggravated by "regular" food allergies. If you have a personal or family history of allergies, it's worth having this possibility checked out. For a list of physicians in your area who can help you with allergy screening, contact the American Academy of Environmental Medicine at (316)684-5500 or www.aemonline.org. There are various ways to determine specific food allergies, but skin testing is not usually an accurate tool in this case.

The $10 osteoarthritis cure

Once you've determined whether or not allergies or sensitivities play a role in your arthritis, you can move on to other natural therapies, starting with glucosamine. By now, even mainstream medical doctors have heard of glucosamine. Research shows that it works by helping to stimulate the growth of new joint cartilage. This is probably why there's usually a three to four week delay after starting treatment for pain relief to begin. I recommend 500 milligrams of glucosamine sulfate three times a day.

There have been some warnings in mainstream medical publications that glucosamine might affect blood sugar control. If you have significant osteoarthritis and don't have diabetes, this theoretical possibility shouldn't be a problem. If you do have diabetes, checking your blood sugar will tell you whether the glucosamine has enough of an effect to warrant not taking it. In most cases, the improvement you'll likely feel will far outweigh the possibility of any slight effect on blood sugar.

Glucosamine is often combined with chondroitin in natural arthritis formulas. But there's enough question about chondroitin and risk of prostate cancer for me to advise all men to avoid chondroitin at this time. Besides, I've observed that glucosamine usually works just as well by itself. So just use "plain" glucosamine until this question is settled for good.

Complete arthritis relief in less than one month

The next natural osteoarthritis remedy on the list is niacinamide. Even many natural medicine doctors have forgotten, or never learned, just how useful niacinamide (not niacin) can be for controlling the pain and swelling of osteoarthritis.

In 1949, William Kaufman, M.D., Ph.D., published his exceptionally careful and comprehensive research about niacinamide and osteoarthritis titled "The Common Form of Joint Dysfunction: Its Incidence and Treatment." Unfortunately, Dr. Kaufman's research came out around the same time that patented cortisone formulas were being heavily promoted, so niacinamide treatment was hardly noticed. But even though it never made much of a stir, niacinamide treatment works very well. I recommend using 1,000 milligrams of niacinamide three times a day (it doesn't work as well if you only take it once or twice daily). You'll probably start feeling results in three to four weeks. Many osteoarthritis sufferers achieve complete relief of pain and swelling as long as they continue on with niacinamide.

Niacinamide doesn't appear to re-grow cartilage, so it's best to use glucosamine along with it. If you have diabetes and are concerned about glucosamine's effects on blood sugar, niacinamide is a good companion for it. Niacinamide also has many benefits for blood sugar problems, and using it with glucosamine is even more likely to relieve your osteoarthritis symptoms.

And a caution: On rare occasion, people who take this amount of niacinamide get low-grade nausea, queasiness, and sometimes vomiting. Although this only happens in less than 1 percent of people who take niacinamide, if you experience any of these problems, stop taking it immediately. The nausea should go away promptly, but check with your doctor before any further niacinamide use.

Three more great remedies to try

Since glucosamine is on the well-known end of the arthritis-relief spectrum, the final two items on the osteoarthritis-fighting list usually slip below the radar of most physicians. But boron and S-adenosylmethionine (SAMe) can both be quite effective.

Epidemiologic evidence shows a greater incidence of arthritis in areas of the world low in boron. A small amount of research shows that boron can relieve many symptoms of osteoarthritis. Since boron is quite inexpensive, is safe in small doses, and is useful in treating osteoporosis and preventing cancer in addition to osteoarthritis, it certainly can't hurt to take 3 milligrams twice daily.

SAMe is quite effective for some cases of osteoarthritis but not so helpful for others. While it's not a surefire cure, it's quite safe and worth trying if the diet changes and supplements noted above aren't helpful. The only drawback is that it's a bit pricey compared with many other supplements. If you decide to give it a try, take 400 milligrams once or twice daily.

Willow bark is actually the all-natural forerunner to aspirin. It's been proven to relieve pain equally as well as prescription pain medications.

The most recent study was published in the journal *Rheumatology* in December 2001. Researchers tested two groups of 114 participants each, treating one group with two to four 240-milligram doses of salicin (one

---

Osteoarthritis relief in one easy-to-use outline

Here's what you need to do:

- Eliminate all nightshade vegetables and other items (tomatoes, potatoes, peppers, eggplants, tobacco, etc.) from your diet for three to four months to see if it helps alleviate your pain

- Have thorough allergy screening done to test for non-nightshade food sensitivities

And here's what you need to take:

- Glucosamine sulfate—500 milligrams, three times a day

- Cod liver oil—1 tablespoon, once or twice daily

- Vitamin E—400 I.U., once or twice daily (along with the cod liver oil)

- Niacinamide—1,000 milligrams, three times a day

- Boron—3 milligrams twice daily

- SAMe—400 milligrams, once or twice daily

- Willow bark—two to four doses per day (of tablets containing 400 milligrams of willow bark extract and 60 milligrams of salicin)

- Myristin—six capsules per day for 80 days

of the main pain-relieving ingredients in willow bark extract) per day and the other with the same number of 12.5-milligram doses of rofecoxib (the generic name of Vioxx). After four weeks there was no difference between the results for the two products in terms of pain, requirement for additional analgesics, or side effects. The only difference in the two treatments is that willow bark extract is much less expensive than Vioxx.

In all the trials done so far, researchers administered two to four high potency willow bark extract tablets per day to each patient. The tablets contained 400 milligrams of actual extract and 60 milligrams of salicin. The 400 milligrams of extract corresponds to 6 to 8 grams of willow bark, depending on the type used. Your local compounding pharmacist can help you make sure you're getting the right amounts. To locate a compounding pharmacist near you, contact the International Academy of Compounding Pharmacists (800-927-4227; www.iacprx.org).

Breast-feeding mothers should use willow bark extract with caution, since the remnants excreted in breast milk may cause rashes in babies. If you are currently taking blood-thinning medications or NSAIDs, be sure to consult your physician before taking willow bark extract. It is much less likely to cause problems with bleeding than prescription medications or even aspirin, but a bit of caution can go a long way in keeping you safe, healthy, and pain-free.

One-time treatment can cure arthritis for good

Back in the 1990s, former National Institutes of Health researcher Harry Diehl became intrigued by the observation that mice don't get osteoarthritis. Working in his home lab, he analyzed literally thousands of mice, finally isolating a type of fatty acid called cetyl-myristoleate (CMO) not found in rats (which do get arthritis) or humans.

He invented and patented the first process to create bio-identical CMO. When he tried the bio-identical CMO on arthritic rats, they were cured. But he couldn't interest any patent-medicine companies in CMO. So he "let it go" until he developed arthritis himself at age 80.

Over the course of 10 days he applied small amounts of CMO (which he combined with DMSO) topically to his hands. Not only did it completely eliminate his arthritis pain, but Harry also reported that it cured a long-standing headache he'd been suffering and prevented any more recurrences of bronchitis which he's suffered on a regular basis.

Harry used CMO only that one time, and never need to take it again. He also made it for friends, who had the same experience.

While Harry's original topical CMO formula isn't available anymore, he developed a capsulized formulation, called Myristin, that appears to be just as effective. You can find Myristin in natural food stores and compounding pharmacies.

I usually recommend taking six capsules of Myristin daily for 80 days. (If it hasn't worked by then, it probably isn't going to.) Although it doesn't work for everyone, the majority of patients who've tried it have had substantial or complete relief.

Chapter 4:

Quit the limping and hobbling and... BANISH knee pain with this time-tested treatment

Remember the good ol' days when you could spring up those stairs two at a time? Now you're holding onto the bannister so tightly, you're practically leaving fingernail marks in the wood.

Let's face it: Your knees just aren't what they used to be.

The moment you get out of bed in the morning, your knees start aching. Getting in and out of the car is like an exercise in torture.

And if you complain to your doctor, there's a good chance you're going to end up with a prescription for an addictive pain reliever that could damage everything from your liver to your gut.

Worse yet, you could end up trading in your old knees for some new ones—and, with surgery, you'll face scary health risks while you're laid up for months, going through painful physical therapy.

All that, for just a 50-50 chance of any meaningful improvement!

Well, there's another, different kind of treatment for your knee pain... something that doesn't require you to swallow a single pill...or get any replacement parts.

All you have to do is close your eyes and let a few tiny needles work their magic in the ancient healing practice known as acupuncture.

After thousands of treatments performed on hundreds of patients in my practice over the course of 30 years, I can promise you won't feel anything but better.

A simple, proven way to relieve twice as much knee pain

I have written, taught, and practiced acupuncture since I was first trained in the early 1980s. But I used to keep my status as a medical acupuncturist secret from my colleagues in conventional medicine, who'd give funny looks any time you mentioned something that didn't involve drugs and surgery.

"It's unproven," they'd say.

Aside from the fact that it's been used with great success for centuries, there is now plenty of scientific evidence supporting the effectiveness of acupuncture—especially where osteoarthritis of the knee is concerned.

Some of the most extensive studies on acupuncture have been conducted by the German government and their public health service. They involved training hundreds of family physicians in acupuncture and treating large numbers of patients with knee osteoarthritis, as well as a variety of other conditions.

One of the first such studies of acupuncture for knee pain was published in the prestigious medical journal *The Lancet* in 2005 and involved 296 patients with knee pain from arthritis, with a control group of patients who were on a waiting list without treatment. After eight weeks, the treated group's knee pain significantly improved over the waiting list group.

For those of you who follow statistics, the P value was <0.0001 which means this study's findings are highly reliable.[1]

In a subsequent study, 498 patients with osteoarthritic pain of the knee and hip were treated by over 200 acupuncture physicians in Germany. Again, the treated group improved over the group that received no treatment, but not just in pain management.

The group treated with acupuncture showed improvements in their quality of life (as determined by their answers to a standardized questionnaire both before and after treatment)…and actually got a bigger bang for their buck with acupuncture versus other treatment options.[2]

In addition, a larger trial was also performed, as part of a huge trial called German Acupuncture Trials or GERAC that were started in 2001 and published in 2006. In this trial, 1,007 patients were randomly assigned to acupuncture treatment or "usual care" (physical therapy, medication). After 26 weeks, the acupuncture group improved *twice* as much as the usual care group![3]

The key fact is this: *Being treated with acupuncture needles improved the symptom of pain in patients with knee arthritis, measured over literally thousands of acupuncture treatments, in hundreds of medical offices.*

Imagine if a prescription drug was found to be twice as effective as taking no medication! The FDA would immediately green-light it, and it would soon become "all the rage" among physicians.

So, the next time one of my patients asks me, "Does it work?" I can tell them about the number of studies that show that the answer is a resounding "YES!"

From ancient Chinese medicine to mainstream medical miracle

Fortunately, there has been a slow shift over the last decade: Mainstream docs have started asking questions about acupuncture out of curiosity, and some of them even refer patients to me for the treatment!

One nice thing about osteoarthritis pain of the knee is how easily it can be treated. The treatment of knee pain is usually done with needling around the knee...and some points on the forearms, hands, and feet...so there's no need to disrobe. In fact, in sessions sometimes called "community acupuncture," several patients can sit in comfortable chairs together in a large room, while the clinician treats them all simultaneously. This helps bring the cost down over the one-on-one sessions.

However, if the acupuncturist needs to target points on your torso as well—usually if you've been experiencing long-term arthritic pain—you'd be better off getting treatment in a separate room with some privacy.

As far as safety goes, there's no evidence that acupuncture causes side effects beyond the sensation of the needle itself—which is a vast improvement over the cardiovascular risks, serious skin reactions, stomach bleeding, and ulcers that come with over-the-counter and prescription pain relievers.

Acupuncture, in fact, is *remarkably* safe, so if you've had chronic knee pains—particularly those caused by knee arthritis—it's definitely worth a try.

Some insurance policies will even cover it with a referral. I recommend seeing a certified medical acupuncturist like myself if you're treating any kind of specific pain or condition. Come see me at the The Rothfeld Center for Integrative Medicine in the Boston area, or find another one near you through the American Academy of Medical Acupuncture www.medicalacupuncture.org.

Chapter 5:

Feds order crackdown on prescription painkillers! Here's what it means for you— and your doctor

By the time you finish reading this chapter, another American will have died from an overdose of opioid painkillers like morphine, Vicodin, or OxyContin.

It's become an epidemic. In 2014, nearly 30,000 people died from opioid overdoses, half of whom had legitimate prescriptions.

Now, the FDA is trying to get control of the problem with some very serious changes. They instituted stricter guidelines to deter doctors from liberally and haphazardly prescribing these addicting medications to patients with pain problems.

They make it very clear that opioid-based pain drugs should be used as a "last resort"—and only for short periods of time. And they're insisting on some new—and pretty bizarre—testing requirements for both doctors and patients.

On one hand, you have to give the FDA some credit for finally acknowledging how serious this issue has become. But... and this is a big "but"... our government has botched these regulations pretty badly.

And if you're in chronic pain, these new rules could leave both you—and your doctor—in the lurch.

Refusing to treat pain won't make it go away

Under the new regulations, doctors who prescribe pain medications must operate under what's called an "assumption of suspicion." In other words, they have to conduct regular urine testing on their patients.[1]

But it's not to keep you from taking too much of the drugs—it's to confirm that the drugs _are actually in your system_. Because if they're not, the theory is that you must be selling the meds on the black market.

And then, the drugs are taken away from you, despite the fact that you might have just been taking a couple of days off.

What kind of heath care system FORCES people to take a drug _every day_... or _not at all_?

In many ways, the new guidelines tie doctors' hands behind their backs, imposing a system of bureaucracy that includes contracts, checkpoints, reports, and a whole lot of red tape—none of which do anything to LESSEN PAIN.

It's no wonder that nearly half of doctors who were surveyed said that these new rules would force them to stop prescribing narcotics like opioids, or at least reduce the amount that they're going to prescribe.[2]

But there are 100 million Americans in chronic pain. And if primary care doctors are going to shy away from prescribing morphine-based medications, then we are on the verge of a crisis of massive proportions.

There's about to be a huge problem—and there are going to be some very confused and cranky patients who are going to be in a lot of pain and have nowhere to turn.

Yes, there are doctors who specialize in pain, and these doctors provide some interesting treatments (mostly epidural injections of steroids in to the spine). But there aren't many of these doctors around now, and most of them have been booked solid for weeks to months (at least in my neck of the woods) even BEFORE these new regulations were announced.

So, if nearly half of doctors are going to reduce or eliminate the number of pain medications they prescribe… and it's very difficult to get an appointment with a pain doctor… what the heck are all these patients currently on painkillers going to do?

And what happens if you aren't in pain *now*, but you *are* in the near future?

Caught between a rock and a hard place

While I applaud the FDA's bold move in admitting that these prescription drugs are causing serious harm to the American public, I'm saddened that they didn't reach out to the alternative medical community first to get some *other* strategies for pain control that aren't "medication-based."

If only they would've just asked for our help!

In fact, I am shocked at their total lack of any backup plan. The new guidelines mention *some* alternatives for people in pain, but here's where I really take issue. They want you to take *other* drugs—NSAIDs like ibuprofen or aspirin, Tylenol, antidepressants, or seizure drugs—that carry a host of their *own* risks!

NSAIDs like ibuprofen lead to 18,000 deaths per year and 100,000 hospital visits due to their obvious damage to the gut lining and kidneys.[3] And as you know, aspirin has its risks and benefits, too—but when you take it for pain control (meaning higher than the "baby" dose of 81 mg.), you run a high risk of intestinal bleeding.[4]

Tylenol (acetaminophen) has less gastrointestinal side effects, but it stresses your liver and severely depletes the all-important glutathione levels in your body[5]… which leads to a whole host of other severe medical issues.

Antidepressants and seizure drugs numb your pain receptors—but they also come with a laundry list of side effects and can actually leave you feeling numb all over!

So what kind of ultimatum have the Feds given us, then? We can:

- Continue to have thousands of people die each year due to opioid-related overdose and have many more addicted;

- Increase the number of NSAID-related deaths from 18,000 to who-knows-what and/or increase the long, slow death from the use of Tylenol; or

- Just leave everyone "numb and tired" from antidepressants and seizure drugs

Come on! We're talking about people on morphine and other opioids, dealing with serious pain.

Not one of these is a good short- OR long-term solution.

Quite frankly, I think these recommendations are laughable. If NSAID's, Tylenol, antidepressants, and seizure drugs truly worked on *that* level of pain, doctors wouldn't have had to turn to such powerful drugs.

Let's face it: One of the reasons that we got in to this conundrum to begin with is that the conventional medical community hasn't had any great pain options.

Pain is a physical problem that needs something WAY more than a Band-Aid. But we can't just pop these pills to make the pain go away unless we're willing to accept these dire side effects and risks.

Don't just clear the smoke—extinguish the fire

What's amazing to me as an integrative physician is the multitude of other options that exist that conventional doctors either don't know about, don't believe in, or don't want to recommend.

Granted, some of these options aren't as easy as popping a pill… and most aren't covered by health insurance. But they ARE effective for a large percentage of people, and they're actually "good for you"—because first and foremost, this alternative approach to pain control is to find the ROOT CAUSE of the pain.

And there are four culprits that are often to blame.

1. Food sensitivity: You'd be amazed at what certain foods can do to your joints! The most common offenders are gluten and casein (the main proteins found in wheat and dairy), but sugar isn't far behind.

Conventional doctors often miss food sensitivities as a cause of pain because they aren't quite as obvious as food allergies. In the case of a sensitivity, the foods don't cause an immediate response. Instead, they start wreaking their inflammatory havoc about two hours (or so) after you eat the offending food. It could even take up to 72 hours before you feel any effects! An integrative physician like me can perform a food sensitivity test to find out which foods you should avoid.

2. Toxins: Exposure to heavy metals such as mercury and lead can cause pain from a slow, insidious process of damage to your nervous system. And other toxins, like mold, can cause some unusually severe inflammatory reactions.

You can work with an integrative doctor to help determine your toxic load and work out a potential detoxification process. I'm a fan of oral detoxification supplements such as chlorella or PectaSol, as well as sauna therapy to sweat toxins out right through the skin.

3. Chronic infections: If the pain and inflammation is infection-related, there are some amazing herbs (such as garlic and cat's claw) with anti-inflammatory properties that can work really well.

4. Misalignment of the body: You can take all the morphine you want to forget that your body is out of whack, but the only way to actually get rid of the pain is to put everything back in its right place.

Easing pain shouldn't lead to something worse

If you've been on opioids for weeks... or months... or even years, work with your doc on addressing the root cause of your pain rather than covering it up.

Keep in mind that your body may be physically dependent on the drugs, so it's important to wean off them slowly to minimize any symptoms of withdrawal (which can range from agitation to vomiting).[6]

Now, addressing the root cause of pain isn't a "quick fix"—so while you're healing, you'll probably still experience *some* pain, at least for a while.

But you don't have to just bite the bullet for the rest of your life... and you don't need to take addictive drugs...or ones that might make your stomach bleed.

First of all, you could do what I call a "detox week," when you eat only organic vegetables, fruits, and protein—basically, the Paleo Diet—for seven days. So many of my patients have seen their chronic pain turn around miraculously when they make this dietary change, which reduces foods you may be sensitive to AND your exposure to toxins.

As far as straight pain control and anti-inflammatory treatments, I'm a fan of supplements like curcumin and boswellia, both of which are available at reasonable prices at your local health food store.

I've been seeing some amazing success with a proprietary extract blend in the form of a medical food called Limbrel. It's stood toe-to-toe with NSAIDs in clinical studies and come out equally as effective in alleviating pain.[7]

I'll admit that these alternatives aren't as powerful as morphine—but they're a LOT safer for you to take, without risk of addiction, overdose, or death.

And you can try different ways of combining these therapies to get the pain control that you need.

There's a legion of other alternative and complementary therapies that you can try as well—and they go way beyond the ones your doctor may have suggested (like talk therapy or exercise).

Chapter 6:

In pain? Nowhere to turn? Send even the worst pain packing... without drugs!

I've shared in the past how the federal government is cracking down on prescription painkillers—namely opioids like morphine, Vicodin, and Oxycontin.

That means lots of people on pain meds are going to be left in the lurch—and looking for alternatives.

That's going to be new territory for many mainstream docs. For years they've just been dashing off prescriptions for these powerful drugs that should really be a last resort.

The good news is that there are plenty of drug-free pain-relief options in the integrative medical community—including eight I'll introduce you to in just a moment.

But first let me get you caught up on where things stand on federal regulations, and how you or someone you love could be affected.

Oh, those fumbling Feds...

FDA Commissioner Robert Califf, M.D. stated last spring, "The FDA remains steadfast in our commitment to do our part to help reverse the devastating impact of the misuse and abuse of prescription opioids."[1]

I do applaud the FDA's bold move in admitting that these prescription drugs are causing serious harm to the American public. But the options that the CDC and the FDA actually DID recommend for these poor patients in pain boiled down to just cognitive behavioral therapy (CBT) and exercise.

I'm not saying that they don't have their merits. But if you've ever been (or are now) in the relentless pain of a chronic condition like fibromyalgia... or severe pain from a surgery or injury... you know that being told to go see a shrink, join a gym, or chant a mantra just isn't going to cut it.

In fact, it's sure to drive a patient away—straight to the office of *another* doctor who WILL give them some pain relief.

To their credit, the CDC recommendations do briefly mention integrative medicine, but they only discuss therapies such as talk therapy, yoga, Qi Gong, touch therapy, creative arts therapy, biofeedback, meditation, and hypnosis. And even those options were buried deep in a link in their report—and I don't think there are nearly enough of them there for the type of pain that people out there are dealing with.

Fortunately, there's some relief that we can offer, without the dangers of addictive and possibly deadly prescription drugs—and they're sure to come in handy, especially if you can't even get your hands on these recently-restricted opioids.

Change your body, change your pain

I've seen one strategy ease the pain of many of my patients: losing weight. It can take the pressure off sore knees, alleviate a bad back, and make chronic pain conditions easier to cope with.

But I know that's not what you want to hear. And since significant weight loss can happen over a prolonged period of time... and you need help NOW... here's a plentiful assortment of eight drug-free options for you to try:

1. Acupuncture and Acupressure: Both of these therapies from ancient Chinese medicine have been around for centuries and are proven to have a host of health benefits—not the least of which is the management of pain. While they each target channels of energy in the body called "meridians," acupuncture is the only one of the two to use tiny needles in the process. As a medical acupuncturist, I've found that it can lessen inflammation and relax muscles—but it can also affect your nervous system, your endocrine system (including endorphins), and your immune system. Visit www.medicalacupuncture.org/ to find a practitioner near you.

2. Physical Therapy: PT is so widely used and accepted, it's funny to think of it as being "alternative"—but it *is* a vastly effective and affordable alternative to more drastic measures, like surgery.[2] And, as we know, even minor surgical procedures are sometimes the gateway for people to unintentionally get hooked on (or overdose on) opioids. It might even be already familiar to you, if you ever had something like a sports injury... a joint replacement... or mobility issues from polio, Parkinson's, or a stroke. The exact nature of the PT sessions will depend on what issue is being treated, but the focus will be on making it easier for you to move—ideally without pain, but at the very least with less pain. This can complement other pain management strategies very well—and what's more, some insurance companies will cover at least part of it.

3. Massage: There are MANY different forms of massage, but on the most basic level, this is a therapy that focuses on manipulating your muscles. It's known to release endorphins, a group of hormones that are known as your body's own natural pain relievers—and some people find it very relaxing, especially when combined with essential oils and aromatherapy. And it's been shown to be equally as effective as exercise in relieving lower chronic back pain.[3] The effects of massage tend to be cumulative, so get into a regular routine with it if you can.

4. Rolfing: This therapy, which started in the early 1970s, manipulates the soft tissues of your body in a sort of hybrid between massage and assisted yoga, working specifically on your body's alignment. While the practice is generally considered gentle, it can go pretty deep... and therefore become a bit intense for some people. It can help with posture problems and stress-induced pain, but it may not be the best option for very serious cases of chronic pain.

5. Chiropractic: While massage focuses on your muscles, and rolfing focuses on your connective tissues, chiropractic treatments focus on your bones—particularly, your spine. It's used to treat low back pain, headaches, neck pain, and a variety of other painful conditions including fibromyalgia and even whiplash.[4] The pressure is generally moderate, and patients can experience some relief after just one session. No two chiropractic sessions are alike, but generally the pressure is moderate and it's considered safe.

6. Craniosacral Therapy: Also known as "Cranial Sacral Therapy," this is another form of "bodywork," and it's considered one type of Osteopathic manipulative therapy (which also includes visceral manipulation and lymphatic drainage).[5] A practitioner focuses on your skull, manipulating the joints of your cranium with a relatively soft touch. Some people find it relaxing enough to ease anxiety and improve quality of life, as shown in a 2011 study on fibromyalgia patients.[6] A recent study in the *Clinical Journal of Pain* found it effective for relieving chronic neck pain after eight weeks of treatment—an effect that lasted for three months after the sessions were over.[7] And while a brand new study out of Spain found that 10 sessions improved pain intensity better than the same number of traditional massage sessions,[8] another study from this year out of Poland showed that craniosacral therapy was at least as good as traditional massage in relieving pain in the cranial part of the spine.[9]

7. Reiki and Therapeutic Touch: Although they're two different practices, both Reiki and Therapeutic Touch are healing therapies that don't necessarily require the practitioner to actually touch you. And that can be good if you don't like the idea of being massaged by someone you don't know. Like massage, some people find these practices incredibly relaxing—especially since they're meant to heal your energy, which, theoretically, allows your body to heal itself. Studies have shown a significant reduction in pain in knee osteoarthritis with Therapeutic Touch.[10] And even *Newsweek* reported that Reiki's "results are hard to deny."[11] Neither one is likely to do you any harm,[12] since most of the time the therapist's hands are hovering over your body rather than actually manipulating your tissues. At the very least, a session may put you at ease... or help you sleep... and when you're in pain, that can be priceless.

8. Portable / Wearable Therapies: If you're less of a "people person" and would prefer your pain relief to come in the form of a machine, there's a growing number of sophisticated "microcurrent" devices out there that have been shown to reduce pain and inflammation through either an electrical current (for example, TENS and MENS) or electromagnetic pulses (PEMF). They come in a variety of formats, from pads you lie down on to knee cuffs, patches, and electrode pads wired to a little machine that you can carry around. Between the adhesives and the "shock" you may feel, these methods can be a bit irritating—especially if you've got sensitive skin or are sensitive to the touch. However, they've been shown to decrease swelling, increase circulation, and actually reduce your perception of pain.[12] These methods are often incorporated into chiropractic treatment visits, and they can get you through the gaps between appointments.

There are too many pain management alternatives to explore exhaustively here, and not every therapy is well-suited to every type of pain... so experiment with an open mind to figure out what works for you. Not everything works on every person.

Imagine: no pain, no drugs needed

As with any complementary therapy, consult your doctor before trying any of the above alternatives to manage your pain. Although they're all considered safe, they may not be recommended for you under certain circumstances.

If you feel anything more than a little soreness a day or two after your sessions, seek medical help right away.

A holistic doctor can help you sort out your options in your battle with pain—especially to make sure you don't do anything to make it worse. I recommend a member of the American College for Advancement in Medicine www.acam.org.

Chapter 7:

Banish pain, inflammation— and even asthma—with this "suction secret"

I f you watched this summer's Olympic Games, you know they provided plenty of breakout moments for top athletes around the world.

But they also provided a breakout moment for a powerful and effective therapy I've been using at my clinics for years. I'm talking about cupping—the practice of applying glass or plastic cups and suction to different areas of the body.

Athletes like swimmer Michael Phelps use cupping to relieve muscle pain and to speed healing. And the telltale round, bruised marks on his body drew lots of attention and discussion during the Olympics.

But, believe it or not, pain relief is just one of the many ways that cupping can improve—and even revitalize—your overall health.

Cupping has a long (and VERY surprising) history

Cupping is taught at modern acupuncture schools, and many acupuncture clinics will offer cupping as well. That's led many people to think that cupping, like acupuncture, originated from ancient Chinese medicine.

But that's not entirely true.

The fact is, cultures all around the world have a history of "sucking out the bad stuff," according to Dr. Paul Unschuld.

Ancient Chinese medicine was not alone in utilizing cupping. Centuries ago, Hippocrates, Galen, and Celsus, all of whom played a role in the development of Western medicine, used cupping and wrote about it. One thousand years ago, the Persian physician Avicenna described a technique for using cupping to disperse inflammation in the body.

So what kind of cupping is right for you?

Depending on where you go for treatment, you'll see lots of different types of cupping performed. Cupping is actually the name given to a variety of techniques, all of which involve round glass or plastic "cups" put on the body in such a way as to cause suction.

The suction can frequently leave some bruising on the back or wherever the cups are placed.

The three many types of cupping are:

Dry cupping: This is the most widely used today. The open end of the cup is placed over the portion of the body to be treated. A small hand pump removes air from the cup, and sucks the skin and tissue up into the cup.

Everything is kept in place for 5 to 20 minutes, sometimes longer. At the end of the treatment, a valve is opened to release the vacuum, and the cup comes off naturally.

Fire cupping: With fire cupping, the cups are made of glass and have no valve—just a round, open end. A flame is introduced into the cup, which creates a momentary vacuum.

Then, when the cup is placed on the body, the skin is sucked up into it. There is a sensation of momentary heat, but it's done very rapidly and without burning.

In the case of fire cups, when the treatment is finished the vacuum is broken by inserting the tip of the finger underneath the cup.

Wet cupping: Wet cupping is done similarly, but first a tiny pinprick or stab through the skin is produced, and then the cup goes over that area. A bit of blood is frequently sucked into the cup by the vacuum, creating the "wet" part. Although this type of cupping is still used in places, I'm going to guess most Olympic athletes don't prefer it.

Watch pain, inflammation, and tight muscles disappear

Millions of people swear by cupping for relieving pain and inflammation. But, believe it or not, there's actually been a healthy amount of debate around exactly how cupping works.

Here's what we know. Cupping produces a negative pressure in your underlying tissues. This negative pressure brings blood and immune cells to the area (called hyperemia), which improves circulation and promotes healing.

In addition, when your muscles are in spasm, they can actually block your blood from flowing through your capillaries. Tiny clots can form throughout the capillary system.

The application of negative pressure through cupping pulls some of these micro-clots to the surface. That can cause some superficial bruising, but it allows for better circulation and the relaxation of your muscles.

But tight muscles are not the only problem that responds to cups. One randomized control study, reported recently in *The Journal of Pain*, showed that cupping helped improve carpal tunnel syndrome, a problem related to tendons and nerves in the wrists.

Postherpetic neuralgia, a painful condition that is a result from getting shingles, also seems to respond to cupping.

A 2012 meta-analysis looked at over 100 randomized controlled trials on cupping and listed facial paralysis, acne, and cervical spondylosis (wear and tear on the spinal disks) as other possible uses for cupping.

Can cupping help you beat asthma?

One of the most remarkable uses for cupping that I've seen is its ability to improve asthma symptoms. And that makes sense, considering the connection between asthma and inflammation.

I had a patient in her upper 80s who had severe asthma. She also had heart disease, so the medications for asthma were dangerous for her.

I started performing cupping on her back, every two weeks. She told me this was actually a familiar therapy, as her "Nonnie" (she was of Italian ancestry) used cups on family members when they were ill or injured.

My patient lived another seven years, with no further need for asthma medications, other than the biweekly cupping. Since then, I have treated a number of other patients with asthma preventively, using nothing but the simple treatment.

And I wasn't exactly the first to discover that cupping can be effective for breathing or lung conditions. In 1931, Sir William Osler, a famous physician, indicated cupping in his textbook for the treatment of bronchopneumonia.

PART V

Diabetes

Chapter 1:

The hidden link between digestion and diabetes

It's embarrassing. Most of us don't even want to admit it, let alone talk about it. But trust me, with potentially millions of adults suffering from digestive troubles, or lactose intolerance, you're far from alone.

They say misery loves company, and with so many experiencing this gut-wrenching misery you're definitely in good company. But the truth is you share something else *far* more sinister with all those folks. Because, believe it or not, if you're lactose intolerant… or have a hard time digesting your food… then you have *at least* a 50-50 chance of developing diabetes in your lifetime.

Shocked? Let me explain.

Tummy troubles are a ticking time bomb

A study published in April 2014 linked lactose intolerance to a *significantly* higher risk of type 2 diabetes. An earlier—and even more convincing—study published in 2000 revealed that over 50 percent of people with type 2 diabetes had issues fully digesting their food. Combined, these two eye-opening studies provide good solid evidence of the connection between digestion and blood-sugar issues.

Of course, having spent 37 years practicing medicine as a holistic doctor this "revelation" didn't come as a big shocker to me. I made the connection between diabetes and digestion long ago.

When the majority of my type 2 diabetic patients complained of digestive disturbances I quickly began to put two-and-two together. I soon realized that their sluggish pancreases were likely to blame. They simply weren't producing enough digestive enzymes to fully digest their food.

And the proof was in the cure. When I had these patients take digestive enzymes with each meal, their tummy troubles vanished almost like magic. That's when I began to realize that digestion problems in an otherwise healthy person could be an early warning sign of future blood-sugar issues. Meaning that being aware of, and treating, these types of tummy troubles (and undiagnosed blood-sugar issues) *early*, could help head off further pancreas troubles—and perhaps even full blown diabetes—at the pass. More on that a bit later.

Connecting the dots... the link between digestion and diabetes

Symptoms of poor digestion are...

- getting full early

- feeling bloated after meals

- seeing undigested food in your stool (corn gets a free pass) and

- increased gas

But despite this obvious connection, and the research, many docs don't take digestion troubles seriously. Unless there's extreme weight loss, severe abdominal pain or a frank case of pancreatitis few doctors even bother to test for pancreatic digestive enzyme efficiency/output. So the problem typically remains hidden, until one day diabetes rears its ugly head, of course.

The good news is that there's a stool test that you can request from your doctor that measures the output and effectiveness of your digestive enzymes. It's called the fecal elastase level and all major labs and hospitals are capable of doing this test. If you're experiencing lactose intolerance, or general digestive troubles, and suspect your pancreas may be falling down on its job, don't be afraid to talk with your doctor about having this simple test done.

Putting the cart before the pancreas

When you think of type 2 diabetes, most of us—doctors and lay-people alike—automatically think of roller coaster blood sugars and the damage those elevated sugars do to blood vessels, organs or nerves. And for good reason, of course. The damage can indeed be devastating. But the truth is by ignoring, or underestimating, the influence the pancreas has on type 2 diabetes we're putting the cart before the pancreas. And we're missing a golden opportunity to break that run-away diabetes horse before it's too late.

The pancreas has two main functions in the body:

1. To make insulin, which is called the endocrine function.

2. To make digestive enzymes, which is called the exocrine function. And this small but powerful organ can only take so much abuse before it starts to give out and become unable to keep up with the workload.

Lighten the load on your overworked pancreas

Luckily, there's one incredibly simple step we can all take right away to start to turn things around. We can dial back the severe stress we're putting our pancreas through on a daily basis. We can ask it to do less.

Westerners—Americans in particular—eat too much.

If you overindulge, even if it's good low-glycemic food you're eating, you're forcing your pancreas to work extra hard to digest all that food. And when you continue to stress this critical organ, over time you end up depleting its precious reserves.

After years of going the extra mile to digest those mountains of food, you essentially end up with a tuckered out pancreas. Not only does the over-worked organ have a hard time keeping up with producing the digestive enzymes you need, your damaged pancreas eventually has trouble producing enough blood-sugar regulating insulin too. The result is wildly fluctuating blood sugars (often referred to as pre diabetes or metabolic syndrome), and eventually, if the tide isn't turned, full-blown type 2 diabetes.

Small steps, BIG rewards

After slashing those portion sizes there are some *other* small steps you can take to help ease the pressure on your overworked pancreas. Chew your food more thoroughly and consider incorporating more foods into your diet that are naturally high in enzymes, such as papaya and pineapple

If you're lactose intolerant switch to Lactaid-containing dairy products, and try taking a lactase enzyme supplement. And if you get bloated and gassy after eating certain foods like beans go ahead and give Beano, or a similar product, a try.

If those changes don't do the trick, and you still find you're suffering with digestive distress, then you can take supplements or medications that help your pancreatic exocrine function. Head to the health food store and pick up some digestive enzymes. These enzymes are broader spectrum and plant-based (usually derived from aspergillus). They tend to be stronger than papaya or pineapple enzymes, and work in a broader variety of foods.

But if your digestive issues are much more serious, there are prescription strength digestive enzymes available as well. These enzymes, called Creon or Zenpep, are derived from the pancreases of pigs, and are significantly stronger than their over-the-counter counterparts.

When we give our pancreatic digestive enzymes the attention they deserve we naturally ease the stress that we're putting our pancreas through. And pampering your pancreas is one sure way to reduce your risk of ever developing type 2 diabetes.

Chapter 2:

Maintain "perfect" blood sugar, blood pressure, and cholesterol levels naturally

Barely a day goes by that I don't find myself talking some poor souls down off the ledge. A doctor has bullied them into believing that if they don't get their blood sugar, blood pressure and cholesterol numbers down (and fast) they're going to drop dead at any moment.

They end up on my doorstep because they don't want to die, but they also don't want to spend their lives chained to dangerous prescription drugs.

They find themselves stuck between a rock and side effect, and they're hoping I can help.

And the good news is I can. I usually start with a quick lesson on those bogus benchmarks they're being asked to meet—and then tell them the real blood sugar, blood pressure and cholesterol numbers they should be shooting for.

Bait-and-switch con sets you up for failure

My patients' jaws drop when I explain that lots of what we call "good" or "normal" health numbers today are nothing but a con. One dreamed up by drug company execs, dutifully carried out by their government pals in DC and reinforced by the lemmings in the mainstream media.

It's no accident that what are considered "good" cholesterol, blood sugar and blood pressure numbers have dropped so dramatically over the years (and we're certainly not any healthier to show for it).

Once Big Pharma has just about everyone in their potential pool of users signed up for a monthly prescription to the latest drug du jour, it's time to find new customers. They do that by funding biased studies, applying political pressure, and demanding that the ranges be lowered.

Before you know it the media is reporting on some new drastic change to the guidelines that are almost impossible to meet without prescription drugs.

In the last 10 years alone, the cholesterol guidelines have plummeted from a total cholesterol of 220 and a LDL ("bad") cholesterol of 120 to a needlessly low 200 and 100. Blood pressure goals have dropped from 140 systolic and 90 diastolic to 120 over 80. And three month blood sugar averages, measured using a test called the Hemoglobin A1C, have now started heading south too.

That may not seem like much of a difference, but the effect is enormous. It makes millions of new customers eligible for cholesterol, blood sugar and hypertension drugs practically overnight.

Suddenly your perfect 220 LDL cholesterol level is considered sky high. Time for a statin!

Or your normal blood sugar numbers now put you into the prediabetes zone and it's time to get you on a blood-sugar-lowering drug before you have "complications."

Or your borderline blood pressure is no longer treatable with diet and lifestyle changes and you need to start popping a blood pressure pill to avoid keeling over from a stroke.

Beware: The prescription drug gold rush can kill

Now don't misunderstand me, I'm certainly NOT against instituting some standard guidelines for these important numbers. But they just need to be reasonable and not driven by the very industry that stands to profit from them.

And for people who really do need to bring their blood sugar, blood pressure or cholesterol numbers down (more on that in a moment) immediately turning to drugs could be a big mistake.

Prescription meds are the third-leading cause of death in the United States, according to a study published in the Journal of the American Medical Association. And, in fact, medical treatments and drugs kill more people than strokes or diabetes!

In some cases the drugs could turn out to be far worse than the condition they're supposed to be treating. Or you could be trading one problem for another such as with cholesterol-lowering statins which have been linked with diabetes.

So what is "problem blood sugar" anyway?

Many of my patients are eager to avoid prescription diabetes drugs. And they want to know whether there is a magic blood sugar number or "tipping point" beyond which some type of intervention is necessary.

I believe a 6.0 three-month average on a Hemoglobin A1C test is high enough that we should pay attention to diet, exercise and natural blood sugar remedies.

But it's not high enough where I'd encourage the use of the potentially dangerous prescription drugs that are now being pushed for patients at that level.

Keep control NATURALLY

If you're concerned about your own numbers, simple diet and life-style changes are almost always the best first steps.

For elevated blood sugar levels talk with your doc about testing you for digestive and pancreatic enzyme deficiencies. If you're running low—which is often the case with pre-diabetes—it could be a sign of an over-loaded pancreas.

Supplementing with digestive enzymes like lipase, protese and amy-lase could give your pancreases the support it needs to help bring your numbers back down naturally. And natural supplements like berberine have been proven just as effective as the drug metformin in maintaining blood sugar control.

To lower your cholesterol think "fat," but NOT low fat.

America's obsession with low-fat (and high-carb) eating is what got us into this mess in the first place. Instead concentrate on eating plenty of natural fats and proteins such as beef and poultry which actually sup-port heart health.

Monounsaturated fats such as olive oil can help naturally lower your LDL (or so-called "bad" cholesterol) levels. And cold water fish such as salmon are packed with omega-3 fatty acids, a natural blood-clot fighter.

I highly recommend you give the Paleo Diet (also known as the Caveman Diet) a try. This healthy approach to eating—which focuses on natural proteins, fruits and vegetables while eliminating processed foods—can help improve your blood sugar control, reduce your blood pressure and lower your triglycerides. It may even help you effortlessly drop a few stubborn pounds.

Chapter 3:

WARNING: Could you get diabetes just from drinking water?

When I was a kid knowing someone with diabetes was pretty rare. But now over 29 million Americans have the devastating disease. In fact, the number of people with diabetes has essentially doubled in the last two decades... and the rise doesn't show any real signs of stopping.

Our waistlines have exploded right along with the rise in diabetes cases. And while everyone can tell you that being overweight is a leading factor in developing the disease, very few people are aware of another hidden cause of diabetes that many of us are accidently exposing ourselves to every day.

I'm talking about the toxic heavy metal arsenic. The same arsenic we regularly find in well water, food, and lots of other places.

Without realizing it many of us are coming into contact with heavy metals several times a day. And there's very good evidence that arsenic is one of the root causes of diabetes. Research has revealed that both high levels of exposure to the metal as well as chronic low level exposures are linked to the disease. And I've seen evidence of the connection between heavy metals and diabetes in my clinic, finding elevated arsenic, lead and mercury levels in a number of my own diabetic patients.

Arsenic is a known carcinogen which is most associated with bladder, lung and skin cancers. The metal has also been linked to immune deficiency, heart disease, hypertension and, as I have now revealed to you today, diabetes.

Countries with serious water contamination issues have taught us even more about the devastating effects of chronic arsenic exposure. The water supply in Bangladesh, for example, is heavily laced with the toxin, which means the people are literally drinking their way to diabetes and plenty of other health problems. A study published in 2010 in the *Lancet* concluded that a staggering 24 percent of all chronic disease deaths in Bangladesh could be attributed to drinking the arsenic-contaminated well water.

Arsenic picks on your pancreas

Shockingly, arsenic appears to cause diabetes by actually destroying beta cells in the pancreas. And these arsenic-linked cases are unlike the other insulin-resistant diabetes cases that we're used to seeing. The damage is often more severe and, even worse, reversing the disease with our typical weapons including supplements, drugs and even weight loss is difficult—and in some cases may even be impossible.

This is why limiting your exposure to arsenic in the first place is absolutely critical. And I can help you do just that by addressing the three main sources of arsenic exposure here in the United States; drinking water, rice and chicken.

Avoiding a drinking water disaster

Many of us are exposed to arsenic through our own drinking water. Currently there's no federal regulation for private wells and it's estimated that 13 million Americans are drinking contaminated well water. The aquifers that supply these wells have been contaminated by the bedrock or the soil. If your home or business is supplied by well water and you want to find out if you're living in an arsenic contamination hot spot you can check the USGS "Arsenic in groundwater of the United States" website at: www.water.usgs.gov/nawqa/trace/arsenic.

While most municipal water is being screened for arsenic the EPA does still allow a certain amount of the metal to be present in our water. The government admits that arsenic exposure is a problem and in 2011 they lowered the limit in drinking water from 50 ug/L all the way down to 10 ug/L. And when sky-high levels of arsenic were found in apple juice the FDA introduced new regulations on the amount of the heavy metal that was acceptable in this childhood favorite.

If you suspect your well water is contaminated with arsenic, or tests have confirmed it, you should switch to bottled water for drinking and cooking in the short term. And then consider a reverse osmosis or distillation water filtering system to help reduce the amount of arsenic in your water. Look for one that's been certified by NSF International (www. nsf.org), a not-for-profit organization that tests home water treatment systems.

Rolling the dice when you eat rice

Although some arsenic occurs naturally in the soil, our food crops, rice included, are doused in pesticides and fertilizers. And they contain a whole slew of sickening chemicals and heavy metals, including arsenic. These chemicals and metals seep into the soil and eventually our food crops absorb some of them. In addition industrial population can drive up arsenic levels in the soil as well.

Rice sucks up these toxins, including arsenic, more readily than some other food crops which is why a report published in 2012, in *Consumer Reports* magazine, found elevated levels of arsenic in rice. And a later investigation by the FDA produced similar findings.

At the current time, there aren't any FDA rules or regulations for the amount of arsenic allowed in rice or rice products. And unfortunately all rice, whether it's organic or conventionally grown, contains arsenic. So we need to take matters into our own hands.

Because arsenic accumulates in rice bran brown rice, which we tend to think of as being healthier than white rice actually has *higher* levels of arsenic in it than jasmine, basmati and pre-cooked instant rice. Also rice grown in California or imported from Southeast Asia tends to have lower arsenic levels than rice grown in other parts of the United States.

Rinsing your rice before cooking it and then cooking the rice in extra water can reduce the amount of arsenic in the final dish. In fact, some research suggests that cooking your rice in a large pot of boiling water, similar to how you cook pasta, could slash arsenic levels up to 40 percent.

But the very best way to reduce your exposure to arsenic in rice is also the most obvious, and that is to limit the amount of rice and rice products your family eats on a weekly basis. For adults one to three servings at most is probably best, and kids should get even less.

Checking on the arsenic in your chicken

It turns out Sunday night dinner could be your family's number one source of arsenic every week. Chicken is one of our biggest exposures to the heavy metal here in the United States because since the 1940s our government has allowed chicken farmers to use certain forms of the heavy metal in their chicken feed.

Why in the world would they do that? Well, arsenic kills parasites in chickens, encourages quicker growth and it helps to make the chicken skin pinker for a more appealing presentation at the grocery store.

Thankfully the FDA is finally phasing out arsenic in chicken feed at the end of 2015. But in the meantime, since studies show organic chickens tend to have much lower levels of arsenic than factory farmed varieties, be sure to choose organic birds until then.

Ditch arsenic to drive down your diabetes risk

If you're worried about your current arsenic levels ask your doctor about running urine and blood tests to check on the amount of the metal in your system. And if your levels are higher than you and your doctor would like a holistic doctor trained in environmental medicine and certified in chelation can use chelation to remove the metal from your body.

They say the best defense is a good offense, and that's true when it comes to diabetes and arsenic too. Armed with this knowledge about arsenic you can limit your exposure to this dangerous toxin and your risk of diabetes at the same time.

Chapter 4:

Get your type 2 diabetes under control…without a single drug

Best known for its natural antibiotic activity, berberine deals a serious blow to common infectious organisms—organisms like "staph," "strep," Chlamydia, diphtheria, salmonella, cholera, diplococcus pneumoniae, pseudomonas, gonorrhea, candida, trichomonas, and many others. Berberine is a component (for the technically inclined, a "plant alkaloid") of the commonly used herbs goldenseal and Oregon grape, and of several other less well-known botanicals. A 0.2 percent solution of berberine has been found effective against trachoma—in "third world" countries, a major infectious cause of visual impairment and blindness, as well as many other types of conjunctivitis.

It's less well known that berberine has been found more effective than aspirin in relieving fever in experimental animals, and is able to stimulate some parts of the immune system. It's also a stimulant for bile secretion.

And it's not at all well known that research published in well-known, respected, "peer-reviewed" medical journals in 2008 found that berberine is just as effective—and of course much safer—than metformin, the formerly patent medicine most commonly now prescribed to help re-regulate blood sugar in type 2 diabetes!

Another cover-up?
That won't stop the truth

Two studies were reported in one of the 2008 research reports.[1] In the first study, 36 adults with newly diagnosed type 2 diabetes mellitus were randomly assigned to treatment with berberine or metformin (500 milligrams of either, three times a day) in a three-month (13-week) trial.

At the end of three months, average fasting blood sugars in the berberine group dropped from 191 to 124 milligrams per deciliter, average post-prandial blood sugar (blood sugar after eating) dropped from 356 to 199 milligrams per deciliter, average hemoglobin A1c (a measurement of longer-term blood sugar control) dropped from 9.5 percent to 7.5 percent, and fasting triglycerides dropped from an average 99 to 78 milligrams per deciliter.

The researchers wrote, "Compared with metformin, berberine exhibited an identical effect in the regulation of glucose metabolism, such as HbA1c, FBG [fasting blood glucose], PBG [blood sugar after eating], fasting insulin and postprandial insulin [insulin level after eating]. In the regulation of lipid metabolism, berberine activity is better than metformin. By week 13, triglycerides and total cholesterol in the berberine group had decreased and were significantly lower than in the metformin group (P<0.05)."

Insulin resistance dropped by 45 percent

The second study in this same publication involved 48 adults already under treatment for type 2 diabetes with diet and one or more patent medications and/or insulin. Despite these various treatments, their type 2 diabetes was still poorly controlled. Diet and all medications had been the same in each individual for two months before berberine treatment was added, and remained unchanged for the three months of this second study.

After just 7 days, the added berberine (500 milligrams thrice daily) led to an average reduction in fasting blood sugar from 172 to 140 milligrams per deciliter, and average post-prandial blood sugar had declined from 266 to 210 milligrams per deciliter.

Are you a type 2 diabetic taking one of these medicines?

The Lancet, considered to be one of the world's "top" medical journals, published an editorial titled "Individualized incretin-based treatment for type 2 diabetes" in the August 7, 2010 edition. The author wrote, "All GLP-1 receptor agonists [molecules which stimulate the receptor for the incretin hormone GLP-1, which helps regulate blood sugar] that are "approved" [quotation marks added] or in development for the treatment of type 2 diabetes cause nausea, vomiting, and sometimes diarrhea in a substantial proportion of patients."

He continued by observing that GLP-1 can help regulate blood sugar without these effects—which should be rather obvious because our own internally secreted GLP-1 doesn't cause any of these problems! But rather than recommend that natural GLP-1—or berberine, which stimulates GLP-1—be used instead of "approved" or "under development" patent medicines, he instead suggests that researchers look into why the patent medications cause these problems, as this would "pave the way to an even more impressive exploitation of the incretin-based treatment strategy."

Exploitation is exactly the correct word to describe this point of view, which ignores completely the much safer and considerably less expensive molecules found in our bodies and in Nature, and continues to pursue the development, sale, and use of prohibitively expensive patent medicine substitutes with much greater incidence of so-called "side" effects—which are actually part of the real effects of these never-before-found-on-planet-Earth (extraterrestrial, space alien) molecules.

But it's your body and your health! If you have type 2 diabetes and are being "treated" with Byetta®—which all affect the incretin-driven blood sugar regulatory system—consider switching to berberine at 500 milligrams three times daily. There's ample scientific evidence to support such a change! Make sure to work with a physician skilled and knowledgeable in nutritional and natural medicine.

During the second week of added berberine, average fasting blood sugar dropped to 135 milligrams per deciliter, and postprandial glucose to 189 milligrams per deciliter. The researchers reported that these improvements were maintained for the rest of the three-month study.

In addition, hemoglobin A1c decreased from 8.1 percent to 7.3 percent, fasting insulin decreased by 28 percent, insulin resistance was reduced by 45 percent, and total and low-density (LDL) cholesterol were both significantly reduced.

The researchers wrote that in their study of newly diagnosed diabetics who took berberine or placebo alone, "[n]one of the patients suffered from severe gastrointestinal adverse events when berberine was used alone."

By contrast, the researchers wrote about the poorly controlled diabetics who added berberine to their on-going patent medication treatment: "Incidence of gastrointestinal adverse events was 34.5 percent during the 13 weeks of berberine…combination therapy."

These adverse events included diarrhea in 10 percent, constipation in 7 percent, flatulence in 19 percent, and abdominal pain in 3.4 percent. The side effects were observed only in the first four weeks in most patients. In 24 percent, berberine dosage was decreased from 500 to 300 milligrams thrice daily because of gastrointestinal adverse events, and all of these side effects disappeared within one week.

The researchers concluded, "In summary, berberine is a potent oral hypoglycemic [blood sugar lowering] agent with modest effect on lipid metabolism. It is safe and the cost of treatment by berberine is very low."

Better blood sugar control
…and a few pounds shed

In a second publication, other researchers described results achieved by 116 individuals with type 2 diabetes and cholesterol and triglyceride abnormalities who participated in a randomized, double-blind trial that compared 500 milligrams of berberine taken twice daily with placebo, also taken twice daily.[2] In the berberine group, average fasting blood sugar decreased from 126 to 101 milligrams/deciliter.

Two hours after a standardized glucose challenge, blood sugars decreased from an average 216 to an average 160 milligrams per deciliter. Average hemoglobin A1c decreased from 7.5 percent to 6.6 percent, average triglycerides decreased from 221 to 141 milligrams per deciliter, average total cholesterol decreased from 205 to 168 milligrams per deciliter, and average LDL-cholesterol ("bad" cholesterol) decreased from 125 to 97 milligrams per deciliter.

These researchers also reported "secondary outcomes." Body weight decreased from an average 151 pounds to an average 146 pounds with berberine, a significantly greater fall (five pounds) than in the placebo group, who went from an average 158 pounds to an average 155 pounds, a loss of three pounds. A greater reduction of body mass index (BMI) was also found at three months in the berberine group than in the placebo group. Systolic blood pressure decreased from an average of 124 to 117 and diastolic blood pressure decreased from an average of 81 to 77 in those treated with berberine, exceeding the fall from 126 to 123 systolic and from 83 to 80 diastolic in those who took the placebo.

Side effects were few and mostly transient in the berberine group. Tests were done for kidney and liver function, as well as blood counts and electrolytes. Mild to moderate constipation occurred in five participants receiving berberine and one participant in the placebo group. Constipation "cleared up" in three of the five taking berberine and the one in the placebo group. The other two in the berberine group reduced their quantity of berberine by half to 250 milligrams twice daily, which relieved the constipation. Three measured liver enzymes (for the technically inclined AST, ALT, and GGT) all decreased to within the normal range.

How berberine does the job

So how does berberine improve blood sugar control? Much of the answer involves the effect of berberine on insulin and insulin regulation.

Some of the rest is explained by berberine's indirect effect on blood sugar regulation through its effect on little-known (to non-researchers) gastro-intestinal hormones termed "incretins."

Berberine improves the action of insulin by activating an enzyme (for the technically inclined, AMP-activated protein kinase, or AMPK) which helps regulate the cellular uptake of glucose, the oxidation ("burn-ing") of fatty acids and the synthesis of glucose transporter 4 (GLUT4), the insulin-regulated glucose carrier found in fat and skeletal and cardiac muscle that is responsible for moving glucose from the bloodstream into cells.[3-6] GLUT 4 is found only in muscle and fat cells, the major tissues in the body that respond to insulin.

Berberine increases the "expression" (number and activity) of insulin receptors.[7,8] The increase in number and activity of course enables the same amount of insulin to be more effective than before. Another way of describing this activity of berberine is "decreasing insulin resistance." Other researchers have reported that berberine inhibits an enzyme (for the technically inclined, protein tyrosine phosphatase 1B, or PTP1B) which in turn inhibits the insulin receptor.[9] When the insulin receptor isn't inhibited as much, it can of course function better, and the net result is that insulin can "work" better.

"Incretins" are hormones secreted by our stomachs and intestines that simultaneously increase the amount of insulin and inhibit the amount of glucagon (a pancreatic hormone which "opposes" insulin) released from the pancreatic islet cells after eating, even before blood sugar levels rise. (It's like an "anticipatory" action so more insulin—and less glucagon—will be immediately available when the glucose starts to rise in the blood.) Incre-tins also slow the rate of absorption of nutrients into the blood stream by slowing stomach emptying; this may indirectly reduce food intake. An-other way in which berberine regulates blood sugar is by increasing the secretion of one of the major incretins, glucagon-like peptide 1 (GLP-1).[10]

However, the actions of GLP-1 and other incretins to increase in-sulin release, lower glucagon release, and help regulate blood sugar are normally rapidly negated by another enzyme called DDP-4 (for the technically inclined, dipeptidyl peptidase 4). Yet another aspect of the blood sugar regulating action of berberine is its ability to inhibit DDP-4.[11] When DDP-4 is inhibited, GLP-1 and other gut-secreted incretins aren't broken down as rapidly, so they can continue to stimulate insulin and inhibit glucagon release significantly longer.

Thousands of years of use, and still largely ignored

Berberine is a major active component of the herb Coptis chinensis (Huang-lian), which—according to one research group—has been used in China to treat what is now identified as type 2 diabetes for literally thousands of years.

According to another research group, its blood sugar lowering effect was noticed when it was given to type 2 diabetic individuals to treat diarrhea. After the isolation of the berberine molecule itself, one of the first publications describing its use to lower blood sugar in type 2 diabetics was published in China in 1988.[12] This and two subsequent research papers published in 2004[13] and 2005[14] found significant reductions in fasting and after-eating blood sugar control, and one also found significant reductions in cholesterol and triglycerides. Only one case of constipation (but no other adverse effects) was reported.

However, despite the safe and effective results reported, these studies suffered from the "defect" of not being placebo-controlled, and were (and are presently) only available in Chinese, so no one noticed them—with the possible exception of patent medicine companies working to make a patentable un-Natural molecule "analog" to berberine, and they won't tell!

But the research studies you've already read about were "controlled," and compared berberine directly with placebo or the number one established patent medication, metformin (Glucophage®, Glucophage XR®, Glumetza®, Fortamet®, Riomet®), or used berberine in addition to patent medication treatment—and all proved berberine to be clinically effective.

If you have type 2 diabetes and are using any patent medication, consider consulting a physician skilled and knowledgeable in natural and nutritional medicine and switching to berberine. Of course, there are many other natural techniques which can also be used to regulate and even normalize blood sugar in type 2 diabetes, including diet, exercise, vitamins, minerals, and other botanicals. It appears, however, that berberine can be a major tool, with fewer and less severe adverse effects than patent medications.

I personally recommend Berberine Plus™ (True Botanica™), 500 milligram capsules, each of which contain 485 milligrams of berberine itself. They are available at natural food stores and compounding pharmacies.

Thank you to Ronald Steriti, N.D., who researched and organized the material used in this report!

Chapter 5:

Is it Alzheimer's—or is it "Type 3 diabetes"? Learn the three ways diabetes is costing you your precious memories

Remember the good old days, when your brain was like a steel trap? You could rattle off names, dates, facts and figures with just a snap of your fingers.

But these days you have enough trouble remembering where you parked the car. And as those "senior moments" start to pile up, you start to worry more and more about Alzheimer's disease.

The good news is that there's a way to predict—and stop—Alzheimer's disease year before it strikes. And it's as simple as getting your blood sugar and diabetes under control.

Because research has proven that metabolic disorders like type 2 diabetes and Alzheimer's are often caused by the exact same problems. The two diseases are so linked that some forward-thinking scientists are even calling Alzheimer's "type 3 diabetes."

And they're saying that by preventing diabetes—or by getting a better handle on the condition, if you already have it—you may be able to stop Alzheimer's from *ever* taking root.

The stunning links between diabetes and Alzheimer's

Researchers argued for years about the relationship between diabetes and Alzheimer's. But, if you ask me, the science is settled by now.

Don't misunderstand me. There are other ways to get Alzheimer's, such as over-exposure to toxic metals like aluminum and mercury. But once you've been diagnosed as diabetic, you're sending your risk of Alzheimer's through the roof.

Ten years ago, researchers looked at the brains of deceased Alzheimer's patients, and they found up to 80 percent less insulin and insulin receptors. They dubbed this Metabolic Cognitive Syndrome or MCS—the first concrete link between diabetes and Alzheimer's.[1]

And in another study, researchers injected a drug that's known to cause diabetes (called *Streptozotocin* or STZ) into lab animals' bloodstreams. They found that the drug caused BOTH diabetes and neurological damage.[2]

So how exactly does diabetes end up leading to Alzheimer's? There are at least three links between the diseases that are important to appreciate.

Link #1: Obesity and Alzheimer's

The first connection between diabetes and Alzheimer's is pretty easy to understand. As you know, people often develop type 2 diabetes after years of being overweight.

But what you may not know is that amyloid protein is common in the fat tissue we usually associate with obesity. And amyloid plaques are considered a telltale sign of Alzheimer's.

In short, the more weight you carry around, the easier you make it for these plaques to develop.

Link #2:
Low blood sugar starves your brain

Type 2 diabetes can cause wild swings in your blood sugar levels. And when your blood sugar crashes, it causes damage to your brain.

Your brain, like the rest of your body, needs the right amount of sugar for fuel. But unlike other cells in your body, your brain cells don't store sugar. They need a consistent supply.

So when your blood sugar plummets (a condition we doctors call hypoglycemia), it chokes off a fuel supply to your brain. You get moody and agitated, and have trouble concentrating—some of the same symptoms you'd describe with Alzheimer's.

Link #3:
Insulin problems are like a death
sentence for brain cells

When you develop type 2 diabetes, your cells become resistant to insulin, which regulates your sugar levels. Or your body may not be able to make enough insulin to pull sugar out of your bloodstream and deliver it to your cells.

Both of those scenarios can put you on the fast track to Alzheimer's.

When it comes to your brain, insulin has a very unique job to do. It sends signals that lead to the release of key neurotransmitters, help nerves grow and repair themselves, and keep your brain flexible.

So when you're not making enough insulin—or your brain's cells are resistant to insulin—the effect on your memory and thinking skills can be huge.

And as the damage piles up, inflammation occurs—and your body sends out inflammatory messengers, called cytokines. These cytokines can lead to the formation of amyloid plaques and tau proteins that have been linked to Alzheimer's.

The bright side to the links between brain and blood sugar

Now that we've established the relationship between metabolic disorders like diabetes and Alzheimer's, we can work to keep Alzheimer's from developing.

For years, I've been telling my patients about the lifestyle changes that can prevent diabetes—and now we know that they may help prevent Alzheimer's too (or, at the very least, lessen its effects).

Avoid diets that are high in sugar and starchy carbohydrates like grains and potatoes—they increase insulin levels in the body, not to mention your weight and risk for heart disease, circulatory problems, and neurodegenerative diseases. You'll do better on a Paleo-style diet or even a Mediterranean diet—any diet with a lower glycemic index will help to prevent dementia from Alzheimer's disease.

Part VI

Anti-Aging, Hearing and Vision

Chapter 1:

Put the brakes on aging... and jumpstart your body's natural healing process... with the world's simplest antioxidant

They say that the best answers are sometimes the simplest ones—and that couldn't be more true when it comes to antioxidants.

You've heard plenty about antioxidants over the years, and how important they are to stopping disease and protecting your overall health.

But it turns out that the simplest of antioxidants, hydrogen, may be the most powerful and versatile one around.

Hydrogen isn't just the simplest antioxidant, but also the simplest of all molecules. Containing one proton and one electron, hydrogen is the "H" in H_2O (water) and in HCl (hydrochloric acid); and you can find it in all plants, the human body, and even the sun.

We've learned plenty about how hydrogen can combat oxidative stress and disease in our bodies. And according to a recent review of studies published in the *International Journal of Clinical Medicine,* this simple gas molecule may hold the key to slowing your body's aging process to a crawl.[1]

When inflammation begets inflammation

Because of its small size, hydrogen is able to move anywhere in the body—including across cell membranes, the blood brain barrier, and even into the cell structures that produce energy (i.e. mitochondria).

Because it's able to pass into parts of the cells in the body and the brain where other antioxidants can't go, hydrogen can have a special role in protecting us from potential illness and cell damage.

In order to understand these remarkable effects, we have to understand the nature of aging and inflammation in the body—both of which are largely a result of something called oxidative stress.

Oxidative stress creates "free radicals"—substances that attack and damage DNA (including in the mitochondria), proteins and fats in the cells, or enzyme systems meant to maintain our state of health.

These free radicals in turn create other free radicals in the body, and a cascade of inflammation and tissue damage occurs—a hallmark of chronic disease.

When this damage occurs, the mitochondria in the cells stop functioning properly... and without their "power house," the cells die.

Whether this oxidative stress comes from environment, diet, chemicals and toxins, infections, emotional stresses or injury, the results are the same.

But studies of autoimmune conditions including rheumatoid arthritis have shown that hydrogen therapy lowers inflammation and interferes with the messengers of oxidative stress over a broad range of illnesses.

It's even been suggested that psychiatric illnesses may respond to this remarkable therapy, since illnesses like schizophrenia and bipolar illness involve oxidative stress and inflammation.

Neutralize the damaging effects of radiation

Although the research suggesting that antioxidants can interfere with cancer treatments is questionable at best, many oncologists and patients are wary of taking antioxidants while having cancer therapy—even if the antioxidants would help to modify symptoms.

The answer to this conundrum may very well lie in this simple element, hydrogen.

You see, radiation damages and inflames the body while it does its dirty work, creating something called "hydroxyl radicals."

The hydroxyl radical is particularly damaging to cell tissues, and it isn't easily eliminated by the normal detoxification processes. But because hydrogen gas is a very stable molecule, it's unaffected by most so-called free radicals—and it has the unique ability to turn hydroxyl into harmless water.

And hydrogen water and other forms of hydrogen can neutralize hydroxyl radicals without interfering at all with the cancer-killing effects of radiation.

In one randomized clinical study of people with liver cancer, those who drank hydrogen water (versus placebo water) demonstrated a clear improvement in quality of life and symptom reduction. (Bone marrow, intestine, skin, and brain are some of the other tissues studied for the radioprotective effects of hydrogen.)

What's more, no side effects were reported... and, in fact, very few side effects have ever been reported with hydrogen water therapy.

Hydrogen water can protect against not only the radiation of cancer treatments, but also ultraviolet rays and their damaging effects on human skin.

Your skin changes with the ravages of time and environmental effects—but human studies have demonstrated that applying hydrogen water directly onto the skin both protects the skin directly through its effect on RNA expression and lowers the inflammatory cytokines that can damage the skin long-term.

Some studies have even demonstrated that burned skin heals faster and with less oxidative damage when exposed hydrogen therapy.

In one Japanese study, chronic pressure sores in elderly patients healed faster when the patient was given hydrogen water through their tube feedings.

And in another Japanese study, subjects who bathed daily in hydrogen water showed improvements in wrinkles in just three months.

A cardiac event doesn't have to be a heart-breaker

Multiple laboratory and animal studies have looked at the use of hydrogen therapy to prevent cardiac damage in the event that the heart's blood supply gets cut off temporarily.

This dangerous condition occurs when oxygen is decreased to cells as a result of heart attacks, strokes, or other injuries (ischemia). Blood then sometimes is restored to the tissues acutely (reperfusion) in a way that can actually damage tissues more.

Multiple studies have demonstrated that hydrogen therapy can protect tissues, particularly cardiac tissue, from this type of injury.

Other studies have used hydrogen gas to protect hearts and other organs during transplantation. Still other studies have shown that hydrogen therapy protects the lungs from damage during cardiac bypass surgery.

An interesting possible use of hydrogen therapy is its effect on blood pressure and its consequences. In one animal study, oral hydrogen prevented the development of hypertension and hypertrophy of the heart muscle wall.

In another study, on humans, drinking hydrogen water versus placebo water lowered systolic blood pressure almost immediately.

Stop nerve damage in its tracks

Neurodegenerative illnesses like Alzheimer's disease, Parkinson's disease and ALS offer another area that seems to be amenable to hydrogen therapy.

Several animal models of Parkinson's disease have demonstrated a prevention of further damage to the *substantia nigra* part of the brain—and even some improvement of function.

In one mouse study, a significant reduction of the loss of dopaminergic neurons (which are damaged in PD) occurred with simply putting hydrogen into the drinking water.

Most exciting was a pilot double-blind, clinical trial of humans with Parkinson's performed in Japan. All the patients were on levodopa, a Parkinson's medication, but some of them were also given a liter of hydrogenated water a day for 48 weeks. The rest of the group was given placebo water.

The treated group actually showed improvement on standardized scales of function!

Just add more H to your H$_2$O

Every cell in the body is attacked by free radicals at least 10,000 times a day, so it's critical that we ingest—in our food and in our supplements—powerful antioxidants to offset the effects of free radicals and oxidative stress.

Substances such as vitamin C and E, glutathione and alpha lipoic acid, plant-based flavonoids, and enzymes such as SOD are all antioxidants that can offset the ravages of free radical damage.

I've started to take hydrogen water myself to see if it has an effects on my Parkinson's symptoms, and I've begun to incorporate it into the healing programs of patients who have inflammation and oxidative stress (which is, basically, everyone).

I'm excited to add it to anti-aging protocols as well.

Drinking hydrogen water gets the hydrogen into the bloodstream rapidly and efficiently. Remarkably, hydrogen can be dissolved into water without changing the water itself, nor its taste, color or other properties.

And it's so mild and innocuous that it doesn't affect the normal function of the cells. There should be little or no adverse effects of hydrogen therapies.

We're currently using a GMO-free supplement product called "H2 Absorb" at my clinic. It's a tablet that, when plopped into a bottle of water, dissolves hydrogen into it while it fizzes.

For more information, visit www.RothfeldApothecary.com.

Chapter 2:

The vitamin that erases 20 years of aging in 90 days

By: Michele Cagan, Health Sciences Institute.

Imagine if the fountain of youth really existed. Imagine if you could wash yourself in its healing waters and walk away feeling and looking like you were in your prime again. What if you didn't have to worry about cancer, hypertension, or other age-related diseases?

Just think about it would you live your life differently? Would you spend more time visiting friends, outdoors, or at the beach? Would you get started on all those projects around the house that you never have the energy for? Would you lead a more active love life, take up a new hobby, change careers, or just play with your grandchildren on the floor once in a while?

This doesn't have to be just a fantasy. You can now slow, halt, and even reverse the effects of aging on your body. The Health Sciences Institute has recently uncovered what could be the most powerful anti-aging supplement ever developed. This breakthrough has been proven to literally reverse the body's aging process by rebuilding old, damaged cells. With this powerful, life-changing panacea you can:

- Protect your cells from degenerative ailments like heart disease, MS, and Parkinson's disease

- Improve chronic age-related conditions like arthritis and osteoporosis

- Wipe away wrinkles and liver spots

- Feel an overwhelming sense of well-being throughout the day

- Regain muscle mass and mobility in your limbs

- Improve the luster and vitality of your hair, nails, and skin

- Sleep through the night and wake up feeling alert and energized

- Boost your immune system

Ultra H-3 promises all this and more. It's the next generation of an anti-aging formula developed in Romania almost 50 years ago and heralded by the TV show 60 Minutes back in 1972. The difference is, Ultra H-3 is six times stronger and lasts 15 times longer than the original Romanian formula.

This cutting-edge compound has been developed by a distinguished think-tank of scientists and researchers-including, acclaimed author, and nutritional expert, Ann Louise Gittleman, N.D., C.N.S., M.S. It's just been patented in the United States, so there aren't many clinical studies yet. However, the initial results collected by Gittleman and her associates are so astonishing, we wanted to tell you about it immediately so you don't have to wait years for Mike Wallace to get wind of it.

The Romanian anti-aging miracle similar to an ingredient every dentist uses

The story of Ultra H-3 actually begins almost 100 years ago in Austria. Procaine-the primary active ingredient in Ultra H-3 was first discovered in 1905 by biochemist Dr. Alfred Einhorn while he was looking for a non-toxic, non-addictive anesthetic. At the time, cocaine was primarily used, but its negative characteristics were becoming apparent and its use was going to be outlawed. Procaine (very similar to novocaine) became a safe alternative anesthetic.

Nearly 50 years later in 1949, Dr. Ana Aslan of the National Geriatric Institute in Bucharest, Romania, discovered Procaine's anti-aging properties virtually by accident. Familiar with its anesthetic properties, Dr. Aslan began to inject her elderly arthritis patients with Procaine. To her surprise, not only did her patients experience decreased pain and increased mobility, they also began to experience overwhelming physical and mental improvements.

Dr. Aslan called her new discovery GH-3 and began a massive series of clinical trials that studied the effects of Procaine on 15,000 patients between ages 38 and 62. The study included over 400 doctors and 154 clinics, and at that point may have been the largest double-blind trial ever undertaken.

Procaine repairs the damage of old age, toxins, and disease from the inside out

By the time most of us reach 30, our bodies stop reproducing cells at the rate they once did. We literally lose more cells than we gain. And the cell membranes begin to erode and don't absorb nutrients as efficiently. New scientific evidence even suggests that many degenerative diseases such as cancer, MS, and Parkinson's are manifestations of damage to these cell membranes.

Dr. Aslan and her research team found that Procaine works by penetrating old or damaged cell membranes and repairing the erosion caused by old age, disease, toxins, food additives, and stress. Bathed in this powerful elixir, cells in the body are then able to receive nutrients and vitamins and expel toxins effectively. This makes for a healthier and younger body, from the inside out.

In 1956, Dr. Aslan presented her findings to the European Congress for Gerontology meeting in Karlsruhe, West Germany. While her claims were initially met with skepticism, Aslan's astonishing conclusions could not be ignored for long:

- Close to 70 percent of GH-3 patients never contracted a disease
- Overall, the death rate in the GH-3 group was more than 5 times lower than the placebo group over 3 years
- Patients were less prone to infectious diseases and seasonal influenza
- Reduction of sick days off work by almost 40 percent
- Joint mobility improved in 56 percent of cases2

While not a cure to any single disease, GH-3 was proven to target and improve many common chronic diseases and conditions including:

- Arthritis
- Chronic fatigue disorder
- Depression
- Sleep disorder
- Migraine headaches
- Lethargy
- Multiple sclerosis
- Decreased sex drive
- Poor circulation
- Excessive cholesterol
- Parkinson's disease
- Peptic ulcers
- Heart disease
- Acne
- Osteoporosis
- Hodgkin's disease

- Liver spots

- Failing memory

- Varicose veins

- Hypertension

- Emphysema

- Rheumatism

- Dementia

- Sickle cell anemia

60 Minutes uncovers Dick Clark's anti-aging secret

During most of the 1960s, GH-3 fought its way through U.S. federal regulations. Then in 1972, Mike Wallace of 60 Minutes did an investigative piece on this underground anti-aging formula and much of the western world finally took notice.

Since it was first developed, over 100 million people in more than 70 countries have used Dr. Aslan's formula. Hundreds of thousands of people were treated with GH-3 at her Romanian clinic, including many leaders from around the world, such as Mao Tse-Tung, Charles de Gaulle, Ho Chi Minh, Winston Churchill, and John F. Kennedy. Even many Hollywood stars-including Dick Clark, the Gabor sisters, Marlene Dietrich, Charlie Chaplin, Lillian Gish, Lena Horne, Charles Bronson, Kirk Douglas and Greta Garbo. All traveled to Romania for Dr. Aslan's GH-3 treatments.

Next generation formula is six times stronger than the GH-3 and without the downside

While Dr. Aslan's results were extraordinary, her Procaine formula has its limitations-its beneficial effects wore off too quickly and the market was (and is) flooded by cheap and ineffective imitations. But now you are among the very first in the United States to hear about Ultra H-3, the new and improved Procaine compound.

According to Gittleman, "Ultra H-3 is the most advanced and only patented Procaine formula ever developed. It's so powerful, many people respond to it within the first three days. I have actually had to reduce my dosage to half a pill because it's so powerful."

The secret to the new formula lies in the purification process. Ultra H-3 is run through a highly complex filtering process-making it 100 percent bioavailable. That means all the Procaine nutrients can be absorbed into the blood stream. Otherwise, Procaine leaves the body too quickly, providing only temporary relief.

Ultra H-3 actually lasts 15 times longer and is 6 times stronger than Dr. Aslan's formula, which only delivered 15 percent of the nutrients and costs thousands of dollars to administer.

According to Gittleman, "Ultra H-3 is a potent anti-aging supplement that keeps you feeling energized all day long. We have an enormous number of success stories from people who've felt relief from arthritis, depression, and lowered libido, and other chronic ailments associated with aging. We have even seen a return of some patients' original hair color. But most of all, you feel this overwhelming sense of well-being." Gittleman added, "It's almost like an adaptogenic herb-it seems to provide whatever your body needs."

Ultra H-3 is all-natural, and you don't have to go to Romania to get it

Like the original formula, Ultra H-3 is a completely natural substance, and you don't need a prescription. It comes in pill form and should be taken once or twice daily (six to eight hours apart) with a glass of water, one hour before or two hours after eating. For most people, taking Ultra H-3 twice a day on an empty stomach for three months gets the best results.

Ultra H-3 can be taken with other vitamins and supplements. In fact, your regular supplements may be absorbed more efficiently while taking it. For ordering information on Ultra H-3, go to www.unikeyhealth.com or call Uni Key Health Systems at 800-888-4353.

Chapter 3:

Stop vision loss in its tracks with these 6 "super herbs"

Imagine living out your golden years never watching the sunset ...never seeing a grandchild step up to the plate in the Little League game...and never reading your favorite book one more time?

Believe it or not, that's what an estimated 35 million Americans are facing right now.[1] Because they all have eye diseases that can lead to permanent blindness, like macular degeneration (AMD), diabetic retinopathy (DR), cataracts, and glaucoma.

For years these people have been let down by the mainstream. Most doctors have almost nothing to say about preventing eye diseases, and lots of times will let serious conditions (like cataracts) progress until they're bad enough to require surgery.

When it comes to something as precious as your eyesight, you deserve better. And the good news is that if your vision is getting worse year after year, there are six safe, natural "super herbs" that may help you stop the problem once and for all.

Body chemistry gone haywire
can steal your eyesight

The first thing to realize is that ALL of these vision-related illnesses involve some biochemical process that's gone awry. And one of the biggest is what we call oxidative stress.

Stresses of all sorts (chemicals, environmental stressors like cigarette smoke and radiation, hormonal stressors including high insulin levels, and even emotional stresses) create supercharged molecules known as reactive oxygen species (ROS) that murder our cells through a process called apoptosis.

Now, a certain amount of cell death is normal—our bodies are constantly regenerating, with old cells being replaced by new ones. But, in this process, it's a veritable killing spree.

And while these ROS are attacking our cells, they're also stimulating something called the "JNK signaling pathway." Think of that like a phone line that carries messages calling for your body to kill more of its own cells and to release inflammation.

6 herbs protect your eyes from
inflammation and cell death

Notice that, when I'm talking about cell death and inflammation, I haven't yet mentioned eye diseases specifically. That's because, while these biological processes can unleash damage on your retina, cornea, and other structures of your eye, they're equally destructive for your kidneys, peripheral nerves, joints, heart, and other organs.

In fact, aging is largely a process in which oxidative stress leads to ROS and inflammation and, eventually, to cell death.

And that's what's particularly exciting about the six "super herbs" that can help prevent conditions like AMD, cataracts, DR, and glaucoma. Because they work by stopping inflammation and cell death that can harm your eyes, they can also protect other organs and parts of your body as well.

1: Curcumin

I've talked a bit before about curcumin, the active component of the common kitchen spice turmeric.

One of the reasons that curcumin works so well is that it's stable in stomach acid. That means it doesn't break down as it moves through the digestive tract.

Curcumin helps control some of the enzymes that cause inflammation, and it interferes with the production of something called TNF alpha. That's a messenger in your body that promotes cell death and inflammation.

In rat studies, curcumin has been found to protect against radiation and hydrogen peroxide damage to the retina.[2] Other studies have shown that curcumin can prevent against damage of diabetic retinopathy.[3] Still other animal research demonstrated the protective effect of curcumin against cataract formation, both the diabetic and nondiabetic forms.[4]

The authors of one review study concluded that curcumin's antioxidative and anti-inflammatory properties make it "a compound of choice" in the treatment and prevention of multiple eye illnesses, including AMD, DR, and cataracts.[5]

2: Saffron

Another kitchen spice that has remarkable effects on the prevention and treatment of eye diseases is saffron. Its active ingredients, crosin and crocetin, protect your cells against ROS—and that means they can stop (or even *reverse)* oxidation, cell death, and inflammation.

Saffron actually blocks the action of Caspase-3, the enzyme that leads to cell death, and increases your levels of glutathione, one of the most powerful antioxidants around.

Test tube trials have shown that saffron protects retinal cells against oxidative stress,[6] and animal trials have shown the protective effect of saffron on the formation of cataracts, seemingly by shielding the lens cells against oxidative damage.[7]

But here's the good news, since your eyeballs aren't in a test tube or the body of a rat: human trials have shown benefits of saffron supplements in improving early macular degeneration (AMD).[8]

3: Lutein and Zeaxanthin

Any discussion of plant-based antioxidants for the eye must include the carotenoids lutein and zeaxanthin. These pigments are commonly found in many yellow-colored fruits (peaches, papaya, squash) and green leafy vegetables, and they've been shown to lower your risk of AMD.[9]

A recent clinical study demonstrated that supplementing with lutein and zeaxanthin slowed down the development of AMD and improved vision.[10]

Researchers think that these pigments absorb blue and UV light, which you're exposed to through sunlight and computer screens. Too much blue light reaching the retina has been implicated in the development of AMD.

#4: Quercetin

I've recently written about quercetin's use in prostate cancer prevention and treatment, but it has also been studied for its usefulness in vision disorders.

Found in vegetables, berries, and tea, this remarkable flavonoid is another botanical substance that acts as an antioxidant and inhibits the formation of ROS. In fact, quercetin beat other antioxidants in a 2011 study on preventing cataracts.[11]

Quercetin has also been shown to slow down *angiogenesis*. That's the overgrowth of small blood vessels in the retina, and it can lead to AMD.[12] Other studies have shown a role for quercetin in the prevention of diabetic complications, including retinopathy.[13]

5: Resveratrol

Resveratrol is a micronutrient found in red wine (among other delicious items in your fridge or kitchen cabinet) that's been shown to improve heart health and slow diabetes. But it also helps prevent the development of ROS. Several studies have demonstrated its ability to reduce diabetic complications, including retinopathy.[14]

In animal studies, resveratrol has been shown to increase glutathione and decrease oxidative stress of the lens of the eye, suggesting its potential use in preventing cataract formation.[15]

And human studies have shown that it can prevent damage to optic nerve cells in patients suffering from glaucoma.[16]

6: Danshen

Now, you probably don't have any of the Chinese herb Danshen in your spice rack because it comes from the root of a flowering plant that's native to China and Japan. Also called Salvia or Asian red sage, it contains antioxidants as well as anti-inflammatory micronutrients that can significantly improve eye health.

Due to its inhibition of TNF alpha, Danshen has been shown to protect your retinal cells.[17] In fact, Danshen prevented the loss of vision in mice whose retinal tissue had been injected with it, in a study looking at diabetic retinopathy. And its intravenous form has shown benefit in treating glaucoma.

Preclinical studies suggest that Danshen can also help prevent AMD, but human clinical trials are needed before we can say for sure.

Start protecting your eyes before the damage has been done

There are supplements available that have been designed specifically for vision support (sometimes called "ocular" support). They usually include at least a couple of these great herbal ingredients in a custom blend—which is a good thing if you'd rather not eat curry for three meals a day or guzzle down carafe after carafe of red wine. (You shouldn't do that anyway—it would take more bottles than you could drink to get enough resveratrol to benefit your eyesight in any significant way).

Chapter 4:

Five ways to avoid that hearing aid

I'll be honest with you: There's not much new to say about hearing loss. Mainstream medicine hasn't "discovered" the cause or cure for hearing loss, so they're usually not interested in spending much time on it. If your doctor has bothered to talk to you about it at all, it was probably just to recommend a hearing aid. But that's certainly not your only option.

Most of the research points to a link between age-related hearing loss and low levels of vitamin B12 and folic acid. In one study published in the *American Journal of Clinical Nutrition*, researchers examined hearing in 55 women.[1] They found that the lower the women's levels of vitamin B12 and folic acid, the worse their hearing. Specifically, women with impaired hearing had 38 percent lower serum vitamin B12 levels and 31 percent lower folate levels than women with normal hearing.

It sounds easy enough to correct: Just take vitamin B12 and folic acid supplements. But these results were found in women already taking B12 and folic acid. It doesn't seem to add up: Low levels of these nutrients are associated with hearing loss, so why didn't their supplements help? My guess is that their stomachs had something to do with it.

It all goes back to your stomach

Age-related problems like macular degeneration and hearing loss usually trace back to poor stomach function—especially a condition called hypochlorhydria, or low stomach acid. As you age, stomach function slows down and produces less and less acid. If your stomach isn't producing enough acid, it won't digest your food—or your supplements—efficiently. So even if you're taking the right supplements for the job, they won't help as much as they could if your stomach were functioning properly.

With that in mind, your first step should be to have your digestion tested. Many physicians test this by radio telemetry using the "Heidelberg capsule."

To take this test, you'll swallow a small, plastic capsule that contains electronic monitoring equipment. As it moves through the stomach and intestines, the capsule can measure the pH of the stomach, small intestine, and large intestine. This information can help your doctor determine whether or not your stomach is producing adequate amounts of acid.

If your test results indicate low levels of stomach acid, it's a good idea to supplement with either betaine hydrochloride-pepsin or glutamic-acid hydrochloride-pepsin before meals. To start, I usually recommend taking one capsule (5, 7 1/2, or 10 grains) before each meal. After two or three days, if there are no problems, take two capsules in the early part of the meal, then increase your dose to three capsules per meal several days later. The dose is gradually increased until it equals 40 to 70 grains per meal.

Hydrochloric acid should never be used anti-inflammatory medications. This method should only be used when testing indicates a need for it and should always be carefully monitored by a physician.

Your step-by-step supplement guide for fighting hearing loss

If you do have hypochlorhydria, even correcting the insufficient levels of acid and pepsin may not be enough to help you absorb vitamin B12.

So in this case, it's a better idea to take this nutrient by injection. I usually recommend injections of 1 cc of vitamin B12 (containing 1,000 micrograms) and 1/2 cc of folic acid (containing 2.5 to 5 milligrams).

Sublingual vitamin B drops are worth a try, but the absorption is variable from person to person. In other words, they may or may not help you.

In addition to vitamin B12 and folic acid, zinc has also been linked to hearing—especially tinnitus, a condition characterized by ringing in the ears. In a study, researchers found that patients with tinnitus had significantly lower levels of zinc than controls.[2] In another study, researchers found improvement in 46 percent of tinnitus patients taking 50 milligrams of zinc per day for two months.[3]

And last, but not least, on the list of nutrients to combat hearing loss is vitamin D. I know this vitamin keeps popping up over and over again, but that just goes to show you how important it is. Several studies have suggested that vitamin D deficiency might play a role in hearing loss.[4,5]

So make sure you're getting enough vitamin D—2,000 to 3,000 IU is a good general range.

I can't promise that following the steps outlined above will cure or reverse your hearing loss. But all of these recommendations are as good for your overall health as they are for your ears, and if they help keep you from ever needing that "doctor-recommended" hearing aid too, all the better.

Chapter 5:

Don't go deaf, blind or lose your mind! Natural strategies for keeping your hearing, vision, and thinking sharp well into old age

Eh? What's that you say? Louder, please. No, don't bother writing it down, can't see very well, either! Oh, never mind…I probably won't remember it, anyway!"

If you chuckled when you read that, it's probably because it sounds familiar—whether it's something you remember your parents or grandparents saying, or whether you've uttered similar things yourself. And while it sounds funny on the surface, the unfortunate truth underlying phrases like these is that varying degrees of failing hearing, vision, and mental function are still considered to be "normal" with advancing age.

But they need not be "normal" for you! In this chapter, we'll cover prevention and treatment of "age-related" hearing, vision, and cognitive functions, while you—and I—can still remember how to lower your chances of going deaf, blind, or losing your mind!

The hormone deficiency that could be destroying your hearing

Dennis Trune, Ph.D., of Oregon Health Sciences University, pioneered the research showing that the naturally occurring adrenal steroid hormone aldosterone can often reverse hearing loss in animals.

Based on Dr. Trune's work, many physicians have tested aldosterone levels in individuals with hearing loss (most of them "older"), and a significant number turned out to have low or "low normal" measurements. But after taking bio-identical aldosterone in "physiologic" quantities—amounts that would normally be present in adult human bodies—more than half of these individuals have regained a significant proportion of their "lost" hearing.

There are two surprising aspects of bio-identical aldosterone treatment for hearing loss. First, when it works, it works relatively rapidly, restoring a significant degree of hearing within the first two months. In fact, some people have literally heard improvement within just two to three weeks.

The other thing that's surprising about aldosterone therapy is that it's capable of restoring a significant degree of hearing even years after the hearing loss initially occurred. So far, one of the longest intervals was in an 87-year-old man who'd lost his hearing 13 years prior to regaining a significant degree of it using aldosterone.

Few have had any adverse effects from aldosterone therapy, likely because the use of bio-identical, physiologic-dose aldosterone restores levels to those that would be found in the body anyway.

This treatment is mainly focused on individuals with hearing loss and low or low-normal aldosterone levels, but there is one individual—an M.D.—who decided to try this approach for his hearing loss even though his aldosterone levels were quite normal. His hearing did improve, but unless you too are an M.D., D.O., or N.D. who can prescribe bio-identical aldosterone and order lab tests for sodium and potassium (sodium and potassium regulation are two of aldosterone's major responsibilities), please don't take aldosterone, bio-identical or not, if your measured levels are perfectly normal!

Beat the top 3 causes of blindness— without patent medicine or surgery

Glaucoma, macular degeneration, and cataracts are three very common causes of vision loss—if they're left untreated, that is.

But many cases of these three sight-stealing conditions can be treated by natural means, often avoiding patent medicines and/or surgery entirely. Even better, it's also possible to significantly reduce your risk of developing any of these problems in the first place.

The vision-robbing disease that's actually a symptom in many cases

Let's start with glaucoma. This condition occurs when the pressure inside the eyeball (intra-ocular pressure) rises. If the intra-ocular pressure rises high enough, it can cause blindness. Conventional treatment of glaucoma uses either patent medications (generally called miotics) or surgery to relieve the excess pressure.

But in 1937, Emanuel Josephson, M.D., an ophthalmologist in New York City, published a book titled *Glaucoma and its Medical Treatment with Cortin*. In it, Dr. Josephson reported many cases of individuals whose glaucoma and high intra-ocular pressure improved after treatment with a substance called cortin. Cortin was the 1930s name for entirely natural injectable extracts from animal adrenal cortex—the part of the adrenal glands which make cortisol, cortisone, DHEA, aldosterone, and all other natural adrenal steroid molecules in natural balance with each other. (Later on, Cortin was renamed Adrenal Cortical Extract, or ACE.)

Some of the improvements Dr. Josephson related were quite dramatic, with the patients' intra-ocular pressure dropping over 20 points to within the normal range. Dr. Josephson carefully explained that Cortin produced such impressive results because many cases of glaucoma don't actually originate in the eye, but instead manifest in the eye as a symptom of weak adrenal glands. In other words, Dr. Josephson discovered that, in many cases, glaucoma is a symptom, not an "independent disease."

Injections of Cortin (which was literally "hormone replacement therapy" for weak adrenal glands) would allow the eyes—which apparently depend on normal adrenal function—to normalize themselves in many cases. In fact, Cortin even helped alleviate high intra-ocular pressure in people who hadn't responded to miotics or surgery.

At the time Dr. Josephson was using it in his patients, Cortin was sold by major patent medication companies, including Parke-Davis. While they couldn't patent the extracts themselves (since they were 100 percent natural) patent medicine companies could patent—and make enormous profits from—the extraction process.

Unfortunately, though, in the late 1940s and early 1950s, patent medicine companies discovered ways to make totally unnatural but very powerful and patentable (and therefore much more profitable) versions of cortisone and cortisol. Even though these space-alien versions have an incredible list of adverse effects when used in human bodies—including diabetes, osteoporosis, high blood pressure, cataracts, and stomach ulcers—the patent medicine industry was so successful in blurring the lines between them and bio-identical cortisone and cortisol (which never have these sorts of adverse effects when used in "physiologic" quantities) that they've become the go-to choice for most mainstream physicians. A more recent example of this type of "blurring the lines" is the inability of the FDA, conventional medicine, and patent medicine companies to distinguish between Premarin and other patentable pseudo-estrogens and bio-identical estrogens. And just like the current situation with bio-identical HRT, the Feds used this line-blurring to outlaw Cortin/ACE in the 1970s.

They claimed that it should be banned because, unlike the synthetic version, ACE was "unapproved," and therefore potentially "dangerous"— even though it had been sold and in use for decades with no reported side effects. In an accompanying illogical leap of FDA "logic," after terming ACE "dangerous," they also stated it was "ineffective."

But it has resulted in tremendous success for normalizing glaucoma. Several individuals had decreases in intra-ocular pressure from well above 20 (normal is under 20) to below 20 following a series of intravenous injections of ACE. Many other physicians practicing natural medicine had seen similar results and have protested to the FDA. Unfortunately, the public didn't get involved, and side-effect-free ACE remains illegal today.

However, individuals with glaucoma can still improve and even normalize their intra-ocular pressure by using more general techniques to improve their adrenal function. The very best place to start is with your diet, eliminating all refined sugar and refined carbs and making sure to get adequate amounts of salt.

There are also a number of supplements that can help boost adrenal function, including the sodium ascorbate form of vitamin C, panto-thenic acid, chromium, vitamins A and E, and ginseng. Another relatively subtle but powerful technique for strengthening weak adrenal glands is "cell therapy" using fetal animal adrenal cells with other related fetal endocrine cells. For even more information on strengthening weak adrenal glands, check your local library for the book Adrenal Fatigue by James Wilson, N.D., Ph.D.

As you've likely guessed, adrenal-strengthening treatment is most likely to be successful treating glaucoma in people who have weak adrenal function. The 24-hour urine test for natural steroids and other hormones can help you and your physician make an official diagnosis, but symptoms of weak adrenal function include lower-than-average blood pressure (especially if the "top"—systolic—number is consistently below 110), dizzy spells when standing up rapidly, and being easily tired out. Being underweight for your particular height and difficulty gaining weight are also common with weak adrenal function, but are not always present.

If you have any or all of these symptoms, check with a physician skilled and knowledgeable in natural and nutritional medicine, as well as bio-identical hormone replacement.

If weak adrenals aren't at the root of your glaucoma, there are still a few other nutritional and natural therapies that may be able to help reverse it. Eliminating any food allergies you might have is a good first step. Research has also shown that daily use of fish oil (I recommend 1 table-spoonful daily) and high quantities of vitamin C (10 to 35 grams daily, split into three to four doses) can help reduce high intra-ocular pressure. Thyroid hormone also lowers intra-ocular pressure in some cases.

And both magnesium (250 milligrams daily) and standardized extracts of ginkgo biloba (40 milligrams three times daily) have been found to improve visual field defects for individuals with glaucoma.

The macular degeneration treatment that starts in your stomach

Just as Dr. Josephson found that many cases of glaucoma don't originate in the eye, but elsewhere in the body, many—if not most—cases of "dry" macular degeneration are "symptoms" of digestive malfunction, specifically poor digestion and assimilation of nutrients. So if you're starting to have vision problems, I encourage you to have your digestive function tested. If it's not operating up to par, correcting it (naturally, of course) will go a long way in helping you get the most from the nutrients that have vision-improving potential.

The most useful of those nutrients are lutein and zeaxanthin, which are found in highest concentrations in spinach, collard greens, and other deep green leafy vegetables. Other important nutrients include zinc (found in oysters, fish and other animal protein), selenium (two to four Brazil nuts a day are an excellent source), riboflavin (which comes from brewer's yeast, almonds, mushrooms, wheat bran, and dark green leafy vegetables), taurine (found in organ meats, fish, and other animal protein), and quercetin (good sources include onions, apples, kale, cherries, grapes, red cabbage, and green beans are all good sources). Bilberry and ginkgo are the best vision-supporting herbs.

I encourage anyone with macular degeneration to consider using Ocudyne II capsules (formulated by my colleague Alan R. Gaby M.D. and me), which contain all the nutrients noted above.

Clearing up cataracts, naturally

Another option for treating cataracts is a combination of Chinese botanicals called "Hachimi-jio-gan," or Ba-wei-wan. This treatment has been used for centuries in China to treat cataracts, and even has a bit of clinical evidence to support it: In a human study of early cataracts conducted in Japan, Hachimi-jio-gan was associated with lessening of cataracts in 60 percent of the volunteers. In the USA, Hachimi-jio-gan is available as a (much easier to pronounce) formula called Clinical Nutrients for the Eyes, which is available from natural food stores and compounding pharmacies.

Rounding out the natural treatment options for cataracts is a single, simple nutrient: Vitamin A. Decades ago, an honest ophthalmologist with a sense of humor wrote a letter-to-the-Editor of a medical journal "complaining" that his income from cataract surgery had gone down by over 2/3 since he started recommending vitamin A to all his patients with any degree of cataract at all. I recommend 30,000 IU of vitamin A (not beta-carotene) for anyone who wants to prevent or treat cataracts. In fact, the only people who shouldn't use this amount are very small children (who don't get cataracts anyway) and pregnant women.

And while we're on the topic of cataract prevention, one of the most important things you can do is eliminate all sources of sugar and refined carbohydrates from your diet! Researchers have found that part of the cause of cataracts is the lens of the eye trying to "help" the body lower high blood sugar by "packing it away" within the lens, which gradually obscures the vision. This explains why individuals with type 2 diabetes have a much greater incidence of cataracts than people with normal blood sugar levels. So even though not eating sugar and refined carbohydrates is better for everyone's health, it's especially important for cataract prevention if you have diabetes—type 2 or type 1—in your family. Eliminating all sources of the milk sugar lactose (milk, ice cream, cottage cheese, and many soft cheeses) will reduce your risk of cataracts, too.

In addition to eliminating refined sugar and carbohydrates, you may also want to consider incorporating some cataract-preventing nutrients (other than just vitamin A) into your daily supplement regimen. Riboflavin, vitamin C, quercetin, zinc, and carotenoids have all been associated with cataract risk reduction. And one study found that people with higher serum vitamin E levels had 50 percent less risk of developing cataracts than people with lower levels. (When you're supplementing with vitamin E, remember to use mixed tocopherols, not just alpha-tocopherol.)

As a side note, patent-medicine "cortisone" preparations that are prescribed to suppress symptoms of asthma, severe allergies, rheumatoid arthritis, and other more severe inflammatory conditions always increase cataract risk. So if you're using prescription patent-medicine "cortisone," check with a physician skilled and knowledgeable in nutritional and natural medicine for effective alternatives.

Your guide for beating cognitive decline (a.k.a "keeping your marbles")

According to health authorities, Alzheimer's disease is slated to become the next epidemic. In fact, current estimates state that nearly half of people over the age of 85 have Alzheimer's, whether it's obvious or not. There are non-Alzheimer's forms of dementia, too, most notably "multi-infarct" dementia, which is thought to be caused by a series of small strokes, and mild cognitive decline, which likely has many causes that have yet to be identified.

The best way to combat any and all of these cognitive problems is to prevent them from occurring in the first place. You keep reading about it over and over again, but an excellent diet is truly the most important aspect of preventing most—if not all—health problems, including cognitive decline. In fact, more and more research is being reported linking blood sugar problems (such as diabetes) and potential blood sugar problems (such as metabolic syndrome and insulin resistance) with a higher risk of Alzheimer's disease. So here we go again: Eliminate the sugar and refined carbohydrates! Make sure to eat several non-starchy vegetables and a wide array of colorful vegetables every day, too. (You want a varied palette on your plate because each color signals a different and necessary-to-good-health group of nutrients.)

It's also a good idea to "eat organic" as much as possible, since organically raised foods have significantly more minerals and vitamins than commercially grown varieties, not to mention a much lower risk of being contaminated with pesticides, herbicides, and miscellaneous non-food chemical additives.

When you can, I encourage you to even go beyond organic produce and also opt for organic, free-range meat and poultry as well. The essential fatty acid ratio in free-range protein is anti-inflammatory, while the essential fatty acid ratio found in grain-fed animal protein actually promotes inflammation, and inflammation is also being implicated more and more as raising the risk of Alzheimer's and other cognitive malfunction.

Along these same lines, one of the best "brain foods" you can eat is fish. (Low-mercury fish, that is.) Not only are the omega-3 fatty acids in fish anti-inflammatory, but they're also essential components of the membranes of every brain cell we have. And since our bodies can't make them on their own, it's critical to get enough omega-3s and other essential fatty acids from supplements (like cod liver oil) and foods (like free-range meat and fish).

Phospholipids are another key component of brain cells. While our bodies can make them, as with many other things (co-enzyme Q10 and glutathione are two prominent examples) our bodies make less and less with age. Eggs—specifically the yolks—are excellent sources of phospholipids, as is the lecithin found in soy. Supplemental lecithin—another good source of phospholipids—is available in any natural food store and is an excellent idea for anyone over 40.

Boost your brain—and your sex life

Despite the common belief that testosterone is mostly for sexual function, it's most important job is maintaining cognitive function. The sex part is important, no doubt, but who cares about sex if you can't remember who you're with or what you're doing with her?

Unfortunately, thanks to this misunderstanding, word hasn't gotten around that—just like estrogen replacement for women—bio-identical testosterone replacement for men is extremely important for significantly reducing the risk of Alzheimer's disease and cognitive decline. Here are just a few of the highlights:

- Higher serum estrogen levels in women in their 60s are direct-ly correlated with lower incidence of Alzheimer's in those same women decades later. (And the reverse is true too: Lower estrogens equal higher incidence of Alzheimer's in later years.)

- The 15-year Princeton men's study determined that men who had higher serum free testosterone in 1983 had less risk of Alzheimer's disease in 1998. (Once again, the reverse was also true: Lower se-rum free testosterone corresponded with higher risk of Alzheimer's.)

- Researchers observing neurons found substantially less accumu-lation of beta-amyloid, neurofibrillary tangle, tau protein, and other "neuronal garbage" associated with Alzheimer's when those neurons were exposed to "physiologic quantities" of either estro-gen or testosterone (depending on whether the neuron was from a woman or a man).

- In numerous controlled experiments, elderly men without Al-zheimer's disease do better on tests of cognitive function when given testosterone than men given placebo.

- Testosterone for men and estrogen (that's real, bio-identical estro-gen —not horse estrogen) for women is very protective for the en-tire cardiovascular system, including the blood supply to the brain. (Remember that cognitive decline due to repeated small strokes?)

The bottom line is, if you want to "keep your marbles" for as long as you live, consider bio-identical hormone replacement when it's appropri-ate for you. Just make sure to be working with a physician who is skilled and knowledgeable in all aspects of this therapy. If you're not sure if your doctor is, one way to find out is to ask the physician's office whether they do routine monitoring of therapy with the 24-hour urine steroid deter-mination. This test is the very best way to check not only the levels of the bio-identical hormones being replaced but also their metabolization (the natural transformation of the starting hormones into pro- and anti-carcinogenic metabolites). Blood and/or saliva testing just doesn't cut it when it comes to bio-identical HRT.

Small dose, big protection

No matter what neurotoxin your brain is exposed to, lithium protects against it.

Not only that, but lithium actually promotes the growth of new brain cells, even in individuals past age 50. So far, no other nutrient has been found to do that.

Yes, high-dose prescription lithium can be toxic, but low quantities like the ones used for boosting cognitive function and protecting brain cells (20 milligrams daily and under) are not associated with toxicity. It's very rare to have a negative reaction to low-dose lithium. Some people have claimed experiencing a slight tremor, but it went away when the lithium was discontinued. On the flip side of that same coin, it's much more common to report improvement in benign tumors with the use of low-dose lithium.

Even though risk of toxicity from low-dose lithium is very small, I always recommend working with a physician skilled and knowledgeable in nutritional and natural medicine if you decide to supplement with lithium. And to be on the extra-cautious side, it's important to use supplemental essential fatty acids when using even low-quantity lithium supplements. Essential fatty acids are the primary treatment for toxicity caused by high-dose prescription lithium, so using them in conjunction with low-dose treatment helps avoid that possibility altogether.

Spicing up your brain-boosting regimen

There are many, many more supplemental items that can help you maintain cognitive function, but we're quickly running out of space, so I'll just mention two more: Curcumin and Ginkgo.

Although no one is entirely sure how it works, the research on curcumin's ability to protect against Alzheimer's (as well as its many other beneficial effects) has been more than a little exciting. Areas of the world in which the spice turmeric (which has a high concentration of curcumin) is routinely used have very little—if any—Alzheimer's compared with areas that don't. Perhaps the best aspect of curcumin is that you don't need to take yet another pill to get its brain-boosting benefits. Just use turmeric in your cooking, perhaps an average of 1/4 to 1/2 teaspoonful daily. (For those of you who just can't stand the taste of turmeric, it is available in capsules, too. If you're using it for long-term cognitive maintenance, consider taking two 200-milligram capsules a day.)

Ginkgo has been used for the brain for thousands of years, and (like lithium) has been found to be neuroprotective.

We all know that none of us will live forever, but there's no reason not to live as long as our "genetic programs" will allow—and keep all of our faculties while we're here. If you can do all of the things outlined above (or at least come close), you'll have a much better chance of living as long as your oldest known relative, getting to know your great-grandchildren, and hearing, seeing, enjoying, and remembering those years of life so much better!

Part VII

Digestion and Weight Loss

Chapter 1:

The "youth hormones" that make weight loss nearly effortless!

By: Dr. Mark Stengler, Health Revelations

Are you fighting a weight-loss battle? By eating a healthful diet and exercising regularly, you can shed some weight—but then it's common to "get stuck." No matter how you modify your diet and exercise regimen, the pounds just stop coming off. What's going on?

Your hormones may be the key. They influence appetite (when and to what degree you desire food)… *metabolism* (how you convert food to energy)… and *insulin sensitivity* (the degree to which your cells respond to insulin, which allows your body to use glucose).

If you have hit a plateau—or even have had a reversal—in your weight-loss efforts, it may be time for you to look more closely at your hormone levels.

To start, have them tested by a physician. Hormone levels can be detected from samples of blood, saliva and urine. A knowledgeable holistic doctor will help you interpret the results and choose supplements or other natural solutions that will allow you to lose those additional pounds.

Important factors to consider...

How active is your thyroid?

Your body depends on thyroid hormones to regulate your metabolism. These hormones are produced in the butterfly-shaped gland just below your voice box. If thyroid hormones are in short supply, you can expect to gain weight. Assuming that your physician has ruled out any serious thyroid disease that must be treated in its own right, you can start to beat your weight problem by optimizing your thyroid function.

Natural solutions: For mild deficiencies—perhaps your levels are just a little off or are normal but you still have classic low thyroid symptoms, such as weight gain, fatigue, cold hands and feet, poor memory—look into one of these daily supplements or, even better, a formula that combines several of them. Take them until symptoms are better, and then taper off. If symptoms return, start taking them again—or have a doctor monitor you. If there is no improvement within four weeks, stop taking the supplements.

• **Bladderwrack** (a type of algae) contains iodine, which the thyroid requires for optimal functioning.

Typical dose: Two or three 500 mg capsules, in divided doses, for a total of 1,000 to 1,500 mg per day.

• **L-tyrosine** (an *amino acid*) helps the thyroid to manufacture hormones.

Typical dose: 500 mg twice daily on an empty stomach.

• **Homeopathic thyroid** (a minute dose of thyroid hormone or animal thyroid gland) stimulates your thyroid gland to produce hormones. Follow label directions.

• **Thyroid glandular** (an extract derived from animal thyroid tissue, typically that of a sheep) contains amino acids, vitamins and minerals that stimulate hormone production.

Typical dose: One to two capsules or tablets twice daily on an empty stomach.

Best formulas: I recommend Thyroid Support Liquid Phyto-Caps containing Bladderwrack and L-tyrosine from Gaia Herbs (800-831-7780, www.gaiaherbs.com) or Solaray's Thyroid Caps, which has L-tyrosine, iodine and thyroid glandular (800-669-8877, www.nutraceutical.com).

If your lab tests reveal a severe deficiency, you will be prescribed a thyroid hormone replacement program. Ask your doctor about natural thyroid replacement treatments, such as Armour Thyroid, Westhroid, Nature-Throid and compounded thyroid tablets.

The power of DHEA

Dehydroepiandrosterone (DHEA) is an adrenal hormone that enhances metabolism. DHEA levels naturally decrease with age. A study of 56 men and women at Washington University School of Medicine found that those who took 50 mg of DHEA daily for six months experienced a reduction in belly fat and visceral fat—the fat that builds up around internal organs—both of which are associated with heart disease, diabetes and other serious illnesses. Insulin levels also dropped significantly, indicating better blood sugar control and insulin sensitivity.

Natural solutions: If testing indicates that your DHEA level is low—less than 100 mcg/dL—take DHEA. If not, take one of the other supplements described below. Get your levels checked every six months.

• **DHEA supplements** increase DHEA levels.

Typical dose: Up to 50 mg once per day. DHEA is available over the counter, but its use should be monitored by a physician. Potential side effects include facial hair growth in women and prostate enlargement in men.

• **Sterols and sterolins** are plant fats that are chemically similar to animal fats but have different biological functions. Sterols and sterolins support DHEA production by the adrenal glands. Moducare Capsules (877-297-7332, www.moducare.com) contain both nutrients.

Typical dose: Two capsules in the morning and one before bedtime on an empty stomach.

• **Cordyceps sinensis** (a medicinal mushroom) also helps support DHEA production.

Typical dose: 2,400 mg of a standardized water and ethanol extract of Cordyceps sinensis strain Cs-4.

The cortisol factor

Prolonged elevation of the stress hormone cortisol can contribute to weight gain. High cortisol levels can interfere with normal thyroid function and decrease insulin sensitivity, both of which lead to weight gain.

Natural solutions: Stress-minimizing techniques curb your production of stress hormones. My favorite stress relievers include regular exercise, positive mental imagery and prayer.

Your doctor can order a saliva test to measure your cortisol level. *If yours is elevated, consider…*

• **Ashwagandha** (an herb) reduces cortisol levels when taken daily. Look for products containing the patented ingredient Sensoril, which offers optimal concentrations of ashwagandha. Widely available products are Liquid Anti-Stress Plus Adrenal Support from Life Solutions Natural Products (a company in which I have a financial interest, 800-914-8771, www.lifesolutionsnp.com) and Tribulus Complex with Ashwagandha by Jarrow Formulas (310-204-6936, www.jarrow.com).

If cortisol levels have not come down after two months of taking ashwagandha, try…

• **DHEA**, described above, which also can reduce cortisol levels.

Typical dose: Up to 50 mg daily, taken under a doctor's supervision.

Estrogen dominance

Most women understand the importance of *estrogen*, but they might not realize that excessive amounts of this hormone can increase body fat and promote fluid retention. Estrogen in women needs to be "balanced out" with *progesterone*, which has a *diuretic* (water-excreting) effect. Perimenopause, menopause and any health condition that interferes with ovulation (such as polycystic ovarian syndrome) will reduce levels of progesterone and give fat-building estrogen the upper hand. This is one reason why some women gain weight for no apparent reason.

Natural solutions: The nutrient *indole-3-carbinol* helps the liver metabolize estrogen. It is found in cruciferous vegetables—broccoli, cauliflower, cabbage and kale. I recommend eating at least one plentiful helping of any of these foods each day.

If a saliva, blood or urine test shows that your estrogen level is elevated even after you adopt an indole-3-carbinol–rich diet or if you just don't like to eat the above foods, try these daily supplements…

•**Indole-3-carbinol** helps the body metabolize estrogen.

Typical dose: 300 mg to 400 mg a day.

•*Vitex* (also called *chasteberry*, derived from the berries grown on the *Vitex agnus castus* tree) has been shown to improve the regularity of ovulation and raise progesterone levels.

Typical dose: 120 mg of a product standardized to 0.6 percent *aucubine* or 0.5 percent *agnuside* twice daily… or 800 mg of a nonstandardized supplement. Vitex is available from Nature's Way (to find a retailer, call 800-962-8873 or go to www.naturesway.com) and Enzymatic Therapy (800-783-2286, www.enzymatictherapy.com).

•**Natural progesterone cream** should be used as directed by your doctor for extreme progesterone deficiencies.

Typical dose: One-quarter teaspoon (20 mg) applied to the skin one or two times daily for two weeks before menstruation (stop when menses begin) or, if menopausal or postmenopausal, applied once per day. Consider Emerita ProGest (to find a retailer, call 800-888-6041 or go to www.emerita.com), a good brand that is commonly available in health-food stores.

The testosterone factor

Testosterone, a powerful hormone found in women and men, affects the body's ability to maintain lean muscle mass. It is primarily produced by the ovaries in women and the testes in men. A low level makes it more difficult to tone muscles and lose weight.

Natural solutions…

• **DHEA** is converted by women's bodies into testosterone. If a woman has low DHEA and low testosterone levels, then doctor-supervised supplementation of DHEA, as described previously, may improve both levels.

• **Panax ginseng** may help boost slightly low levels of testosterone in men and women.

Typical dose: 200 mg daily of a product standardized to five percent *ginsenosides.*

• **Tribulus terrestris** is a plant whose extract may increase testosterone amounts in men and women. So far, research has been done mainly with animals, but this herb appears to be safe. Tribulus by Source Naturals (for a retailer, call 800-815-2333 or log on to www.sourcenaturals. com) is a good choice, as is Life Solutions Natural Products' Liquid Natural Libido Enhancer (800-914-8771, www.lifesolutionsnp.com), which contains ginseng and, for a calming effect, the herb passionflower.

• **Natural testosterone** is available by prescription only and should be used when there is a moderate to severe deficiency. I prefer the transdermal gel or cream form, which is applied to the skin, because it requires less metabolism by the liver than pills.

Is insulin on your team?

Blood sugar (*glucose*) is terrific fuel for an active person, but you need the right level of insulin to transport the sugar from your bloodstream into tissue. A condition known as insulin resistance occurs when cells become less accepting of glucose and insulin levels spike. It is one factor that sets the stage for weight gain.

Natural solutions…

• **High-fiber diet** that includes seven to nine daily servings of fresh vegetables as well as three servings of whole-grain breads and cereals. Nuts, seeds and raw vegetables are especially good to help balance insulin levels. Stay away from simple-sugar food products, such as white breads, pasta, soft drinks, cookies and other sweets. For protein, avoid fatty red meats and favor quality sources, such as legumes, nuts, eggs, fish and poultry.

• **Help yourself to some cinnamon!** Studies show that it helps balance blood sugar levels.

• **Eat smaller servings** throughout the day rather than three big meals, so your body metabolizes food more effectively.

• **High-potency multivitamin/mineral supplement**. Everyone should take one daily for general health—it provides nutrients that, among other things, balance insulin levels.

If tests for fasting blood glucose and insulin indicate that you have insulin resistance, try taking all three of these additional supplements daily…

• **Chromium** (a mineral) is particularly important to balance blood sugar levels.

Typical dose: 400 mcg.

• **Alpha lipoic acid** (an enzyme that acts as a powerful antioxidant) reduces levels of insulin and blood sugar.

Typical dose: Up to 200 mg.

•**Fish oil** (an essential fatty acid supplement) improves insulin sensitivity.

Typical dose: One teaspoon daily or a one gram capsule, three times a day. Nordic Naturals fish oil supplements are widely available and free of mercury and other toxins (to locate a retailer, call 800-662-2544 or go to www.nordicnaturals.com).

Caution: If you are taking a blood-thinning medication, such as warfarin (Coumadin), check with your doctor before taking fish oil.

Root causes of weight gain

- Poor diet.

- Lack of exercise.

- Genetic predisposition.

- Hormone imbalance.

- Neurotransmitter imbalance, such as serotonin deficiency.

- Side effects of drugs.

- Toxins, such as chemicals (pesticides).

- Psychological reasons, such as stress, anxiety and depression.

Chapter 2:

Is this hidden illness leaving you tired, bloated and in pain? Cure it for good with a simple diet trick!

He's best remembered for setting the health industry on its ear with his revolutionary "Atkins Diet." But many people forget that Dr. Robert Atkins was a holistic doctor, just like me.

And when he introduced his new eating philosophy—when he fought back against the anti-fat mainstream and declared that carbs were the real health enemy—Dr. Atkins was just a physician trying to help his patients. He understood that a protein-rich diet that avoided health-destroying added sugars could help the people he treated lose weight, improve their heart health, control their blood sugar, and even sharpen their brains.

He saw the results at his thriving Manhattan clinic every day.

But decades later, we're learning an amazing new secret about Dr. Atkins low-carb movement—one that may turn out to be his greatest discovery yet. Because research is now proving that a high-fat, low-carb diet may help millions of people conquer a debilitating digestive condition that's been making them sick for years.

An illness you might not even realize you have.

Change your EATING and change your LIFE

I regularly "prescribe" a low-carbohydrate diet to my patients. (I specifically recommend Paleo, and I'll tell you more about it in just a few moments.) And the reason why is simple; it works! In fact, hardly a day goes by that I don't see the dramatic results of a patient heeding my advice, cutting out the bread and slashing the "white carbs."

They soon start to look great… but more importantly they FEEL great. And that's because when you change your eating you change your life.

But it's not just the weight loss that's making the difference. Adopting a low carb way of living doesn't just help you shed pounds, although it does that INCREDIBLY well. It has another huge side benefit that I don't believe even Dr. Atkins anticipated.

This hidden sensitivity could be why you feel so sick

It turns out the low-carb diet is an accidental diagnostic tool. Going low carb can reveal your undiagnosed gluten sensitivity because when you drop the carbs in your diet you're also dropping the gluten and that change can have dramatic effects for a significant number of us.

Gluten, a protein that's found mostly in bread, can be damaging to essentially every part of the body. In certain people who are particularly sensitive, the gluten protein acts like a toxin causing…

- joint pain

- fatigue

- bloating

- nerve pain

- muscle pain

As well as, literally, dozens of other troubling symptoms you may be feeling every day.

Gluten-free goes from fringe fad to mainstream acceptance

When gluten sensitivity first started to come to light, many in the mainstream refused to acknowledge it even existed. If you weren't suffering from celiac disease—a condition that makes you 100 percent unable to process gluten—then they insisted you could eat all the gluten you want.

But those of us in the trenches who were effectively eliminating a huge variety of troubling symptoms by putting our patients on low-carb/low-gluten diets knew different. When they stopped eating wheat, barley and rye they suddenly felt better than they had in years. It was, in effect, what we doctors like to call "an elimination diet," which is often used to diagnose allergies and sensitivities.

I'm happy to say, the tide is finally starting to turn and gluten-free diets are losing their "fad" status. I'm even starting to see some straight-laced conventional gastroenterologists admit that gluten sensitivity is real. Some are even advising their patients who were once diagnosed with irritable bowel syndrome that they might, in fact, be gluten sensitive instead.

Now THAT'S progress. And an incredible legacy for Dr. Atkins whose pioneering work laid the foundations for the sea change.

Shed that spare tire AND eliminate gluten problems

Believe it or not, Dr. Atkins' low-carb message stretches all the way back to the mid-60s. In fact, he appeared on the Tonight Show in 1965. That was 27 years before his second book Dr. Atkins' New Diet Revolution, published in 1992, sold 15 million copies worldwide.

At the time America was smack-dab in the middle of a misguided low-fat brainwashing campaign—the devastating effects of which are

STILL being felt today. As Americans desperately tried to stick to the bland, unhealthy low-fat, high-carb lifestyle their doctors insisted was good for them, they grew fatter and fatter and got sicker and sicker.

Dr. Atkins' eating plan changed—and saved—lives. And over the years, the low-carb diet has evolved (or, depending on how you think about it, devolved). The Paleo Diet is the logical next step in low-carb eating, and it's the diet I typically recommend to my own patients.

Today's modern diet is full of processed refined foods, sugar and fats. The Paleo Diet, sometimes called the Caveman Diet, is based on the way our ancestors, early humans, ate. The diet is naturally low carb and low gluten and consists mostly of delicious fresh foods including meat, fish, vegetables, fruits, nuts, seeds and healthy oils. Dairy, grains, refined sugars and oils, potatoes and processed foods are all avoided.

If you suspect that you might have an undiagnosed gluten sensitivity I suggest you give the Paleo Diet a try. You might notice a change almost immediately.

Chapter 3:

Cure this weird digestive disorder and watch years of brain fog vanish

You have brain fog that seems to follow you around all day. You can't seem to think straight or concentrate—you're even slurring your words.

If someone didn't know any better, they'd swear you were drunk.

Well, believe it or not, thanks to an increasingly common digestive disorder, you may be.

Even if you haven't had a drop to drink.

The booze that brews in your gut

A couple years ago, a woman in New York was pulled over with a blood alcohol level that was *five times* the legal limit. Exactly the kind of person we should be throwing the book at, right?

Well, not so fast. She hadn't been drinking.

Believe it or not, this woman had her case thrown out when her lawyers found out she has a condition known as auto brewery syndrome.

If you often suffer from brain fog or a feeling of mental confusion...

like you would if you were drunk...you could have auto brewery syndrome, too.

Yes, that's a real, known medical condition!

If you've got it, so much yeast builds up in your intestines that if you consume any sugar, your body will brew an alcoholic cocktail so strong that it could make you fail a Breathalyzer.

Think about it: How do you make alcohol? You feed sugar to yeast and then wait. And then before you know it...you've got alcohol.

The same thing happens right inside our bodies. In the case of the New York woman, a medical team monitored her blood alcohol level all day. The more she ate, the more it went up—and by 6 p.m. she was a whopping four times the legal limit—*without touching a drop of alcohol!*

Auto brewery syndrome can affect anyone— including you

The most interesting part of the case is that this woman— and other people afflicted with the same issue—are almost always walking, working, raising children, and driving (as scary as that is) as "functional alcoholics." They're just used to having this high level of alcohol in their blood, and they've adapted to it to the point that they can be over four times the legal limit and still appear at least *somewhat* normal.

They certainly don't seem blackout drunk—they just come across as brain fogged, or maybe ditsy, confused, or even depressed.

This overgrowth of yeast can cause a host of other very common symptoms, but the two main areas that are affected are the brain and the gut.

The mental and neurological symptoms, as I noted, can range from brain fog to depression, anxiety, fatigue, and headaches. Excessive yeast and their byproducts of fermentation can also cost a host of gastrointestinal complaints, which include gas, bloating, diarrhea, and irritable bowel syndrome.

When yeast goes wild

There have been some well-documented and proven cases of auto brewery syndrome in scientific literature—including a 2013 case study of a 61-year-old male out of Texas and a 1984 study out of Japan, which was able to replicate the phenomenon in the laboratory in two different individuals.

There also have been a few studies done with children that undoubtedly get "drunk" when they eat too much sugar and carbohydrates—but in their case, it's because of a gut disorder called short bowel (or gut) syndrome.

But, the important lesson from these fascinating cases is that this condition—also known as "gut fermentation syndrome"—is not as _un_-common as you would think.

Brain fog itself is a very common complaint in my office, and many times the patient's "fog" isn't coming from "old age" or that dreaded diagnosis of dementia—but, rather, from an overgrowth of yeast!

Some of my patients will claim that they feel "drunk," and you know what? They're right; they are basically inebriated.

Of course, I'm not routinely doing Breathalyzer testing or blood alcohol levels in my office, but I AM testing patients' stool samples for yeast. I find an overgrowth of it on a routine basis. And what's really cool is when I treat the yeast in their intestines...and poof! The brain fog goes away.

In most of the severe cases, the patients have usually figured out by trial and error that their worst enemy is sugar. Within minutes of eating sugar or a sugar-laden meal, they feel downright poorly and become brain-fogged, tired, and lightheaded.

Most of them have figured out that they can't tolerate large amounts of carbohydrates, as well.

Some patients even come back to be treated again because the symptoms returned after excessive sugar intake...or a round of antibiotics.

Killing off your good gut flora paves the way for fermentation

Aside from carb and sugar addiction, one of the main causes of auto brewery syndrome is taking too many antibiotics, and too often. It's an accumulation of damage from antibiotics over the course of your life-time...since you were a little kid.

Antibiotics kill the good, healthy bacteria in your gut right along with the bad. And when that happens, it's very easy for yeast to grow in the place of the good bacteria...especially in a damp and moist environment such as the intestines.

There's always supposed to be SOME yeast in the mix in your intestines, and most of it is considered "good" yeast. But when antibiotics kill off a fair amount of the good bacteria (and you fail to take probiotics while on the antibiotic), these yeast species will start to grow like wildfire in place of the bacteria.

The analogy that I use in the office is that you want a lot of grass and a few mushrooms on your lawn, but after you take antibiotics, the mushrooms will take over—and that's when problems ensue.

When you are on an antibiotic, you should not swallow the probiotic at the same exact time as the antibiotic, because the antibiotic will kill the probiotic. I have my patients wait two hours after taking the antibiotic to take the probiotic. To make it easy, you could take the probiotic at bedtime, since you must take most antibiotics with meals.

Put your body's microbrewery out of business

Really, anything that disrupts the bowel flora and allows the good bacteria to diminish and the bad "bugs" to flourish can contribute to the alcohol brewing in your body. This includes consuming too much sugar, carbs, and/or alcohol—but also NSAIDs (like ibuprofen and naproxen), coffee, chemotherapy, and even stress—all of which can be avoided or reduced.

The good news is that there are proactive strategies that you can take to start tackling potential auto brewery syndrome or yeast overgrowth. The first step is to eliminate as much as sugar and carbohydrates from your diet as you can. This will at least stop feeding the yeast their fodder! I always recommend the Paleo Diet, which also happens to masquerade as an anti-fungal, anti-yeast diet with very few sugars and carbohydrates.

Then, you can replenish and repopulate the good bacteria in your gut by going on a high quality probiotic.

You also can consider killing some of the excessive yeast with natural germicidal remedies like garlic, oil of oregano, or grapefruit seed extract—but a word of caution: If you start killing the yeast too quickly, you could feel worse before you feel better.

So, if you have undiagnosed mental, neurological, and perhaps gastrointestinal complaints...or if you suspect that you might have this malady of yeast overgrowth...you should seek out a holistic doctor. This condition is so prevalent that almost all holistic doctors are trained and versed in diagnosing and treating the condition.

Chapter 4:

Powerful protein extract fights chronic GI disorders... and you won't believe how much better you'll feel!

I've said it before, and I'll say it again: Your health begins and ends in your gut.

You might not put much thought into it, but your gut is the powerhouse of your body—not only when it comes to digestion, but also mood, weight management, blood sugar control, and even cancer prevention.

And every month that goes by, the medical community learns more and more about the gut lining...how it houses at least 80 percent of your immune system...and how crucial its balance of flora is to almost every disease.

One of the most powerful investments you can make in your health is EnteraGam, a medical food that's got the power to repair damage to your gut AND fight off infections.

Fighting off infections from moment one

I'm a big fan of medical foods. They're the perfect bridge between the holistic medical world and the conventional medical world. Instead of "band-aiding" them, medical foods actually HEAL diseases—without drugs or dangerous chemicals that merely mask symptoms.

And, yes, they're "food," but their healing powers can take hold in very powerful and potent versions—so much so that they require a prescription from a doctor.

EnteraGam is basically a very powerful and concentrated version of something called "colostrum," which is a special form of milk that comes from mammals' mammary glands in the first few days after giving birth. It can be found in the form of human breastmilk as well as the milk of farm animals like horses, sheep, pigs, and cows.

Colostrum is often referred to as "liquid gold" because of its yellowish color...and its amazing healing properties. It's high in antibodies, which helps protect newborns from disease before their own immune system develops.

Colostrum has a long history of use in the holistic medical world, having been used for *thousands* of years in India to treat a varied array of medical issues. Colostrum was one of the only ways we had to kill infections before antibiotics!

In fact, Albert Sabin made his first oral polio vaccine using colostrum from cows because it had polio immunoglobulins in it. In the 1950's, colostrum was also used to treat rheumatoid arthritis.

Despite these historical references...and its anecdotal uses which vary from immune support, gut support, and weight loss, to allergies and even autoimmune support...the regular medical establishment still isn't convinced.

In the 1980s, when studies showed that colostrum doesn't pass through the gut lining of adults,[1] the mainstream medical community immediately dismissed it. They argued that if colostrum just stays in your intestines, taking it would be a waste of time.

Well, in my opinion, that's a GREAT thing! The more "liquid gold" that stays in the gut lining, the better—because THAT'S where the healing occurs. And when the gut lining is healed, the reverberations to the rest of your health are easily ten times the power of absorbing some of it into in your bloodstream!

What's leaking into your bloodstream?

The specific diseases that medical studies have shown EnteraGam to help include HIV-associated enteropathy, pediatric malnutrition, Irritable Bowel Syndrome with diarrhea (which affects close to 10 percent of the population), and Inflammatory Bowel Disease (which includes ulcerative colitis and Crohn's disease).2

IBD is actually one of the most vicious forms of a conditions that's been coined "leaky gut syndrome," or, more officially, "increased intestinal permeability."

Even that name doesn't tell the whole story...because in addition to small "holes" in the gut lining, this condition is also associated with a disrupted gut flora—both of which can be caused by a host of issues, most commonly: NSAID's (like ibuprofen), stress, coffee, alcohol, sugar, poor diet, antibiotics, and chemotherapy.

Not surprisingly, these are also the factors that can throw your ratio of good-to-bad bacteria out of whack—and that imbalance is what causes the excess permeability of the gut lining.[3]

Those "holes" in the gut allow unwanted pathogens to enter the bloodstream... which is why evidence supporting the infectious component of IBD and IBS-D continues to mount,[4] and why colostrum can be such a powerful healing agent for these conditions.[5]

And if your gut lining has taken on the appearance of cheesecloth, you can bet that you won't be able to absorb nutrients from the foods you eat and even the supplements you take.

The cumulative negative effects of the disrupted flora and poor absorption can wreak havoc throughout the entire body.

The gap in your health may be a hole in your gut

EnteraGam contains two types of immunoglobulins—one that addresses each of these issues. The first (type A) can "seal" an adult's damaged and inflamed gut lining, especially one that is "leaky," just like it helps seal the intestines of a newborn baby. The second (type G) binds and neutralizes the "bad" gut bugs to ward off infections.

This medical food version of colostrum is an amazing advancement because it finally gives me the power that I have been looking for to "plug the holes" in my patients' guts as well as improve their immune systems.

As a holistic doctor of many years, I know that fixing a "leaky gut" can aid in the healing of almost any disease. I think that almost every patient who comes to my office with a chronic health condition has some form of enteropathy...and I'm pleased to say that I've been seeing really exciting results with EnteraGam. It's literally one of the best and most powerful gut products that I have ever used.

EnteraGam comes in the form of a powder that you can take with or without food. Most patients find it easiest to stir it into a glass of water.

The process that extracts the immunoglobulins from the colostrum eliminates all of the actual "dairy," which makes it a game-changer for anyone who can't tolerate "dairy" colostrum because of the casein, whey, or lactose.

It's also gluten-free, but since it's been formulated from proteins extracted from the colostrum of cows, it's technically an animal product and wouldn't be suitable for anyone with a beef allergy.

If you'd like to learn more about this breakthrough medical food, visit www.EnteraGam.com and ask your doc about it. The FDA has recognized it as effective and safe, so he should be willing to prescribe it for you if you've been diagnosed with enteropathy (basically any disease that involves the intestines, especially the small intestine).

If all else fails, you can get an over-the-counter version of colostrum in powder, capsule, and even chewable forms at your local health food store. Although these products won't have as much muscle as the prescription-strength medical food version, they're still well worth the investment.

Chapter 5:

Indigestion... Colitis... IBS... Can this ONE "super probiotic" tackle them all?

B eing a doctor comes with its share of tough decisions.

But deciding whether or not to recommend probiotics—those healthy "gut bugs"—for my patients isn't one of them.

Because, sick or not, my patients DO need them—and so do YOU.

Working on your intestines and "gut" will give you the biggest bang for your buck in terms of your overall health.

In fact, when you improve the state of your intestinal gut lining, the health benefits reverberate through your whole body... MANY times over.

When I started practicing many years ago, we doctors felt that we were giving *plenty* of probiotics if we could get 5 to 10 billion live cultures in a supplement. And although that level of probiotic dosage did help patients, the holistic medical community has upped the ante over the years.

These days, a good probiotic at a health food store can have between 10 and 100 billion live cultures.

But now, I've found a new gem in the probiotic world that's up to 100 times MORE potent than the average probiotic.[1]

It's called VSL#3, and its "Double Strength" version (VSL#3-DS) has *900 billion* live cultures! More specifically, it contains eight different strains of live bacteria in very large quantities, including three species of *Bifidobacterium*, four species of *Lactobacillus*, and one species of *Streptococcus*.

It takes the prize for the most potent probiotic that you can find. In fact, it's so powerful that, like the other "medical foods" I've shared with you in the past few issues, you need a prescription from a doctor in order to get it.

And that prescription is well worth getting. Because when I started prescribing VSL#3-DS for issues like Irritable Bowel Syndrome (IBS)—as well as many other gut complaints—they became much easier to treat.

In fact, my patients often beg me for refills.

Taking care of the "good guys"

There are ten times more naturally-occurring "good" bacteria in your gut lining than there are other cells in *the rest of your body*.

It's almost unfathomable! All of your good gut bacteria together weighs more than your brain.

That is, of course, under ideal circumstances. If you want to stay healthy, your main goal should always be to keep as many "good guys" in your gut as you can... and limit the number of "bad guys."

But sometimes, something can happen to throw off that balance and diminish the level of the "good guys" in your gut—and usually, you can blame antibiotics for it.

Even just the word "antibiotic" tells you exactly what it does—it's "against life" (*biosis*). Antibiotics kill ALL life in the gut lining, including the good AND the bad bacteria.

Unfortunately, when everything starts to grow back, the bad bacteria will often flourish unless you restore that optimal balance between good and bad bacteria.

And the best way to do that is by replacing the probiotics—those "good" bacteria that are *for* ("pro") life.

There are 400 species of probiotics—that we currently know of—that work in so many different ways. If you watch any TV, you now know that probiotics can support regular bowel movements and prevent constipation (thank you, Jamie Lee Curtis!). They can even decrease lactose intolerance and improve how you digest other foods, too.

And because probiotics can influence your mood and food cravings, they can help control your weight... and actually *improve your ability to lose weight*!

Probiotics make essential fatty acids—as well as vitamins A, K, and B vitamins—and they've got a strong influence on your immune system. In fact, they actually produce antibiotic chemicals—and, therefore, they can kill infection-causing bacteria naturally.

They can even fight off viral infections... and cancer![2]

You've got a lot of territory to cover in your gut

Some cultures around the world have been using probiotics for centuries, often in the form of fermented foods like kefir, natto, lassi, miso, tempeh, sauerkraut, and kimchi. But the most obvious source to Americans like us is yogurt.

You can pick up any yogurt and see on the side of the container that it "contains live cultures"—and *those* are the probiotics!

Although the probiotic counts in foods are hard to calculate accurately, a good guesstimate is that you're likely to get about a billion colonies from a serving of sauerkraut and 10 to 20 billion colonies from a cup of plain yogurt.

So food sources are a good way to get probiotics, but they're not GREAT—and you can do better.

The 900 billion colonies in VSL#3 may sound like a TON of good guys, but in no way is it too many... especially if you're suffering from one of the many serious gut illnesses.

Considering the fact that your small intestine is about 24 feet long and your colon is about five feet long, you need as many colonies as you can get.

Bottom line: You'll feel better fast

Over 100 medical studies show the effectiveness of VSL#3-DS in the treatment of ulcerative colitis and IBS.[3]

In a 2012 study out of Korea[4] and a 2010 study out of Italy,[5] VSL#3 improved the symptoms of patients with mild to moderate ulcerative colitis—both in just eight weeks. It's even been shown to safely increase the remission rate in CHILDREN with mild to moderate ulcerative colitis![6,7]

A 2010 NIH-funded study also showed that VSL#3 improved symptoms in patients with IBS-D, also after just eight weeks of treatment.[8]

What's more, many of these studies—including in a 2003 study from the Mayo Clinic[9]—have shown that this potent probiotic is well-tolerated by patients of all ages without adverse effects or risk of overdose.

The FDA has even given it the "Generally Recognized As Safe" (GRAS) designation in treating ulcerative colitis as well as irritable bowel syndrome.[10] Ulcerative colitis is a very serious medical disease of the colon, so I'm impressed that even the FDA recognizes that you can treat this condition with a high-powered probiotic!

We've still got a long way to go to convince them of how amazing nutritional remedies are to heal MOST medical issues... but this is a start.

Superior potency, even from the lowest dosage

It is possible your doc won't want to prescribe the Double Strength version of VSL#3 for your gastrointestinal issues, so fortunately there are three other "single strength" versions that you can purchase on your own at www.vsl3.com or your local pharmacy.

Your choices are either packets of flavored and unflavored versions, with 450 billion bacteria each, that can be mixed into cold or room temperature beverages or soft foods, or vegetarian capsules that contain 112.5 billion each.

You can start with as little as one single-strength packet or two capsules a day... and that might be enough to make you feel better after a week or so. If not, you can try gradually increasing, up to eight capsules or single-strength packets a day. It's better to start low and move your way up, since it can take three weeks to really make a change in your gut flora. If you start too high or increase the dose too quickly, you may experience mild belly bloat.

Of course, take the prescription-only Double Strength version as directed by your doctor.

My goal is to introduce you to cutting-edge therapies that I'm using in my own practice—but that doesn't mean that you won't benefit from other probiotics. In fact, my experience with VSL#3-DS has made me even more diligent about having my patients continue their probiotics, whether it is VSL#3 or not.

So, please keep on eating yogurt, sauerkraut, or kimchi... drinking kombucha... and taking an over-the-counter probiotic supplement.

It's especially important to take probiotics while you are on antibiotics—as long as you do it correctly. I recommend that my patients stagger the dosages and take the probiotics either in the late afternoon or bedtime, since most antibiotics are taken with meals.

If you take the probiotics *at the same time* as you take the antibiotic, the antibiotic will just kill the probiotic, like it does everything else in your gut!

PART VIII

Immune System and Autoimmune Diseases

Chapter 1:

Six simple steps to make your body "flu-proof"—no shot required!

Believe it or not, flu season starts up again soon. And that's when our government will start trying to sell all of us one of the biggest lemons on the lot.

After all, would you buy a car from me that only started once out of every five times you turned the key? Of course not! And yet this past year's flu shot was just such a car.

By the CDC's own estimates, the 2014-2015 flu shot only worked 1 out of 5 times! In the end the vaccine was only effective in a dismal 19 percent of the cases. And although the numbers vary from year to year, this is by no means an isolated incident. In fact, in the 2003-2004 flu season the results were even worse.

It's important to understand why our government's vaccine continues to fail us—and the six simple things you can do to stay healthy this season. No shot necessary.

Blind guessing can lead to big failures

Why are these statistics so low for a drug that conventional medicine feels so strongly about? First, influenza viruses are notoriously hard to replicate. There are many strains of the virus, and the flu vaccine manufacturers, in cahoots with government scientists, have to quite literally guess which strains will appear in a given year.

That's right, the contents of each year's flu vaccine is actually nothing more than a crap shoot. In some years, the major strains of influenza virus were missed entirely, leading to a situation in which millions of vaccines were given without any positive effect, even though there's some evidence that the CDC knew ahead of time that they were guessing wrong.

Mutations mean even correct flu shots can still fail

But bad or good guesses aren't the end of the story. Even if the strains are guessed right, the vaccine can lose effectiveness due to something called antigenic drift. The virus itself can mutate as it goes through the population. It remains the same virus, but looks different enough so that our immune systems don't recognize it as the same virus that was contained in the flu shot.

This is what happened when the H3N2 strain was the prevailing influenza virus strain causing the flu, but was altered enough so that the flu shot was ineffective. And this antigenic drift isn't always a natural phenomenon either. In 2012-2013, in the process of creating the vaccine the drug manufacturers actually introduced mutations of the H3N2 virus into the vaccine.

And then there's the problem of actually evaluating the vaccine's ability to do the job. When my patients get sick during the winter months, they tend to report it as "the flu." This is despite the fact that the most common flu symptoms are fever, muscle ache and (sometimes) a cough. On the other hand a stuffy or runny nose, bronchitis symptoms, stomach aches or sinus issues are far less likely to be influenza, and more likely to be triggered by a different virus or bacteria. And, of course, the flu tends to be more severe and last longer. By one FDA estimate, only 20 percent of so-called cases of "flu" actually turn out to be the influenza virus.

Follow the money

Up until a few years ago, annual flu shots were generally only recommended for the elderly, people with severe respiratory illnesses and children. But then, with zero hard evidence that the vaccine had more widespread applications, the recommendations were suddenly extended by the CDC. Now, the flu shot is recommended for everyone, and we are pummeled by ads trying to shame us into rolling up our sleeves for it every time we turn on the TV or go to a grocery store, pharmacy or doctor's office.

So why are we being harassed to get the shot for months on end? Well, to paraphrase the bank robber Willie Sutton: it's where the money is. Producing a different flu vaccine every year is expensive and the pharmaceutical companies are hard-pressed to make the profit they want if only those people who truly may need the shot get it. So they started calling in favors in DC, and have been heavily lobbying Congress for years to expand the flu shot mandate. And it worked. Their profits have ballooned into the tens of billions of dollars, and there's no end in sight.

At the same time, another factor is at work. Doctors are trained to believe that vaccinations are ALWAYS good medicine, and that even includes dubious ones like the flu shot. And most of them simply choose to ignore serious issues like occasional neurological problems linked to the vaccine; questions about the dangers of contamination and preservatives used in the shot; and whether our immune systems may be overstimulated by the sheer volume of vaccinations we're receiving these days.

Six steps to foil the flu

Getting a flu shot is, of course, a personal decision. But if you do decide to not get one this year that doesn't mean you need to remain unprotected. The flu can be a serious illness in some people, and even life-threatening to those at the highest risk. So it's important to take measures to avoid catching the bug. And I have six drug-free steps that can help you stay flu-free this season.

Foil the flu step #1: The flu virus is a "droplet" virus, meaning it spreads in droplets when people cough and sneeze, or from exposure to nasal discharge followed by touching the mouth or nose. To combat this you should wash your hands well and frequently. You may even want to consider wearing a mask if you're going to be in a situation where you might be exposed. (And if you get sick you can help stop the spread by always covering your mouth or nose when sneezing or coughing.)

Foil the flu step #2: Watch that sweet tooth. Sugar found in sodas, desserts, ice cream and many processed foods is a well-researched immune suppressor.

Foil the flu step #3: Get plenty of sleep, at least eight hours a night. Sleep is a great immune booster, and can help keep you from getting sick even if you're exposed to the virus.

Foil the flu step #4: Make sure you're getting enough daily zinc. Try a zinc supplement. I typically recommend 25-50 mg a day of zinc citrate, picolinate or other chelated form.

Foil the flu step #5: Stay hydrated by drinking plenty of water. Moist mucous membranes are powerful barriers against viruses and other infections.

Foil the flu step #6: Try homeopathy. Certain homeopathic remedies are designed to be taken at the first sign of the flu. Occilococcinum, the most well-known of these, is as safe as a remedy gets. We use influezinum in our office, and homeopathic formulas like these have been shown in studies to modify the symptoms of infections such as influenza.

Chapter 2:

Everyday exposure to hidden parasites could be making you sick

They're the kind of symptoms nobody ever wants to talk about; gas, bloating, abdominal pain, constipation, diarrhea and rectal itching. Embarrassment keeps a lot of people from ever going to see the doctor about them.

And far too many folks that do build up the courage to make an appointment get handed the catch-all waste-basket diagnosis of irritable bowel syndrome (IBS) for their troubles. The next thing you know, you're put on powerful drugs or restrictive diets that don't do a thing to help your symptoms.

If this sounds like you—and you've battled for years to get your stomach problems under control—the real cause of your troubles may shock you.

Because, believe it or not, many so-called IBS patients are actually infected with hidden parasites. And, these ugly intestinal bugs and worms are far more common than most people think.

And even if you're NOT suffering from any gastrointestinal woes, don't think you're out of the woods yet. Although intestinal parasites can be behind just about any type of tummy trouble you can think of, their reign of terror could extend far beyond the GI tract leading to joint pain, headaches, fatigue, skin issues and even emotional and psychiatric symptoms.

Have you been exposed?!

When most people hear the word parasite they think of South America or Africa. But the truth is you don't have to travel anywhere exotic to be exposed to many of these ugly bugs. As I mentioned earlier, parasites are actually far more prevalent than most people think. And it's really quite common to pick them up right here at home.

The list of common potential parasite culprits may even shock you…

- Pets—"kissing" your beloved dog or cat
- Raw seafood—eating sushi and raw crustaceans
- Uncooked meat—meats served rare or medium rare bring a higher risk
- Water—drinking unfiltered water
- Hygiene—poor toilet habits
- Vegetables—eating certain unwashed vegetables (salad bars at restaurants)

Once you're infected it's relatively easy to infect other people, which can put your entire family at risk. Some parasites lay hundreds—possibly thousands—of eggs a day when they're active, meaning that if left untreated your entire system could eventually be infested with these bugs. And an infestation that lasts for months or even years can become increasingly difficult to fully resolve.

4 common testing flaws

The popular press has most Americans believing that if you're infected with a parasite you have to look as if you're wasting away and literally have—and please pardon the visual—worms coming out of your rectum.

The reality is that's FAR from the truth. But to make matters worse the so-called professionals often don't have a much better grasp on diagnosing parasites than the public does, which is why so many patients are misdiagnosed (usually with IBS) and miserable.

There are four major flaws to the testing methods that conventional doctors typically use that have led to a lot of frustrated and miserable patients:

Flaw #1: Parasites live in life cycles and if you're not collecting a stool sample at the time of the month that the parasites are "active" then the testing is really a waste of time. The trouble is it's hard to predict when the parasites will hatch. This leads to patients who are actually infected being cleared for parasites.

Flaw #2: Parasite eggs will perish when they're exposed to air for more than a few hours. Yet there are no preservatives used in the stool specimen containers that most laboratories use. By the time a pathologist is able to review a specimen it's often long past that short window of time; meaning, of course, that the parasites will be missed by the very test that was designed to find them.

Flaw #3: Many doctors fall for the colonoscopy myth. They believe that they will be able to see a parasite with a colonoscopy. In my almost 35 years on the job I have NEVER seen a colonoscopy reveal a parasite. And there are several good reasons for that.

First, the clean-out process for the colonoscopy is very thorough (if you've had one you know what I mean) and it wipes out any obvious parasites. Even more important, is the fact that parasites actually live INSIDE the colonic wall which will not be seen with the camera.

But the most obvious reason colonoscopies don't work is that many of these parasites live in the small intestine not the large intestine that's viewed in a colonoscopy. The small intestine, which makes up about twenty feet of the gastrointestinal system, is basically unchartered territory where these critters can hide.

Flaw #4: There are many different species of parasites and our current testing simply isn't designed to search for all of them… or even most of them for that matter. Parasites can range from microscopic ameba to large tapeworms. And some don't even live in the intestinal tract—such as a flukes that set up shop in your liver instead.

It's NOT all inside your head

These flaws leave doctors with the false impression that parasitic infections are rare. Even worse, unless a patient has been to a Third World country, or is rapidly losing weight, many doctors simply don't order tests for parasites any more.

They'll just diagnose you with IBS—and if you keep insisting you may have parasites, they may call you crazy. There's even a medical term for it—delusional parasitosis.

But I've had countless patients who had been told they're "crazy," but had their gastrointestinal symptoms clear right up when I treated them for parasites. And I've also treated patients who were told that their gastrointestinal problems were from IBS or stress, who then went on to pass handfuls of worms during my treatment for their parasites!

If you're suffering with mysterious symptoms and not getting anywhere with traditional mainstream medicine, you could very well be suffering from a hidden parasite infection. A holistic doctor should be able to help, or you can try tackling them on your own at home first.

Knock out parasites

If you suspect you have parasites I've got good news. You don't just have to live with them and you don't have to resort to heavy duty drugs to kick them. There are some safe, natural, and proven methods for ridding your body of these bugs.

Food: Let's start with diet. Certain foods could help you rid yourself of these ugly bugs. Raw garlic, carrots, beets, coconut, honey, pumpkin seeds, papaya seeds, cloves and pomegranate have all been traditionally used to kill parasites.

"Sesame seed" stool

Parasites are tough to diagnose. There's seldom any visual evidence to tip you off. However, if you see something that looks like a sesame seed in your stool on a fairly frequent basis, there's a good chance that what you're actually seeing are the eggs of a parasite.

Tips to avoid parasites

Despite what you may have heard, you don't have to do anything exotic to get parasites. In fact, you're being exposed to these hidden ugly bugs every day. But there are some simple things you can do to avoid being infected.

- Cook meats completely and avoid eating raw fish, beef or pork

- Wash all fruits and veggies carefully (even those so-called "pre-washed" ones!)

- Avoid too many simple carbs like those found in processed and refined foods

- Drink only properly filtered water

- Wash your hands frequently and leave your shoes at the front door

- Keep your home mold and bug free (call in experts if you need too)

- Deworm your pets regularly, keep them off the furniture and glove and mask to clean up after them

- Take a quality probiotic from a maker you trust

In one study, published in the Journal of Medical Food, researchers found that a mixture of papaya seeds and honey was a remarkably effective method for killing off parasites. Sixty children with confirmed intestinal parasites were given either a papaya seed and honey mixture or honey alone for seven days and then follow up stool samples were taken.

The samples from 23 of 30 of the children who received the mixture instead of just honey alone were found to be anywhere from 71.4 percent to 100 percent clear of all parasites! Though less effective, the honey alone did manage to clear 5 of the 30 children of parasites as well. And, of course, there weren't any significant side effects from either treatment.

You can try blending fresh papaya, including about a tablespoon of the seeds, into a parasite killing smoothie. (There are also papaya powders on the market if you find that the seeds are a bit too bitter.) Raw pumpkin seeds, shredded coconut, coconut water and a dash of coconut oil and honey all make good parasite-fighting additions. Toss in a little fresh pineapple while you're at it and you'll also get a dosage of healthy digestive enzymes.

Also be sure to eat plenty of fiber rich foods and drink plenty of filtered water, both of which can help flush parasites from your system.

Supplements: Try a good probiotic from a maker you trust to help keep your digestive tract healthy and in top working order. Vitamin C and zinc are both excellent for overall immune system support.

Herbs: There are a number of herbs that have been traditionally used to tackle parasites including black walnut, garlic, goldenseal, barberry, anise, and wormwood.

Don't forget to check with your doctor to make sure that none of these supplements or herbs will interfere with any meds you're currently taking.

Chapter 3:

Stunning research reveals gut bug balance causing everything from diabetes to colon cancer!

There an old adage among holistic docs that says health begins and ends in the gut.

Unfortunately, most of our mainstream colleagues have been a little slow to catch on. When most docs talk about gut bacteria or probiotics, they focus on how they affect digestion and even your bowel movements.

But we're learning fast that there's a whole lot more at stake than an upset tummy. Research is proving that maintaining a healthy balance of gut bugs (I'll show you how in a moment) can help you beat everything from diabetes to depression.

In fact, gut bacteria may even hold the key to beating one of the deadliest cancers around.

Is bad bacteria giving you colon cancer?

A recent study, published in the journal Genome Medicine, found that keeping enough healthy bacteria in your gut may be a powerful secret to preventing colon cancer.

Researchers analyzed the gut bugs in colon cancer patients and found they were far different than those of their cancer-free peers. Those volunteers with cancer had many more bacteria in their stool, including pathogenic—or potentially disease-causing—bugs than the healthy volunteers.

But even more telling was the fact that one of the bacteria the researchers found in greater quantity, Providencia, has been proven to damage the lining of the intestine.

It appears that infections caused by bad gut bugs like Providencia slowly damage the lining of the colon over the years. This damage eventually causes the healthy cells to turn into cancerous ones.

This groundbreaking theory not only provides us with a much greater understanding of how and why colon cancer occurs, it also provides us with a potential path to conquering this formidable foe once and for all. Some simple short- and long-term changes to our diet and supplement regimen could be all it takes to get the upper hand over these bad bacteria.

I'll have more on those changes in just a moment, but first let's take a closer look at what else we know about the connection between belly bugs and our overall health.

Could bacteria in your belly make you fat?

This cause-and-effect connection between gut microbes and cancer isn't as farfetched as it may seem at first glance. In the last decade we've seen a seismic shift in the way we view gut bacteria. Although we're really just beginning to understand the connection between our gut flora and disease, studies from the last several years have already linked the bacteria in our guts to inflammation, diabetes, mood, obesity and more.

In fact, two recent studies found that our gut flora may be at least partially responsible for whether we're overweight or normal weight.

The studies found that obesity is tied to a form of bacteria in the gut called Firmicutes. Obese patients had about 20 percent more of the Firmicutes bacteria on board. While another bacterium, Bacteroidetes, was clearly associated with normal weight, with the obese patients having a shocking 90 percent less of the bugs.

However, when the obese patients lost weight the bacterial balance in their intestines shifted. Suddenly the thinned down patients had less of the fat producing Firmicutes in their guts and far more of the Bacteroidetes bacteria. Even more incredibly, when the obesity-linked Firmicutes species was implanted into "skinny" mice they actually gained twice as much fat as a control group of mice. It turns out the Firmicutes bacteria are apparently far more efficient at extracting calories out of food and depositing them in fat.

Belly bug balance linked to diabetes risk

In another study out of China in 2012 researchers revealed the link between the balance of bacteria in the gut and diabetes. Scientists looked at more than 60,000 markers associated with type-2 diabetes and found that people with the disease had an overabundance of bad bacteria and a lack of the helpful bugs in their guts.

And of course antibiotics, which use a scatter approach that kills off both good and bad gut bacteria, are associated with insulin resistance and diabetes. In fact, one recent study found that the more often you take the drugs the higher your risk of the disease rises. Downing an antibiotic just five times within 15 years can cause your diabetes risk to skyrocket by 50 percent compared to someone who took the drug just a single time or never.

Probiotics blow away anxiety

UCLA researchers have even found a link between gut bugs and how we think and feel. Within just four weeks of taking a probiotic supplement there were measurable changes in the brains of women who took them.

The areas of their brain that effect cognition and emotion and sensory stimuli were all affected, according to the study published in the journal

Gastroenterology. In the real world that means that the probiotics could help improve mood, reduce anxiety and perhaps even relieve depression. In fact the women in the study were subjected to tests designed to make them feel uncomfortable and those who received the probiotics were measurably less anxious than their peers.

Putting probiotics into action

So how do you keep yourself healthy and maintain your balance of gut bugs? Here are some simple things you can try:

1. Start with a quality probiotic supplement from a maker you trust. Look for one that contains several different strains of bacteria.

2. Limit the amount of sugar and processed foods you eat. They provide fuel for bad gut bugs. I recommend the Paleo Diet which focuses on the meats, vegetables, nuts and other natural foods that our ancestors would have eaten.

3. Next, beef up the number of fermented foods in your diet which will naturally help raise your good gut bug levels. Some good ones to try are non-sugar sweetened yogurts and kefir. In general you should limit the amount of dairy you eat, but dairy that's been fermented long enough to eat up the majority of lactose in it, in moderation, is fine.

You can also try homemade "pickled" fruits and vegetables such as sauerkraut, dilled cucumbers and gingered carrots (there are lots or recipes online, search for "homemade fermented foods").

4. Work with a holistic doctor to test your gut flora and to get advice on achieving an optional gut bug balance.

Stick to this simple plan and before you know it your gut will be the picture of perfect health—and so will the rest of you.

Chapter 4:

Fight infections... eliminate toxins... and stop disease with your body's "secret system"

You might be inclined to think that flushing the toxins and waste out of your body is what happens when you go to the bathroom.

But the entire process doesn't start with the toilet—it actually ENDS there.

No, where it *starts* is at the cellular level... when toxins and infectious agents move out of cells and into something called "lymphatic fluid."

That fluid is your body's wastewater, and it gets circulated away from your vital organs and "locked up" to be dealt with later.

To be honest, I'm not sure if most people even know that there's a "system" of lymphatics inside our bodies—it's a great secret to many. There's a common misunderstanding that the lymph nodes are just stand-alone "glands" in the body that get swollen when you get a sore throat.

But the lymphatic system is of far greater import, with far-reaching effects throughout your body!

Because if that stuff doesn't get picked up and moved out of the cells, it opens the door for disease to come walking right in.

Thus, keeping the lymph moving on a daily basis is crucial to a healthy body for many potential reasons—including immune support, infection control, as well as toxin removal.

Send your disease risk down the drain

I believe that all diseases are, in some way, caused by toxins and infections—and so I've learned to have an incredible respect for the lymphatic system, which can make sure these toxins are efficiently excreted and infections are efficiently killed.

The lymphatic system is the body's drainage system. It's responsible for taking the "excess" fluid that's generated every day from the organs all over the body (even including the 30 feet of the intestines) and forcing it out.

This is your body's *true* waste removal mechanism—not the final stage of "evacuation" that you're probably far more familiar with.

The lymph system plays an integral role in contributing to a free-flowing and flawless working immune system. It involves a ragtag team of organs, including the spleen, thymus, tonsils, adenoids, and parts of the gut.

These organs aid in the process of providing ammunition and protection from the infections that are found in the excess fluid, by signaling a "call to arms" in the form of white blood cell soldiers called LYMPHocytes.

Lymphocytes are transported through the bloodstream to help whichever area of the body is overwhelmed with infection. They have an easier time destroying these harmful organisms once they're trapped in the 500 to 600 lymph nodes in the body—which is why they swell up when you're battling an infection.

If you could imagine what this system might be like, it would resemble the underground pipes of our homes and cities. The human body has set up check points along the way to slow down, analyze, and process certain crucial elements of these "excess fluids" (that is, infections or cancer cells).

These small check points are the lymph nodes; and if there's too much infection to process, they'll swell for a period of time—and that's when you finally notice it.

But don't let your drain get clogged

When things are bad with your lymph, they're *very bad*.

There are a ton of consequences and symptoms of sluggish lymph that can range from fatigue, swelling, weight gain, weak immune system (repeated infections/colds/flus), joint pain, nausea, breast swelling or tenderness, and an overall feeling of un-wellness (toxicity).

It's obvious when the lymph in the head and neck is overwhelmed, because the lymph nodes in the neck and throat area get swollen. But the scary part is that you could have *slightly* swollen lymph glands in your arm pits, groin, or even your stomach... and never feel them.

But you don't have to wait till the waste has built all the way up and your glands are "swollen"—because just like a lot of things with the human body, glands swell when the worst situations are occurring, like an infection or cancer.

And if the lymphatic system is *already* overwhelmed or sluggish, it makes my job of killing infections and dredging the body of "gunk" (toxins) almost impossible to do without side effects.

Move around, or the waste won't move out

As with most processes in the human body, an ounce of prevention is worth a pound of cure. That's why it's so important to have a clean and freely flowing lymphatic system.

And I've learned that giving this system even just *a little attention* will go a long way in preventing and treating disease, as well as promoting wellness.

It's important to note that the lymphatic system does not an official engine or "pump," the way your heart moves blood throughout your body.

Instead, the lymphatic system's movement and flow is dependent upon motion and movements that are only under your control—like walking, exercise and deep breathing.

Actively moving lymph is of paramount importance, because things are much more likely to get backed up if you lead a sedentary life. But all it takes is getting your body moving for at least 20 minutes of exercise, a few times a week.

Here are some other simple things that you can do to ensure a clean lymphatic system:

Rebounding: You can buy a cheap mini trampoline and lightly bounce up and down a few times a week. This is one of my favorites, because it can work wonders to efficiently move lymph and blood while sparing your joints the pounding on the pavement.

Sweating: Removing toxins by sweating will give the lymph a break. Some people use sauna therapy to get the body to perspire, but working up a sweat by exercising will kill two birds with one stone.

Deep breathing: Just taking long, slow deep breaths through your nose, holding your breath for a second or two, and then slowly releasing the air through slightly pursed lips can force the lungs and muscles of the chest to move the lymph in the entire chest area.

Contrast showers: You can force fluid shifts in the body by taking a hot shower for a few minutes, abruptly changing the water temperature to cold for few minutes, and then alternating back and forth a few times.

Lymphatic massage: Some massage therapists specialize in moving the lymph in the whole body by gently massaging over and with the flow of lymph in the body. After a mastectomy, for example, lymph can build up in the arm of the breast that was operated on, which can cause infection. LDM can help relieve the discomfort in breast cancer patients, and it can help other areas or other health issues as well.

Herbal supplements: My two favorite secret weapons for lymphatic flow come from a company in Florida called Nutramedix. You can find their liquid products Pinella and Burbur, which are both great lymphatic "movers," at www.nutramedix.com.

Really, *anything* that speeds the lymphatic drainage process up—or eases it—is a positive momentum builder for your system.

One of the most intriguing contributors to the lymphatic system is the fact that the gut contributes its own huge load to the drainage system, with a special kind of lymph called "chyle."

In fact, the lymphatic system of the gut it is so special, important, and unique is that it has its own name: the GALT (Gut Associated Lymphatic Tissue).

What you eat... how you digest... and the balance of your good versus bad gut "bugs" are all huge contributors to the lymphatic system and to "freeing" your lymphatic "flow."

Finally, make sure that your immune system is strong, and decrease the toxic load in your body, liver, and colon so good health can prevail.

Chapter 5:

5 ways to make sure you've had your last bout with the common cold— And 3 cures you never knew could work so well

If you, your children, or grandchildren never get colds or the 'flu, then you can safely skip this chapter. Still reading? I thought so. But there's a lot you can do keep yourself and your family from catching those occasional—or not so occasional—colds. In fact, there's a good chance that if you follow the steps I'm going to outline you may have had your last bout with these all-too-common nuisances.

And if you do come down with one at some point, there are several research-proven things to do to make colds go away a lot more quickly. Some of them, like vitamin C and zinc lozenges, are things you've likely heard of and probably even tried at some point or another. Whether or not they were effective, though, depends on some important details.

But before we get into the details that will help make those old standbys work as effectively as they should, let's talk about how you can keep from needing them in the first place.

Give your white blood cells a (germ) fighting chance

The first step in beating cold and flu season once and for all is the same first step for preventing many illnesses—get rid of the sugar!

Decades ago, Professor Emanuel Cheraskin and his colleagues demonstrated that refined sugar significantly impairs the ability of white blood cells to fight germs. To reach this conclusion Professor Cheraskin drew blood samples from research volunteers, and then observed under a microscope how many germs the average white blood cell could destroy per minute. One hour after each volunteer swallowed approximately 1 teaspoonful of refined sugar, his or her white blood cells could only destroy half as many germs as before. And the white blood cells didn't recover their full "germ-eating" capability until four to five hours later.

So as Professor Cheraskin observed at subsequent lectures, if an individual ate a sweet roll or doughnut for breakfast (or even just sweetened his or her coffee or tea with sugar), then had a soft drink or candy bar at lunch, ate a piece of pie or other sugared dessert at dinner, and perhaps had some ice cream before bedtime, the only time he or she should ever expose him or herself to germs should be between 2 AM and breakfast time. Otherwise the likelihood of catching an infection would be significantly greater since the person's white blood cells would be impaired from sugar all day long.

Granted, the "germs" Professor Cheraskin's team observed were bacteria, not "common cold" viruses. But it's been my experience in over many years of practice that eliminating refined sugar (as well as refined carbohydrates) is absolutely necessary to minimize or eliminate colds.

Uncovering and eliminating (or desensitizing) allergies is a close second to eliminating sugar when it comes to cold prevention. Many family health practitioners have seen this in children with recurring colds, sore throats, ear infections, bronchitis, and 'flu. If the recurring infection hadn't subsided after the parents got rid of all the refined sugar in the child's diet, they would then check the kids for allergies, particularly food allergies. Every single one of these children had significant food allergies, and if the offending foods were eliminated (or in the long run, desensitized), the recurrent colds and infections always vanished (or nearly so, except perhaps for the very infrequent case of sniffles).

The same strategy applies with adults, although in general adults have a greater proportion of inhalant allergies than children, which can only be dealt with by total removal from the environment, or desensitization.

Build your body's store of "natural human antibiotics"

Taking care of sugar and allergies will give your immune system a solid foundation for fighting all kinds of infections, including colds and the flu. But there are also a few supplements that can support your efforts even further.

Some of the most exciting recent vitamin D research has demonstrated its ability to prevent viral and other infections by stimulating the production of "natural human antibiotics" in your body. (For the best discussion of recent vitamin D research available anywhere, see www.vitamindcouncil.com.)

For adults, I recommend 3,000 to 4,000 IU of vitamin D daily, for children, from 1,000 to 3,000 IU, depending on size. (It's certainly best to check with a physician skilled and knowledgeable in natural and nutritional medicine for recommendations for children.)

Many people still believe that long-term use of Echinacea can have adverse effects. The truth is that there is solid evidence showing this herb's ability to increase the production of natural killer (NK) cells in the body. NK cells are a critical part of fighting off any type of infection. To help prevent colds Kerry recommends 1 to 3 grams of dried Echinacea root per day. Echinacea is available in all natural food stores, compounding pharmacies and even many national supermarket and pharmacy chains.

A product called "Cold-fx," a standardized extract of American ginseng (panax quinquefolius) was touted as the "official cold and flu remedy of the National Hockey League and the National Hockey League Players Association." Double-blind, placebo-controlled research showed that regular use of a single 200-milligram Cold-fx capsule daily significantly reduced the incidence of colds, and that when colds did occur, their duration was significantly shorter.

The evidence is convincing enough that the Canadian equivalent of the FDA recently "approved" Cold-fx and allows it to bear the therapeutic claim that it "helps to reduce the frequency, severity, and duration of cold and flu symptoms by boosting the immune system."

Cold-fx is available at some compounding pharmacies, natural food stores and in some national pharmacy chains.

The germ-killing duo you need at the first sign of a sniffle

One of the things that makes Cold-fx unique is that it works for both treatment and prevention. Most people think that the next item on the list does so as well. But research on vitamin C done decades ago showed that this nutrient doesn't actually help prevent the common cold. It does, however, reduce the severity and duration of colds that do occur.

At the very first sign of a cold, I recommend taking a minimum of 1 gram of vitamin C four times daily, and if the vitamin C is tolerated well (meaning it doesn't cause loose bowels or diarrhea), considerably more is safe and even more effective.

Next to vitamin C, one of the most effective germ- and infection-fighting treatments available is something known as, colloidal silver, but I prefer to use a slightly more technical name, nano-particulate silver. The "nano-particulate" part is very important because the smaller the

---

Keeping it real with Korean ginseng

Korean Red ginseng (also known as Panax or Asian ginseng) shouldn't be confused with Siberian ginseng. The Siberian variety doesn't contain the ginsenosides that scientists believe are the active, and therapeutic, ingredients found in the other ginsengs. So be sure to read the label to make sure you're getting the right kind.

particle size of the silver, the greater the germicidal effect.

I recommend Argentyn 23™ and Sovereign Silver™, both of which are available at natural food stores and compounding pharmacies. At the first sign of a cold, use 1 tablespoonful to start, and then continue to take 1 teaspoonful on an empty stomach every 3 to 4 hours while you're awake until the infection is gone.

Unlike vitamin C, nano-particulate silver should not be used every day (unless recommended for a very particular reason by a physician skilled and knowledgeable in nutritional and natural medicine), but reserved only for treatment of active infections.

Forget what you've heard: Zinc can knock out colds in half the time

Some individuals with have sworn that zinc lozenges are "almost miraculous" for treating colds. Others swear they're useless. Research studies have been equally conflicting. The answer to this apparent contradiction is that *certain types* of zinc lozenges are indeed very effective, while other types are not very effective at all.

Ananda Prasad, Ph.D. (professor at Wayne State University School of Medicine) is widely recognized as one of the leading researchers and authors on zinc. Recently, he gave a presentation at the meeting of the International Society for Trace Element Research in Humans (ISTERH) about a randomized, double-blind, placebo-controlled study he and his colleagues conducted to examine the effects of zinc acetate lozenges against the common cold.[1]

Fifty research volunteers took either zinc acetate lozenges (which contained 13.3 milligrams each of elemental zinc) or placebo every three hours while awake, starting within 24 hours of the onset of cold symptoms. In the zinc acetate lozenge group, the subjects' colds lasted an average of 3.5 days versus 7.4 days in the placebo group. Coughs lasted a mean 2.1 days and nasal discharge 3.0 days in the zinc acetate lozenge group versus 5.3 days and 4.7 days in the placebo group. In essence, the zinc cut the amount of time the subjects spent sick in half—that's quite a significant reduction (just ask anyone suffering a cold).

This was actually Dr. Prasad's second positive research report about zinc acetate lozenges shortening the mean duration of the common cold and its symptoms. Seven years ago, he published similar results in the *Annals of Internal Medicine*.[2]

As in his recent study, Dr. Prasad enrolled 50 volunteers who each took zinc acetate lozenges (these ones containing 12.8 milligrams each of elemental zinc) or placebo, every 2 to 3 hours while awake, within 24 hours of the onset of cold symptoms. Compared with the placebo group, the zinc group experienced results similar to those seen in the recent study: Shorter overall duration of cold symptoms (4.5 vs. 8.1 days), cough (3.1 vs. 6.3 days), and nasal discharge (4.1 vs. 5.8 days) and decreased total severity scores for all symptoms.

A tasteful solution to zinc's spotty reputation

But despite the fact that Dr. Prasad's two research reports (as well as several others) have been very positive, there have been almost as many negative reports about zinc lozenges' ability to treat colds—including first-hand accounts from many people who have tried them and say they had no effect. So what's the real answer?

The real answer is that the zinc itself isn't what's contributing to the conflicting results: Zinc has been proven to interfere with virus replication by direct contact, as well as in other ways. So there's no doubt that the zinc itself works. To sort out which zinc lozenges are actually effective, you have to look at the "rest of the story," meaning all the other things going into the various zinc lozenge products that have been put on the market since the first positive research on zinc and colds was published back in 1984.[3]

When you buy a mineral supplement, you never just buy just the mineral itself. The mineral is always attached to something called a "binding ligand" which makes it stable, and (in some cases) easier to absorb. For example, calcium tablets or capsules don't contain just calcium; they contain calcium carbonate, calcium lactate, calcium citrate, or some other "form" of calcium. Similarly, magnesium is sold as magnesium oxide, magnesium citrate, magnesium glycinate, magnesium taurate, and many other forms. Zinc is sold as zinc picolinate, zinc citrate, zinc aspartate, and—in lozenges—zinc acetate.

Making zinc lozenges to treat common colds is particularly tricky for manufacturers. First, the goal of the zinc lozenge isn't absorption of the zinc as it is with capsules or tablets. The goal of the zinc lozenge is to rapidly release the zinc so it can come into contact with both the cold virus itself and the mucous membranes of the mouth, throat, and surrounding areas.

But while it's doing that, the zinc lozenge must also achieve its second goal—to taste good, or at least acceptable, even to small children. Unfortunately, anyone who's ever tasted an "elemental" liquid zinc solution in chemistry class (usually zinc chloride) knows that zinc tastes terrible!

As George Eby, one of the original zinc lozenge researchers, explained: "[Manufacturers] found that zinc gluconate forms very bitter complexes with all sweet carbohydrates (except fructose) upon aging for a few days to a few months, depending on the exact formulation… Manufacturers and researchers alike in desperation to solve the taste problem added metal chelators, reduced [zinc] dosage or used other non-ionizable zinc compounds, resulting in a loss of $Zn2+$ ions and efficacy, with at least two formulations actually making colds worse in clinical trials; reports of which temporarily discredited this major medical discovery."[4]

But sometime before 1990, Mr. Eby found that zinc combined with acetate could be made into compressed tablets or hard candy lozenges that were both stable and pleasant tasting. When the lozenges dissolve, the zinc and acetate rapidly break apart, releasing the ionic (positively charged) zinc to come into contact with both the viruses and mucous membranes where it can "do its job." Research continued until zinc acetate lozenges were proven to be effective when mass produced. And this technology still holds today: As noted above, Dr. Prasad's very positive work used zinc acetate lozenges.

At present, to make certain of effectiveness against the common cold virus, I recommend only the zinc acetate lozenge formula designed by George Eby, called Zinx™. You should start taking it within 24 hours of the onset of cold symptoms, and continue with another dose every two to three hours while you're awake until the cold symptoms are completely gone.

Zinx™ lozenges are available through a few natural food stores and compounding pharmacies)

How to juggle that ounce of prevention and pound of cure

Obviously, prevention is always best. Your chances of eliminating or at the very least minimizing your bouts with the common cold are excellent if you follow the preventive measures noted above. But just in case, and particularly if you have children at home, it's a good idea to have some nano-particulate silver (Argentyn 23™/Sovereign Silver™) and zinc acetate lozenges (Zinx™) in your pantry, along with a powdered form of vitamin C, which can be stirred into liquids to make it easier to take larger doses.

Of course, while getting better as quickly as possible is the ultimate goal when you come down with a cold, there are a couple of precautions to bear in mind before bombarding your system with all of these treatments at once.

Certainly eliminating sugar and allergies, and taking vitamin D, Echinacea, and Cold-fx are all compatible with each other and can be taken together safely. Vitamin C can be used with all of these, too, but at higher (treatment) quantities it's best taken with food to reduce chances of gastric irritation. By contrast, nano-particulate silver should be taken on an empty stomach, with no food for at least one hour before or after. And, as I mentioned above, nano-particulate silver isn't a preventive measure to be used on a daily basis. It should only be used when you're actually sick.

And last but not least, make sure you don't swallow those Zinx lozenges. To get the germ-killing effects, you should let the lozenge dissolve completely under your tongue. After that, you might gargle the resulting liquid or otherwise "swoosh it around" your mouth to try to contact as many infected surfaces as possible. If there's any liquid left after doing all this, it won't hurt to swallow it—after all, it's a low quantity of zinc—but it does the most good against the "common cold" by contacting the lining of your mouth and throat.

Chapter 6:

Tired of the sneezing... sniffling... and sinus pain? Relieve stubborn seasonal allergies with these all-natural cures

Autumn is here—and you know what that means, right?

The trees are shedding their leaves... the nights are cool... and the ragweed is doing a number on your sinuses.

Popping antihistamines and other allergy meds is practically a way of life for many people this time of year. And that can be incredibly dangerous.

Some of the most popular prescription and over-the-counter allergy drugs can cause an irregular heartbeat, leave you in a permanent brain fog, and even contribute to dementia.

You shouldn't have to accept those risks to keep your allergies in check. And, as I've shown many of my patients over the years, you *don't* have to.

Because there are safe, proven herbal remedies that can help you overcome even the most stubborn allergy symptoms—and that can have you feeling better quickly.

Powerful herbal allergy fighters

When you have an allergic reaction, your immune system has essentially shifted into overdrive. The symptoms you experience, such as heavy mucus or inflammation, are basically your body responding to a perceived threat.

That's why I recommend herbs that can soothe your symptoms while also strengthening your immune system.

To reduce mucus accumulation

Goldenseal (*Hydrates Canadensis*): Also known as yellow root, goldenseal dries up and soothes the mucous membranes throughout the body. This quality makes it useful in alleviating congestion and excess mucus, both in the respiratory system and in the digestive tract.

Prescription and preparation: Goldenseal is usually sold as capsules (taken 2 to 5 times a day) and a tincture (½ to 1 teaspoon a day). You also can get it in powdered form, from which you can make a tea by pouring a cup of boiling water over about ½ to 1 teaspoon of the powder (taken twice a day).

Red Sage (*Salvia officinalis*): Red sage is a classic remedy for inflamed and congested mucus membranes. It may be used internally and as a mouthwash (if your throat and mouth are also sore).

Prescription and preparation: You can use about 1 teaspoon of dried red sage leaves to make a tea to drink up to three times a day. Red sage tincture is also available. You can take about 2 to 4 milliliters, three times per day.

To reduce bronchial and nasal inflammation

Cayenne (*Capsicum minimum*): Cayenne, which we Americans know as hot red pepper, is one of the most useful herbal remedies available. Its active ingredient, capsaicin, is a strong anti-inflammatory and thus helps to soothe burning nasal passages, bronchial tubes, and lungs.

Prescription and preparation: Cayenne is readily available in powdered form and can be used in food, drunk as a tea (a cup of boiling water over 1/2 to 1 teaspoon of cayenne), and taken as a tincture (0.25 to 1 milliliters, three times daily).

Yarrow (*Achillea millefolium*): A powerful anti-inflammatory, yarrow is useful in treating fevers. It also reduces blood pressure, stimulates digestion, and reduces swelling of bronchial tissue.

Prescription and preparation: You can use dried yarrow leaves to make a tea, or you can consume it in tincture form (about 2 to 4 milliliters, three times a day).

To strengthen the immune system

Astralagus (*Astralagus memebranceus*): This ancient Chinese herb is used to increase resistance to disease. It has a warming effect on the body and soothes the digestive tract and other organs.

Prescription and preparation: Astragalus is most commonly available in commercial form as capsules (1 400-miligram capsule up to three times daily) and tinctures (1 teaspoon, three times daily).

Echinacea (*Echinacea angustiolia*): Also known as purple coneflower, this plant is a traditional Native American remedy known to have extraordinary immune-boosting qualities. Many clinical and laboratory studies document the ability of echinacea to strengthen the body's tissues and protect you from invasive germs and allergens.

Prescription and preparation: You can buy echinacea in any number of different forms: Capsules (1 capsule up to three times a day), tinctures (1 teaspoon up to three times a day), and extracts (mix 15 to 30 drops in water or juice and take up to four times a day).

Remember, herbs are drugs and may have serious side effects if not taken properly. It is best to devise an herbal prescription plan with a trained professional.

Chapter 7:

Get control of your Parkinson's symptoms with these simple (and fun) programs

More than 10 years ago, my life changed forever. That's when I was diagnosed with Parkinson's disease—and I've been constantly on the hunt for new treatments that are safe, natural, and effective.

I've been able to keep my Parkinson's from advancing for a decade, and it's thanks to these new breakthroughs that I've been discovering and sharing with patients just like you.

And one of the most exciting breakthroughs in Parkinson's treatment today has to do with exercise and stabilizing our muscles.

You may think that Parkinson's is a condition of *too much* movement—you know, those uncontrollable tremors—but actually, INACTIVITY is a big problem with PD patients. If you have Parkinson's, exercising might be the LAST thing you want to do when you're feeling fatigued and...well, *impaired*...but getting up and making some deliberate, rigorous movements might be just the thing to help you regain some control over your body.

And the best part? These are all remedies that you can explore *without* going to the doctor's office, physical therapy, or the hospital.

Picking up good vibrations

One of my patients made me aware of the benefits of Full Body Vibration, or FBV, where you do exercises on vibrating plates. The theory behind it is that, when your balance is thrown off by the vibrations, multiple muscle groups throughout your body respond by contracting and relaxing in an attempt to stabilize your posture. The result is a whole body workout utilizing most of the muscles in your body.

Working out on these plates has been shown to improve mobility and posture in several studies using patients with Parkinson's—and other neurological diseases that affect posture like multiple sclerosis are also obvious choices to apply this technology to.

Modern research on FBV first started in the 1970s, when Russian Olympic athletes who exercised on metal plates that vibrated rapidly reported great improvement in their workouts.

And believe it or not, it was also used on Russian cosmonauts to improve their bone density and strength while in space! NASA is now doing their own research into this for use on our own country's astronauts.

The vibrational exercises are painless, easy to do at home, and really give a sense of working out fully, even for patients who are pretty impaired physically. I urge all my Parkinson's patients to consider adding this to their plan to reverse the disease. If you're curious about picking up some of your own good, good, good vibrations, read the research for yourself on the websites www.fullbodyvibration.com and www.powerplate.com.

Ramp up your pedal power

I ran across some other fascinating research about exercise and Parkinson's, and the story is incredible.

In 2003, Cleveland Clinic biomedical researcher Dr. Jay Alberts undertook a 200-mile ride on a tandem bike with a partner who had Parkinson's disease. As they pedaled together, his partner got up to 80-90 rpm, which is MUCH faster than she could've ever pedaled normally.

And you know what? Shockingly, her tremor disappeared.

Eventually, after more preliminary studies were positive, the Cleveland Clinic initiated an NIH-funded study of "forced exercise" in PD[2] with a stationary bike called Theracycle, which has an assist motor. The person with PD slips their feet into pedals with toe straps sets the motor's speed, up to 90 rpm. The result of the study (and others[3]) is that the person using the Theracycle regularly had statistically significant improvements in both manual dexterity and motor functioning, when compared with PD patients doing regular aerobic activity when they could choose how fast to go and whether or not to stop.

You can find Theracycle at some physical therapy facilities, or you can get one to use in your own home. I've got a Theracycle in my family room, and I find that 20 minutes per day at around 90 rpm makes a huge difference in my function during the entire day. Visit www.theracycle.com to learn more.

Fill your dance card

If you have PD, though, you might not want to stay at home for all of your exercise. It might be nice to have an activity companion other than your physical therapist.

So, if you're looking for a more social form of exercising and movement, how does ballroom dancing sound?

There's a whole body of research demonstrating the ability of "music-based movement therapy" (um, *dancing*) to slow down the progression and even reverse the symptoms of Parkinson's and other movement disorders!

Just this past year, a large review of the existing studies supported dance as a demonstrable treatment for PD—and it doesn't have to be just ballroom style, either. In fact, tango dancing has garnered the most studies of its usefulness in PD, while salsa and even Irish set dancing have also been studied.

Multiple studies have also shown that there are many benefits to community-based dance workouts, so dance clubs and classes specifically designed for Parkinson's patients have popped up throughout the U.S. as well as Canada and Europe.

Regardless of your particular taste in music and style, choreographed dancing is great fun, really good for your heart health, and helps you work on your physical balance, your mental agility, and your state of mind. Learning something new as you get older is always a good idea.

Work on your right hook

Finally, if you're looking for an activity that will help improve your mobility and function AND let you get your frustrations out at the same time, try doing a little dance around the boxing ring with Rock Steady Boxing.

Since vigorous exercise—preferably rhythmic and emphasizing core strength and balance—can reverse the scourge of Parkinson's disease, this program puts people with PD through the same rigorous workouts as boxers go through.

No, you don't get to spar with each other, so this isn't the time to live out your *Rocky* fantasies—but they do try to make sure you're having fun, no matter what your fitness level is or how much your PD has progressed.

The results have been so promising that mainstream medicine has even begun to embrace it. The National Parkinson Foundation is helping fund an expansion of the program—and it has already spread to 11 states and three foreign countries from its origins in Indianapolis, just in the past year.

To find a class near you and try it out for yourself, visit www.RockSteadyBoxing.org

These are just a few examples of how exercise can work as a complementary therapy for a movement disorder like Parkinson's. Other studies have looked into the benefits of yoga, video game systems like the Wii Fit, and even virtual reality. Even if their benefits haven't been scientifically proven yet, these activities have shown to do no harm to patients with Parkinson's...and trying them might actually give you a good time.

Chapter 8:

Real cause of dozens of autoimmune diseases revealed: Simple three-step plan treats everything from rheumatoid arthritis to Crohn's disease

I call them the Big Four—cancer, heart disease, type 2 diabetes and Alzheimer's. And it feels like just about every research dollar in America (and every health care discussion) is directed at these killers.

But there's another group of diseases affecting 24 million Americans right now—maybe even you or someone you love. These are chronic autoimmune diseases that can cause progressive pain, disability, and even death—and we hardly hear anything about them.

There are more than 80 different illnesses that can be classified as autoimmune diseases, and just about anyone can be at risk. In fact, one out of every nine women will get an autoimmune disease sometime in her lifetime.

Some of the most well-known autoimmune diseases include:

- Graves' disease;

- Hashimoto's thyroiditis;

- type 1 diabetes;

- rheumatoid arthritis;

- celiac disease;

- Crohn's disease

- ulcerative colitis; and

- multiple sclerosis.

There are even some lethal but rare autoimmune diseases like sclero-derma, myasthenia gravis and autoimmune hepatitis.

But the good news is that no matter which autoimmune disease you have, the causes are essentially the same.

And that means we can use the same three-step process to help conquer literally dozens of autoimmune diseases and get you feeling better than you have in years.

Autoimmune diseases are a vicious (and painful) cycle

When you have an autoimmune illness, your immune system can't tell the difference between your own cells and foreign invaders. So your immune system forms antibodies that literally attack your own tissues, causing damage, stiffness, and inflammation.

Even worse, your body begins to form fibrous tissue to "heal" the inflammation, and you end up with more pain and disability. If you have a condition like rheumatoid arthritis, you know all about this cycle.

There's a scientifically proven link among many different autoimmune diseases. In fact, once you have an autoimmune disease your risk of getting another one in your lifetime is around 25 percent.

But conventional medicine insists on treating each illness as a separate problem. Ulcerative colitis is treated by a gastroenterologist; psoriasis by a dermatologist; rheumatoid arthritis by a rheumatologist; and so on.

Instead of taking a bigger picture, comprehensive approach, each doctor works in isolation treating the one illness and ignoring the others.

Worse still, autoimmune diseases are frequently treated by what I call cross-your-fingers medicine. Patients are loaded up on heavy-duty medications such as:

- corticosteroids like prednisone;
- anti-inflammatories such as indomethacin and diclofenac;
- metabolic poisons such as methotrexate; and
- biological response modifiers or TNF blockers such as Enbrel, Remicade and Humira.

Each of these medications comes with dangerous—sometimes deadly—potential side effects. And none of them treat the actual underlying *cause* of the illness. Instead they merely suppress the symptoms in the hope that the inflammatory disease burns itself out.

In other words, doctors simply cross their fingers and hope for the best!

Three powerful steps for treating ANY autoimmune disease

While the mainstream is busily trying to treat 80+ individual autoimmune diseases, they're failing to realize what they *really* have on their hands.

And that's a single immune system problem with 80+ manifestations.

Let me explain. If your irritated immune system attacks your thyroid, it causes Hashimoto's or Graves' disease. If it attacks the lining of your bowels, it can trigger ulcerative colitis or Crohn's disease. If it attacks the synovial membrane of the joints, you end up with rheumatoid arthritis.

So the actual cause of all autoimmune diseases (your immune system turning against you) is the same. It's only where you suffer the damage that can vary.

That's why I and other doctors who practice integrative medicine take a broad "systems" approach to treating autoimmune disease. It focuses on addressing the actual underlying causes and effects of the disease using three simple steps:

1. Control your symptoms;

2. Identify and eliminate immune system triggers; and

3. Restore your immune system's health.

Step #1: Control your symptoms

It does no good to try to correct an immune system imbalance while someone's joints are deteriorating, for example.

So the first order of business is always to get symptoms under control. Treatment will depend on which organs are being attacked and may involve both natural therapies as well as, in some cases, short-term medications.

Curcumin (found in the herb turmeric) is an effective anti-inflammatory that can help with everything from bowel diseases to rheumatoid arthritis. In one study, published in the journal *Phytotherapy Research*, rheumatoid arthritis patients were given either curcumin or the anti-inflammatory drug diclofenac. Curcumin beat the drug and had zero significant side effects.

Fish oil, white willow bark, proteolytic enzymes like bromelain and serrapeptase and the herb boswellia are all effective natural anti-inflammatories as well.

To address thyroid issues, I use natural thyroid supplements of desiccated (dried) animal thyroid, such as Armour Thyroid and NatureThroid. Bio-identical hormones like DHEA and pregnenolone can often be used in place of synthetic steroid hormones like prednisone.

Step #2: Identify and eliminate immune system triggers

Next we need to try to identify and remove any triggers that are irritating your immune system. And that can be a bit of a tall order.

The EPA, which is tasked with keeping us safe from environmental toxins, has already approved 80,000 chemicals for use in our environment, and thousands more are being added every year. Our environment is packed with so many immune system irritants that our immune-cell switches are essentially permanently stuck in the "on" position.

But when working with your doctor to try to discover what's triggering your body's immune response, there are some places you should look first.

In a major meta-analysis in 2012, researchers confirmed that there's a significant association between exposure to organic solvents (like the kind you find in many paints, pesticides and cleaning products) and an increased risk of developing an autoimmune disease.

And a stack of credible animal studies have found a link between the chemicals contained in Teflon and an increase in autoimmune illnesses.

So you can start reducing your own exposure to some of these damaging chemicals by replacing any non-stick Teflon coated cookware in your home with cast iron and stainless steel.

Use only *natural* pesticides, weed killers and fertilizers in your garden, and buy organic fruits and vegetables. Also try to use natural or even organic cleaning products when you can.

You should also get comprehensive allergy testing. Allergies are an often overlooked trigger for the development of autoimmune disease. And diagnosing—and successfully treating—an allergy can help turn down the inflammatory response of an autoimmune illness.

Step #3: Restore your immune system's health

Once we've eliminated these irritants, we need to restore your immune system—which has been going haywire for years—to good health.

Balancing your Th1 and Th2 lymphocytes can help. Th1 lymphocytes protect cells against invasion by organisms. Th2 lymphocytes prowl the bloodstream, creating antibodies.

In the case of an autoimmune disease (or allergy) your Th2 lymphocytes are overactive, and your Th1 lymphocytes are likely suppressed. But this isn't the first time your system will have faced this situation. We come into the world in a similar state. But nature provides us with a powerful immune-strengthening substance called colostrum in our mother's milk.

Colostrum contains transfer factors, molecules which boost a newborn's Th1 immunity while quieting down the blood-based antibody response involving Th2. This makes the newborn less vulnerable to cellular viruses, and lowers his risk of having an antibody response to his mother's blood.

We can mimic colostrum's powerful immune-balancing effects by supplementing with transfer factors derived from animal sources. You can find these transfer factor supplements online, and I've used them with success in my own practice.

White peony extracts, called peony glucosides, can also have a balancing effect on Th1 and Th2 lymphocytes.

One extract in particular, paeoniflorin, balances the Th1 and Th2 lymphocytes in much the same way as transfer factors from colostrum. Inflammatory messengers in the immune system (called cytokines) are essentially switched off. At the same time this remarkable herb offers significant pain relief, helping to relieve symptoms *while* helping to cure the disease.

Vitamin D3, fish oil and soy isoflavones can also help rebalance a dysfunctional immune system and put you on the road to healing.

Three other steps to strengthen your immune system include:

1. Taking a probiotic: Remember, a large proportion of your immune cells reside in your gut, and probiotics help maintain a healthy balance of "good" gut bacteria.

2. Switching to a naturally anti-inflammatory diet: I recommend the Paleo or "Cavemen" diet, which focuses on fresh meats and produce and eliminates processed foods and added sugars.

3. Reducing your stress levels: Exercise, yoga, meditation, acupuncture and connecting with your spiritual side can help you de-stress.

Choose whatever methods work best for you.

Chapter 9:

Allergies, asthma, and autoimmune diseases are exploding. Here's why your immune system is broken—and how to fix it

Let me ask you a question that I'll bet you've thought about before.

With all our advancements in modern medicine... with everything we know about how to prevent illnesses... why in the world are we sicker than ever?

The number of people suffering from asthma, serious allergies—and autoimmune diseases like psoriasis and rheumatoid arthritis—is going through the roof.

It's almost like we're *doing* something to ourselves that's making us sick.

And, in fact, we are.

Our obsession with germ-free living is literally destroying our immune systems, causing an explosion in diseases that practically didn't exist a couple centuries ago.

That's something that could put your health—and even your life—at risk.

But the good news is that we caused this problem—and we can fix it, too. I'm going to show you some simple things you can do, starting today, to fortify your immune system and protect yourself from allergies, autoimmune disorders, and other health-wrecking diseases.

An allergy explosion

The numbers speak for themselves.

Allergic rhinitis (a.k.a. "hay fever") currently affects between 10 and 30 percent of the world's population—but it was *unheard of* 200 years ago.

In fact, as far as we know, hay fever was described for the first time ever in 1819 by Dr. John Bostock.[1] That makes seasonal allergies one of the fastest-growing epidemics EVER!

Food allergies are exploding, too, especially in recent years. According to one study, allergies to peanuts and almonds, pecans, and other tree nuts have more than *tripled* in a recent 10-year period.[2]

Other allergic diseases—like those of the skin—have also been on the rise in recent times. From 2000 to 2010, the rate of childhood eczema increased:[3]

- from 9 to 17 percent in black children
- from 8 to 13 percent in white children
- from 5 to 10 percent in Hispanic children

And let me tell you: An increase in five or six percentage points over 10 years is pretty big news.

Let's not forget about asthma, of course, since it also continues to increase steadily—by as much as 16 percent a year, according to some surveys.[4] Black children experienced a 50 percent increase in asthma between 2001 and 2009—when asthma went from affecting 1 out of 14 to 1 in 12 people in the U.S.[5]

That may not *seem* like a big difference, but it means about an extra 5 million people in just eight years.

Is living clean making us sick?

Now, there's a theory as to why we have such an increase in allergic diseases—and it's not just that the world is more polluted today than it was back then. In fact, it's quite the opposite!

Instead, it seems that our sterile, germ-free environments could actually be the culprits (although probably not the *only* culprits) behind the development of asthma and allergic disorders.

Known as the "Hygiene Hypothesis," this theory was first proposed in 1989 by Dr. David Strachan.

He found that the more siblings that children had, the less likely they were to develop hay fever. That led him to hypothesize that older siblings likely expose their younger siblings' developing immune systems to a variety of allergens early in life. This early exposure would make their immune systems less "skittish"—and therefore less reactive to the natural world and the many antigens that it contains.

In the 27 years since Dr. Strachan first proposed it, many other pieces of information have come to light in support of this theory. For example, it's been found that children who are in daycare when young tend to have a lower risk of asthma,[6] and those who grow up on a farm or have lots of rural exposure also have lower incidences of allergic diseases.[7] This is even true if the child is only exposed while in the womb!

One interesting group of studies looked at children born in East Germany versus West Germany. The assumption was that since East Germans had a less "westernized" environment, they would have been exposed to more organisms in early life—and, sure enough, the children raised in East Germany had lower incidences of asthma and allergy.[8]

However, after German unification, they became more like their West German counterparts, with increasing levels of these types of disorders.

The home and living environments aren't the only factors implicated in this explosive increase in asthma and allergy. There's more and more evidence that antibiotic use in early life is associated with the development of allergy and asthma later on. The use of antibiotics in early childhood increased sharply in the late 1980s and early 1990s—and, *at the same time*, the allergy rate started to trend upwards.[9]

And that's simply hard to ignore.

A delicate balance of defense and attack

To understand why this all makes sense, we need to understand how our immune systems work (or are supposed to work).

This gets a little scientific, but hang with me.

The white blood cells that are responsible for most of the "heavy lifting" of the immune system are called "lymphocytes," and, as their name implies, they're found in your lymphatic system. There are different types of lymphocytes—including T cells, B cells, and "Natural Killer"/NK cells—but for this topic, we'll talk about the T cells.

In particular, two subtypes of T cells—T Helper cells and T regulatory cells—make sure that an immune response is initiated when it needs to be, that the immune response isn't too weak or too strong, and that it "turns off" when the danger has passed.

The two subtypes of T Helper cells are TH1 and TH2. TH1 lymphocytes guard against viruses, parasites, and fungi—as well as cancer. This is called "cellular immunity," because it guards the cells themselves.

TH2 lymphocytes, on the other hand, travel in the bloodstream, triggering the formation of the antibodies that go out and attach to antigens, enabling them to be damaged and killed. The TH2 response is considered "humoral immunity" (that is, traveling in the blood), and it's is largely what we think of as allergy.

Now, the TH1 and TH2 cells may do much of the legwork, but it's the dendritic cells—generally found on your skin—that act as a kind of "lookout" and, like Paul Revere and the redcoats, announce that trouble is on its way.

When dendritic cells become activated, they send a message out to not only initiate an immune response, but also to determine how powerful a response it should be.

That means calling upon the T Helper cells, and producing T regulatory ("Treg") cells to modulate the immune response and make sure it doesn't go overboard.

Now imagine a situation where the T Helper cells are activated, but aren't properly kept in check with Treg cells. You'd have an immune response gone haywire.

And that's essentially what's happening when you have an autoimmune disease.[10]

Immunity is a skill you learn

But something else can go wrong with the TH1 and TH2 immune responses, starting with the very first moments of life.

And that's where the Hygiene Hypothesis comes in.

In the womb, the environment is predominantly TH2 by default. If TH1 was predominant, there is a risk that the mother's immune system might reject the fetus and placenta as foreign matter.

By design, this TH2 predominance is temporary. After birth, exposure to environmental organisms outside of the womb (viruses, pollens, food antigens, etc.) stimulates the TH1 response until an ideal balance of TH1 and TH2 is established.

But if the newborn comes into a completely sterile world—or is given antibiotics at or near the beginning of life—there's nothing to wake the dormant TH1 response up, leaving the newborn's T Helper cells way out of balance.

As the TH2 response continues to dominate, the child becomes allergic and is at increased risk of autoimmune responses, candida, and other fungi.

And we don't even know yet how this may affect the child's future risk of developing cancer and possible inability to fight it.

Many studies have shown a correlation between early-age antibiotic use and later-age asthma and allergy.

One study of more than 193,000 children in several countries showed that antibiotic therapy before their first birthday led to higher incidences of asthma and eczema by age 6 or 7.[11]

This conclusion was supported by both a Canadian study of over 215,000 children[12] and a Spanish study of 13,908 children.[13]

Now, it has been argued that antibiotics could have been prescribed to treat the symptoms (like coughing and wheezing) that actually turned out to be early signs of asthma. And, if that were true, the studies would be mixing cause and effect. But I'm inclined to say that although that scenario is possible, it doesn't apply to these studies because it still doesn't explain the correlation between antibiotics and allergic skin diseases like eczema.

At this point, the Hygiene Hypothesis is just a theory. Although many studies seem to support it, it's far from having been *proven*. But there's a lot of new science coming out of places like the Mayo Clinic and Johns Hopkins that's deepening our understanding of it... and it's a real enough possibility that even the FDA has acknowledged it.[14]

Preventing one illness may bring on another

Think about all the things we do to *prevent* illness and death, from pumping antibacterial soap into our hands at the sink to dutifully getting an annual flu shot (even though they largely don't work).

And at the slightest sign of a sniffle, we can get a prescription for an antibiotic filled in two seconds flat.

But all in all, it seems that in our attempts to keep our children free from germs of any sort and free from any and ALL illnesses (even the benign childhood illnesses that *we* all survived), we've helped to create a monster.

On a day-to-day basis, our immune systems have had nothing to do since *before birth*—so by the time we're faced with a *real* threat out in the "real world," our bodies can't quite figure out what to do.

But regardless of what's happened in the past, there are ways to naturally boost immunity NOW... fight off any diseases that may have already developed... and guard against whatever may come in the future.

And that applies to those of us who've got quite a few years under our belts as well as the little ones who haven't made their grand entrance yet.

I've had a lot of success using probiotics with my patients, since replenishing the "good" bacteria in your gut can bulk up your line of defense against any "bad" bacteria. Probiotics have even been shown to relieve hay fever AND eczema!

There's a particularly potent probiotic that can help fight autoimmune diseases like ulcerative colitis.

On a final note, I would never tell you to stop washing your hands... but maybe ditch the antibacterial soaps and wipes. They could be doing more harm than good.

Instead, you can try nature's own vampire repellant and natural germicide, garlic. If you don't love eating it with your food, you can also take it as a supplement, along with other immune-boosting nutrients like vitamin C and zinc.

Zinc deficiency is common among people over the age of 55, and zinc is important for a properly functioning immune system. All it takes is 30 mg a day for 30 days to increase your T-cells to fight off infections—especially if your immune system is already compromised.

PART IX

Energy and Thyroid Health

Chapter 1:

Stomp out chronic fatigue and get back your old get-up and go

If you've been diagnosed with chronic fatigue syndrome, the first thing you should do is take an adrenal function test. This test measures how the adrenal glands respond to stress of any kind, physical or mental. Adrenal glands are stress-response glands and should make considerably more of each steroid hormone when stressed. It wouldn't be normal for our hearts to beat at the same rate or even a little slower after exercise than before, and it isn't normal for adrenal glands to make the same amount of hormone after stress as before. When they make less, weakness becomes a serious problem. They "go all out" just to keep you walking around. When they're called on to do more…exercise, working hard…they just can't do it.

If your adrenal glands are overstressed, stress reduction is a necessary part of recovery. But even though it's necessary, it can't usually do the job on its own. So you'll want to begin taking a number of supplements to combat weak adrenal glands, beginning with cortisol, DHEA (15 milligrams per day), and salt. Extra salt is important in the production of a hormone called aldosterone. The main function of aldosterone is to regulate minerals like potassium and sodium, and it is a major factor in enabling our bodies to retain salt. You couldn't survive if your body didn't retain salt. If you're not eating much salt, your body has to make more aldosterone to make up for it. But if salt intake is high, it's actually normal for your adrenal glands not to make any aldosterone at all. So, if you eat enough salt, your adrenal glands don't need to make aldosterone, and that saves them some work.

Extra salt, cortisol, and DHEA help to rest the adrenal glands so they have more energy to repair themselves. But, you can help the repairs go even faster with the right diet, nutrients, herbs, and other supplements.

People with weak adrenal glands should never follow a low-carbohydrate diet. Weak adrenal glands are among the causes of low blood sugar levels, and a low-carbohydrate diet is meant to control blood sugar. Perhaps the most surprising nutritional recommendation given for strengthening adrenal gland functioning is incorporating six or more pieces of licorice (with no added artificial color or sugar) into your diet daily. Licorice contains substances that slow the liver's breakdown of steroid hormones.

In addition to these dietary modifications, vitamins A, E, and the entire B complex are thought to help the functioning of the adrenal glands. Usually, any good multivitamin and B-complex supplements from a natural food store will contain enough. Other supplements found to be helpful in treating weak adrenal glands are "Adren-Plus" and an "adrenal glandular." Adren-Plus is a combination of botanicals that have been shown to improve adrenal health. Adrenal glandulars are whole, dehydrated, animal adrenal cortex.

Chapter 2:

Keep your energy levels from sagging with this (seriously) misunderstood vitamin fix

Over the years, treating fatigue has become a big part of my practice.

Every day, I have patients in my waiting room with the same complaint—their "get up and go" has "got up and went."

Their energy levels are tanking. Getting out of bed in the morning is a struggle—and they've lost the pep they need to play with the grandkids, work in the garden, or enjoy their other favorite activities.

Sounds familiar, right?

But when I recommend a vitamin B12 injection—or advise my patients to start a supplement program—often they'll object. And it's because some mainstream doctor has tested their B12 levels and claimed they were fine, or even elevated.

I've even had some patients who had doctors warn them about "poisoning" themselves with B12.

It's a load of nonsense based on a seriously flawed testing system. And, unfortunately, too many doctors are using it to deny patients a life-changing vitamin treatment that could help protect their hearts and brains, and give them more energy than they've felt in years.

What your B12 test *isn't* telling you

As a doctor, it pains me to admit this—but the medical world got really dumb when lab testing was invented. Doctors stopped using their brains!

Conventional doctors tend to use lab results as "gospel." They'll tell a patient she doesn't have a disease or vitamin or hormone deficiency, even if she has EVERY symptom of it, just because the blood work came back "normal."

And it's the same deal with B12. If your results come back within the normal range, doctors will steer you away from shots or supplements.

But what they won't tell you is that there's a BIG problem with how they define normal.

The conventional medical community has devised those "normal" lab values by taking a population of patients and taking the AVERAGE of them. That's it.

The established norms aren't even CLOSE to being based on perfect people with perfect energy levels, so I don't think the bar has been set high enough.

Because when you're my patient, I want you to live a life that's MORE than average...and BETTER than normal.

Are you getting ENOUGH of this monumental nutrient?

If there were a Mount Rushmore of vitamins, B12 would be on it.

It always amazes me how many biochemical processes are tied to B12. It's responsible for the repair and upkeep of the nervous system and the refinement of every red blood cell your body makes.

B12 also lowers your levels of homocysteine, an amino acid that's been implicated in stroke and cardiovascular disease.

And B12 helps provide you with energy and stamina and even helps your body produce serotonin, a brain chemical that regulates your mood. Even better, you feel the results very quickly.

Its incredible breadth of responsibilities in the human body—and amazing healing properties—make B12 a staple of my practice.

In fact, I'm adamant about maintaining my patients' B12 levels to be in the upper end of normal—and even getting in to the elevated levels—because I'm looking at B12 for its therapeutic purposes.

You can't get too much of this good thing

Now, because B12 is a water-soluble vitamin, your body absorbs some of it to use for its healing purposes...and then urinates the rest out.

So you wouldn't get the maximum benefit of B12 unless you SATU-RATE the body with it via a shot or high-dose oral supplements.

Supplementing with B12 can help ward off disease and restore your energy levels, but only if you're getting ENOUGH of it.

Some studies do show that certain diseases are linked to having nat-urally-elevated levels of B12 in your bloodstream WITHOUT the influ-ence of vitamin supplementation;[1] but by and large, the scientific com-munity agrees that this age-old treatment has stood the test of time and is a very safe therapy...even at high levels.

Unlike the prescription drugs that have countless side effects and have been linked to some pretty scary risks, there's scant if any data show-ing any real dangers of taking too much B12.[2]

But to get more B12 than what's available in one of those supermarket vitamin brands, you might need to get a very different kind of prescription from your doctor. Some supplements are so strong that they require a pre-scription. They're called "medical foods," and I'm a fan of them.

Metanx has methylated versions of B12, B6, and folic acid. In fact, this FDA-regulated medical food will likely raise your B12 level to the upper echelon on the B12 laboratory spectrum...if not make your B12 level appear to be "elevated," according to their established norms.

But don't worry about those elevated levels. Because aside from giving you an energy boost, Metanx is a wonderful tool in the healing of the nervous system, having helped ease the discomfort of peripheral neuropathy (numbness and tingling in the extremities—often, the feet).[3] You can find out more at www.metanx.com.

Chapter 3:

Sluggish and suffering? Doc says you're fine? Take a closer look at your thyroid function with this commonly overlooked test!

Nearly every day, I hear patients complain that they have symptoms of low thyroid.

They've gained weight... feel tired all the time... are constipated... and just can't stand the cold. They may even experience some swelling.

Yet, they've been told by their doctors that their thyroid test results were "normal."

Well, the truth is most mainstream doctors' standards don't even come close to mine.

I want my patients' levels to be more than "normal" or "average." I don't want you to feel "OK" or "fine"—I want you to feel great!

Thyroid function in particular is more complicated than a single blood test result.[1] To make sure you're getting the optimum performance out of this critical gland— which can stimulate metabolism, lower cholesterol, and improve healing—it's important to explore other ways of testing for thyroid issues.

And it may involve a lab test that I'm betting your physician has barely heard of—but that you can ask for!

The usual test performed by doctors is a TSH (thyroid stimulating hormone) test. This test is fine if you're looking specifically for low thyroid due to thyroid damage (mostly due to an autoimmune condition called "Hashimoto's Thyroiditis").

But to get the real story of what's going on with your thyroid—especially if you've been experiencing weight gain, fatigue, and other "classic" symptoms—you may need a lab test called "Reverse T3," or rT3 for short.

Peel back the layers of how your thyroid actually works

In order to understand rT3, you've got to understand something of the activity of thyroid hormones in the body.

Thyroid hormones are made up of an amino acid called "L-Tyrosine," to which iodine atoms are added. The bulk of the thyroid hormone released into the bloodstream is T4, or L-Tyrosine with four iodine atoms added.

Many factors are involved in the proper production of T4 by the thyroid, besides the obvious candidates of both L-Tyrosine and iodine. A number of other nutrients are critical to the production of T4 by the thyroid, including:

- Vitamins E, D, and C

- B vitamins (specifically B2, B3, and B6)

- the minerals iron, zinc, and selenium.

If any one of these important nutrients is missing, the thyroid gland is unable to keep up with production demands from the body, and it won't be able to produce enough T4.

Many other conditions in the body will lead to a lessening of thyroid function and slow the production of T4 at the gland site (sometimes referred to as a "down-regulating" of thyroid hormone production).

These include toxins such as mercury, lead, pesticides, and cadmium. Fluoride, a known neurotoxin that interferes with iodine in the body, has also been implicated.[2]

Infections, radiation, trauma, and various medications can block thyroid function. And auto-immune diseases, particularly celiac disease (extreme gluten sensitivity), do the same.

And so can stress.

How "normal" test results happen

It's perfectly common for a patient's thyroid to produce a proper amount of T4. When that happens, the pituitary gland thinks everything is okay and puts out a normal amount of TSH.

The end result is that the patient suffers from the symptoms of hypothyroidism without showing abnormalities of the standard lab tests that measure TSH—because even when your thyroid IS producing enough T4, it isn't very active in the body.

In fact, T4 needs to be converted into T3 (L-Tyrosine + 3 iodines) before it can do much of anything at all.

So, here's yet another stage at which point something can go wrong with your thyroid function—yet most doctors aren't even looking for it. In fact, a number of the same conditions that prevent the thyroid gland from producing T4 can also interfere with the proper conversion from T4 to T3 (like stress), as well as:

- trauma

- inflammation (with elevation of cytokines and other pro-inflammatory messengers)

- infections (including chronic ones like Lyme Disease)

- toxins

- medications, and

- problems with other organs such as liver and kidneys.

And this is where reverse T3 (rT3) enters the picture. In situations of stress to the body, cells convert T4 into a different hormone, called rT3, which is much less active than regular T3.

Even a low-calorie diet will favor the conversion to rT3 over T3. This is why some people have such a hard time losing weight, even when they're on a very stringent diet. Their body metabolism slows down as more T4 is converted to the metabolically less active thyroid hormone, rT3.

Since rT3 looks so much like T3, it actually competes with T3 to attach to the binding sites of the body's cells. And when it attaches, it is much less active in its effects, plus it prevents the regular T3 from performing its duties. The end result is a slower metabolism, even in the face of normal thyroid production of hormone.

Only the complete picture
will lead to a cure

Whenever I'm evaluating thyroid function, I look at a variety of factors.

I do measure TSH of course, as well as T4. Specifically, I look at the "free" T4, which is the one that's unbound to anything.

But I also look at free T3 (fT3) and reverse T3. The ratio of rT3 versus fT3 is a critical measure.

Even if the patient has already been put on a synthetic version of T4 called levothyroxine (commonly known by the brand names Levoxyl and Synthroid), I might give them some T3 if their ratio is off.

I tend to prefer a natural glandular medication over synthetics—so I might recommend Armour thyroid hormone replacement therapy, which contains both T3 and T4.[3]

Nature Throid is another natural alternative to synthetics that also contains both T3 and T4, but it's also gluten- and corn-free.[4]

Both are made from animal products, so they're not suitable for vegetarians or vegans.

You need a prescription from a doctor for either Armour or Nature Throid. You don't want to go trying to fix your own thyroid without the benefit of some knowledgeable medical advice.

But don't forget an ounce of prevention

More critically, their test results will likely lead me to go looking for toxins, infections, deficiencies, and other situations that would lead to this result.

That way, I can address the root cause of the reduced thyroid function.

Needless to say... if stressors can sabotage the proper function of thyroid hormone production, conversion, and attachment... then by all means find a way to reduce or eliminate that stress to your body!

Exercise can give you the extra boost you need, and can help jumpstart your metabolism as well.

I should note that since the proper conversion of T4 into T3—and the proper attachment of T3 to cell binding sites—requires a good amount of zinc and selenium available in your body, you can naturally support your thyroid function with supplements. You can get both of these essential minerals by taking a good multivitamin along with eating a nutrient-rich diet, although they're available individually as well at your local health food store.

While you're at it, make sure you're getting proper levels of vitamin A and B vitamins.

Part X

Women's Health

Chapter 1:

Ladies: Losing your head over your thinning hair? My "Halt the Hair Loss" plan can help!

In my nearly four decades of practice, I've seen countless women show incredible strength and steely resolve in the face of almost any sort of disability or devastating diagnosis you can imagine. But there's one symptom that's practically *guaranteed* to have a women crying in frustration and desperately seeing solutions.

And, believe it or not, that's hair loss.

You see, men are basically conditioned to expect to lose our hair sooner or later. Oh we may not like it, but it doesn't usually devastate us. And if you've ever seen a photo of me you know that I know what I'm talking about.

But for woman it's different. When a woman sees clumps of her hair in the shower drain it can really wreak havoc with her self-image. Women are taught to think of their hair as their "crowning glory." And when a woman starts to lose that crowning glory by the handful it's really no wonder that she'll try practically anything to hold on to as much of it as she can.

Over the years, I've researched strategies to help women ward off... and even *reverse*... this self-esteem destroying symptom. I'll get to those solutions in just a moment. But first let's take a look at what could be causing that hair loss in the first place.

Assessing the damage

Keep in mind we *all* lose anywhere between 50 to 100 strands of a hair a day. This is normal. But if you're losing significantly more than this there's likely a problem.

Hair loss can be caused by either damage to the living, growing hair roots, or to the dead and hardened material of the hair shaft. If it's only a problem with the hair *shaft*, it's usually temporary and can be improved by making some changes to the habits that damaged the hair shaft in the first place.

The most common example of this this type of damage is the breaking of the hair shaft that's seen when a woman uses too much hair dye or other harsh hair products. Once the bleaches and coloring agents that damaged the hair are removed, the new hair should grow in fine.

But damage to the growing area of the hair follicle can be more widespread and a longer-term problem. This kind of damage can be all over the head, which is called *alopecia capitis*, or more at the temples in in a "male baldness" pattern that's then called *androgenetic alopecia*.

To distinguish between normal shedding of hair and these other conditions a doctor may look at your scalp under a microscope. The hair follicles should all look fairly thick and uniform. But if some of the follicles are thin and anemic looking your doctor will likely diagnose you with androgenetic alopecia.

Contributing causes

There's a super long list of toxic and metabolic factors that can contribute to hair loss, but on that list a few that stand out. Hormones, for example, could be behind your hair loss.

Low thyroid or certain kinds of synthetic hormones like those given for menopause can cause your hair to start falling out. (Bio-identical or natural hormone therapy generally *doesn't* cause hair loss since it is typically *synthetic* progestin that leads to hormone-imbalances.) And a profoundly stressful period in your life can alter your adrenal and sex hormones leading to hair loss a month or two later.

Illness can affect your hair and extreme dieting or nutrition can play a role too. In addition, drugs are an often overlooked cause of hair loss. Acid blockers, anti-seizure medications and blood thinners are all notorious for causing thinning locks.

Genetics play an important role too. If your close female relatives lost their hair, you're much more likely to lose your own. In fact, according to the American Academy of Dermatology up to 30 million American women are in this boat.

But the good news is despite your contributing factors, and despite your genetics, you don't have to simply accept hair loss. You do have options.

Over the years I've developed a Halt Your Hair Loss strategy designed to (1) identify the cause, (2) stop the hair loss and (3) in many cases even reverse it. And with the help of an integrative medicine doctor you can put this same strategy to work for you. I'll show you how.

Halt the Hair Loss!

I always start hair loss consultations with taking a good history. This will help you identify what's causing your own hair to fall out. You can do this step with the help of an integrative physician, or prepare your history and take it with you to your next appointment.

Write down any recent stresses, exposures to toxins or any infections or illnesses you have had. Make a list of any medications you've taken recently, keeping in mind there's a lag time so drugs taken three months ago can be affecting your hair now. And write down any close female relatives that have had thinning hair.

Next up is a thorough lab evaluation. Since low thyroid function, even if the numbers look to be normal, is a widespread cause of hair loss a thyroid test is almost always a good idea. There are a number of thyroid tests your doctor can perform, so talk to him about your options.

Ask your doctor about taking a 24 hour saliva assay to look at your cortisol levels as well. Cortisol is the main stress-responding hormone of the adrenal gland and this test can help narrow down if stress is contributing to your hair loss.

An extensive hormone panel that includes a look at sex hormone binding globulin (SHBG), which binds to testosterone and its more active metabolite, dihydrotestosterone (DHT) is also a good idea. When your liver—due to toxins, blood sugar elevations, etc.—fails to produce enough SHBG a lot of the testosterone and DHT becomes free and penetrates the follicular cells causing male pattern baldness. In fact, thyroid stimulates the production of SHBG in the liver, which is thought to be why *low* thyroid causes hair loss.

A test for heavy metals, usually through a urine collection after a "challenge" with a chelating agent, can reveal if these toxins are playing a part in your hair loss. And tests that evaluate the status of a number of important nutrients should be considered as well. In my clinic we look for an overdose of vitamin A and deficiencies of biotin, zinc, iron and ferritin, all of which can lead to hair loss.

Roll out the remedies

Once the cause of your hair loss is pinpointed it's time to remedy it. This can include stress reduction, changing medications, treating adrenal exhaustion or combatting a heavy metal problem.

In almost all the cases I've worked on I find some sluggishness of the thyroid gland. This can be reversed using small doses of desiccated thyroid hormone or the active thyroid hormone T3.

Hormone imbalances can also be remedied using bio-identical hormones, usually low doses of estriol, estradiol and progesterone. The herb saw palmetto can help block the conversion of testosterone to DHT. And if more intervention is needed the hormone spironolactone, which blocks the DHT from getting into the cell and doing its damage, is another effective option.

A mixture of nutrients can be used to strengthen your hair and encourage new hair growth. I typically recommend...

- **biotin** and **zinc**, both of which are essential for proper follicular hair generation,

- the amino acid **L-Lysine**, which has been shown in studies to play a role in hair-growth factor (possibly due to its role in iron utilization), and

- **methylsulfonylmethane** (MSM), an important metabolic factor in the body.

If more help is needed I usually turn to a compounding pharmacist. I have the pharmacist make up a hair cream in a base that penetrates the scalp and into the hair follicles. Typically the cream contains saw palmetto, a small dose of the thyroid hormone T3 (usually about 1 mg) and biotin. In women who have documented high DHT a small dose of natural progesterone is added.

If all of the natural options are exhausted and you're still having trouble it could be time to consider a pharmaceutical medication. In particularly stubborn hair loss cases I sometimes add the DHT blocking drug Minoxidil (typically 5 percent) to the hair cream.

Remember hair loss typically takes months to develop and you should expect it to take several months to reverse it. But with some time and patience I've found this treatment plan does the trick for most women, restoring their crowns of glory.

Chapter 2:

Warning: Unsightly varicose veins could be sending you warning sign. Try these 4 simple steps to send them packing

You name it, and I've seen it. Patients with just about any disease or dysfunction you can imagine have walked through the doors of my busy practice at some point. I'm kind of a last resort for a lot of people. They come to see me after conventional medicine has failed them.

But surprisingly it's not always the patients with critical health issues who are the most desperate—or that have been let down the most by conventional doctors. In fact, one of the most common issues that bring patients—women in particular—to see me is the appearance of varicose or spider veins.

If you're 65 or older, you have a greater than 75 percent chance of developing the bluish, swollen lines in your legs that signal you have varicose veins. Spider veins—the varicose vein's smaller and more superficial cousin—are equally as common. Both of these unsightly conditions can occur anywhere from your upper thigh down to your lower leg and ankle.

But these swollen and poorly functioning vessels don't discriminate; they can appear in much younger women as well. It's quite common for them to pop up during pregnancy or soon after childbirth, with up to 40 percent of pregnant women reporting them.

If you have a job that keeps you on your feet all day, or you're carrying around some extra pounds you're at a higher risk for varicose veins. Circulation issues, cigarette smoking, wearing high heels, chronic constipation, long-term bedrest or the weakening of leg muscles can all contribute to the condition as well. And heredity plays a part too, since the condition has a genetic component and tends to run in families.

Unsightly and embarrassing

Varicose veins are rarely dangerous. In fact the main complaint patients have about them is that they're just plain unattractive. Many women find their swollen corkscrew appearance embarrassing and they avoid wearing skirts, shorts and bathing suits, preferring to hide them under long pants no matter the weather or occasion.

But for some unlucky women they can be uncomfortable. The swollen veins can become warm and sore, and in some situations downright painful. In extreme cases the small clots in the vessels can become inflamed, causing something called superficial thrombophlebitis. Superficial thrombophlebitis can be treated with warm compresses, elevating the

---

Varicose veins don't discriminate

Varicose veins can strike women of any age regardless of their lifestyle, even athletes. Summer Sanders, the most medaled US swimmer of the Barcelona Olympics in 1992, is a good example. Summer, who became a television sports correspondent following her wins at the Olympics, participated in a campaign to raise awareness about varicose veins. Despite her incredibly active lifestyle, Summer developed varicose veins on her legs during her first pregnancy.

legs to reduce swelling, and by taking aspirin or, preferably, white willow bark and clot-busting enzymes such as bromelain.

Varicose veins are a warning sign

But varicose veins aren't always just simply a cosmetic issue. They can also be a warning sign of a far more serious deeper circulation problem called chronic venous insufficiency, or CVI. More on CVI in just a moment, but first let's take a quick look at how veins and circulation work.

When we walk our calf and leg muscles act like pumps sending blood upwards into our body and towards our heart. Throughout our veins there are a series of valves that prevent that blood from flowing backwards.

Both spider veins (which are essentially a smaller version of varicose veins) and varicose veins occur when those valves in our veins stop working efficiently or fail. Poor blood flow... otherwise known as venous insufficiency... causes the blood to collect in the small vessels in your legs.

Eventually the pooling blood begins to clot causing the inflammation and bluish color we see through the skin. The clotting causes even more pressure to build up on the remaining working valves and vein walls leading to even more damage. Over time venous insufficiency can lead to deep veins starting to break down, the condition I mentioned earlier known as CVI.

Blood clots can kill

When you're suffering with CVI your legs become weak and heavy, and they swell with fluid. Areas of your skin, particularly around the ankles, can break down and form dangerous hard to heal ulcers. And most dangerous of all, the chronic swelling and poor circulation can cause a blood clot in the deep veins of your legs leading to more severe inflammation and pain.

This potentially life threating situation is a condition called deep vein thrombosis, or DVT. The blood clot can easily break off and travel either to your heart where it can obstruct blood flow, or to your the lungs where it can cause a pulmonary embolism or PE. Either scenario can be deadly.

Although not all people with varicose and spider veins go on to develop CVI, they're a warning signal that shouldn't simply be ignored. In the Edinburgh Vein Study 880 adults were followed for 13 years, and nearly half of those with CVI had their condition worsen. But even more telling was that around 1/3 of the people who only had varicose veins at the start of the study showed the skin changes and other signs of CVI by the end of the study!

4 simple steps to prevent bulging veins

Although varicose veins tend to run in families if you don't have them yet, want to prevent more from forming, or want to improve the appearance of the ones you have, there are some simple diet and lifestyle steps you can take.

Lighten the load: As I mentioned earlier, carrying around extra weight puts increased pressure on the blood that's trying to re-enter your body from your legs. Over time this added pressure causes venous breakdown.

Some simple changes in your diet can help you shed those extra pounds. Start by reducing the amount of sugars, starches and carbohydrates you're eating. You'll be surprised by how fast the weight will start to come off when you make this one change.

Tweak what you eat: Next make sure you're taking in enough fiber. Constipation causes you to strain whenever you have a bowel movement. This straining adds extra pressure to the veins in your legs which are already working hard against gravity to move blood back up to your heart.

The damage to vein walls, and the skin above them, is caused by oxidative stress on the tissues. Green, red and yellow fruits and vegetables, which are naturally high in antioxidants, can help prevent oxidative stress and the resulting vein damage.

Make a move: Exercise will help keep your blood circulating to prevent it from pooling and clotting in your legs. As I mentioned earlier, it's the movements of the muscles in your legs that keeps blood moving upward out of your legs towards your heart. If you have a desk job, or spend a lot of time sitting, you need to make it a habit to get up and move around more even if it's just taking a stroll around the office or the dining room table every hour to start. And try to find a low impact hobby you enjoy that keeps you active.

Start some supplements: There are several herbs that can help prevent varicose and spider veins, as well as help relieve some of your symptoms if you already have them.

Research on ginkgo biloba suggests the herb may be able to help strengthen vein wall tissues as well as widen and relax blood vessels. I recommend an extract of at least 24% in a dose of 40 mg three times daily.

The antioxidant herb pycnogenol, extracted from a type of French pine bark, has been shown to help with blood flow. In a placebo-controlled randomized study published in the Italian journal Fitoterapia, researchers demonstrated that the herb helps to improvement venous function. I typically advise my own patients to start off on a daily dose of 200 mg for two months.

Butcher's Broom—an evergreen bush native to the Mediterranean—and Horse Chestnut—a tree common in south Eastern Europe—have long been paired together in traditional medicine to treat varicose veins and hemorrhoids. Several studies have shown that Butcher's Broom can help reduce the swelling associated with chronic venous insufficiency. And research has proven that Horse Chestnut is able to help relieve the symptoms of CVI. I typically recommend 40 mg of Butcher's Broom and 100 mg of Horse Chestnut twice daily.

And finally, I recommend good old vitamin C with bioflavonoids. Vitamin C can help strengthen vein walls and keep them flexible. And studies suggest flavonoids may be able to help reduce vein leakage and swelling in the legs. I recommend 500-1000 mg twice daily.

Chapter 3:

Say goodbye to those dreaded "cottage cheese" thighs with my "Beat the Cellulite" plan

If you're at least 30 and female, chances are cellulite is already a reality for you. The appearance of dimpled skin—sometimes described as looking like orange peel or cottage cheese—is a nearly universal complaint for women over a certain age, plaguing at least 80 to 90 percent of women.

Cellulite can appear anywhere on your lower body… on your legs, hips or backside… regardless of your weight or physical fitness levels. And while cellulite isn't an illness, it is the result of the breakdown of healthy fat and connective tissue, much like we see with the breakdown of healthy joint tissues in arthritis.

Although cellulite has been studied quite a bit, it's still poorly understood. It can't simply be exercised away and it doesn't completely disappear with diet. And most doctors will simply shrug their shoulders if a woman bothers asking about how to treat it.

That's why you might be surprised to learn that there ARE some things you can do to reduce the appearance and progression of cellulite.

I'll tell you more about them in just a moment, but first let's take a closer look at exactly what cellulite is.

Connective tissue break down

Cellulite, also known as gynoid lipodystrophy or GLD for short, happens when the normal structure of the connective tissue breaks down, and the surrounding fat cells become water-logged and swollen.

The connective tissues in your body are made up of collagen, elastic fibers, hyaluronic acid containing "goo," proteoglycans and glycoproteins (substances that hold everything together on a cellular level). Together these materials are responsible for the movement of nutrients, fluid, oxygen and waste products in and out of your cells.

But when they become in-flamed and swollen the damaged tissues become less effective at their job. They start to suffer from a lack of nourishment, connections start to fail and eventually the tissues break down. While some of the fibrous connections remain, the cells around them are bloated and swollen producing that classic cellulite appearance.

Exposing the cellulite "curse"

There are several reasons why cellulite first appears, starting with genetics. If your mother had a significant amount of cellulite, chances are you will too.

Estrogen also plays a key role in the development of this unwelcome condition. Since women have more estrogen in their bodies than men, cellulite tends to be more of a woman's problem. Some guys do get it, but it's much rarer.

The last factor is one that you do have some control over, and that's lifestyle. If you happen to be overweight—a common problem as people age—you have a greater number of fat cells. Since fat cells produce estrogen, the more fat you're carrying around the more estrogen you're producing. And the more prone you will be to cellulite.

Losing weight can help reduce your estrogen levels improving the appearance of existing cellulite and discouraging new cellulite from forming.

Turn the cellulite tide

Besides weight loss, there are a number of other tricks you can try to turn the tide against cellulite.

Move every day to keep cellulite at bay: As I mentioned earlier, physical fitness isn't a guarantee that you won't experience cellulite. But, on the other hand, exercise is associated with less inflammation of the connective tissues.

In the real world that means that getting up and moving more can help your healthy connective tissues STAY healthy so they don't break down, leading to more cellulite. I typically recommend yoga or Pilate's to my own patients to keep the blood circulating, and to build the underlying muscle.

Ditch your pro-cellulite diet: Anti-inflammatory foods can help keep your connective tissues in tip top shape. But that's not the only way diet can help.

Eating too much salt, sugar, carbohydrates or unhealthy trans-fats can encourage cellulite to develop; cutting back on all of them can help keep your skin smooth and tight. A great way to do just that is by making the switch to the delicious Paleo diet, which focuses on the natural meats, fruits, vegetables and nuts our ancestors would have eaten. Going Paleo will not only help you get the proper amount of healthy fats and proteins, it can help lower your insulin levels as well. This is key because when your insulin levels drop you will naturally shed some of that excess estrogen-hoarding fat you've been carrying around.

Take toxins out of the mix: Toxins of any sort including food preservatives, heavy metals such as lead and mercury, mold and environmental chemicals can act as irritants on the connective tissues. This can cause those tissues to begin to break down forming the dimpled skin we all love to hate.

But you can help avoid new cellulite from appearing by reducing the toxins you're exposing yourself to by eating organic foods, dropping refined foods from your diet, switching from farmed fish to wild caught and sustain-able seafood instead, stopping smoking, ridding your home of mold and choosing cleaning and body care products that are free of harsh chemicals and metals.

Delve into the drug connection: Certain drugs can cause cellulite to get worse. Chemical—non bio-identical—estrogen replacement drugs are the most obvious culprits. But antihistamines, beta blockers (commonly used for high blood pressure, cardiac problems, and migraines) and thyroid medications can all contribute to tissue breakdown, and cellulite, as well.

If you're on any of these drugs and are concerned about the appearance of cellulite, talk with your doctor about potential alternatives. Reducing your antihistamine use and switching to bio-identical hormones may help.

Consider a nutrient cocktail: Mesotherapy, an injection technique used to direct substances into the mesodermic or connective tissue layer of the body, can be a very effective way to fight cellulite. I was first trained in the technique in 2004 in Southern France and in my clinic we use an injection gun to assure that we're getting exactly the right amount of nutrients into each injection.

In the case of cellulite, we inject a cocktail of nutrients including phosphatidylcholine (the critically important phospholipid that lines our nervous system and much of our connective tissue), caffeine, vitamins A and C, various amino acids, and an herb called butcher's broom.

After several mesotherapy sessions women typically find that the dimpled skin on their legs, thighs and buttocks is noticeably smoothed out. But keep in mind that mesotherapy isn't a quick-fix technique, it can take some time and it can also be pricey.

Try a topical instead: If you're having trouble finding someone to administer mesotherapy in your area, or you find the price is too steep for your pocketbook right now, a topical approach might be just what you're looking for.

In my own clinic we have a compounding pharmacy where we produce a cream with hyaluronic acid that penetrates into the tissues delivering vitamins, caffeine, and phospholipids directly into the damaged connective tissue.

A holistic medical doctor in your area can help tailor a topical cellulite-fighting formula for you, or you can try one of the cellulite creams on the market. There are several natural ingredients that show great promise in the fight against those dreaded cottage cheese thighs.

Vitamin A is involved in the formation of those glycoproteins I mentioned earlier. These important proteins help to hold everything together on a cellular level and play a critical role in the health of connective tissues. Vitamin A may be able to help build collagen and restore elasticity to skin. You'll find vitamin A added to a number of skin products designed to improve skin appearance and reduce cellulite.

Caffeine helps break down fat tissue while enhancing the tightening of underlying connective material. Most topical cellulite formulas contain caffeine.

Both butcher's broom and forskolin, the active ingredient in the herb gotu kola (Asiatic centella), can stimulate blood capillaries and improve microcirculation within tissues. This means they can help reduce the fluid retention that's seen with cellulite improving the appearance of the skin. These herbs are often included in over the counter and compounded cellulite products.

Silicon is one of the building blocks of connective tissue and plays a critical role in the formation and reformation of the proteoglycans I mentioned earlier.

A personalized plan

In my clinic we will often combine a number of these techniques to tackle their cellulite. We work with people on their lifestyle issues such as reducing stress and adjusting their diet and exercise, and we utilize a number of topical, injectable and oral natural remedies to strengthen underlying tissues.

We carefully evaluate the buildup of various toxins in the fat cells in the body and create a plan for reducing each person's toxic burden. (You can start reducing your own toxic load using some of the tips I shared above.) And we perform hormone testing and work to restore your hormone balance. You can talk with your own doctor about having your hormones tested.

Manual therapies such as heavy kneading of the affected tissues, and mechanical treatments such as laser therapy and ultrasonic therapies can have their use in addressing cellulite, but they don't get at the root of the problem and should generally be considered only after all the other avenues have been explored.

Chapter 4:

Forget your annual mammogram! New tool offers better, earlier breast cancer detection (and it's pain-free, too!)

Over the years, I have heard from many women who have reservations about mammography for breast cancer, and some who just refuse to get mammograms altogether—especially every year for a decade or more. Their concerns are understandable: While it's true that mammograms have increased the detection of breast cancer, more and more flaws associated with this screening tool have come to light too.

Some studies have found the sensitivity of mammography to be as low as 25 percent. In other words, it only detects about one quarter of breast cancers. Mammograms' "specificity" (accurately identifying an area as cancerous) is even worse: It can be as low as 17 percent—which means that as many as 83 percent of areas deemed "suspicious" from mammogram images actually turn out not to be cancerous after further checking. Obviously, this puts many women and their families through a great deal of unnecessary worry and emotional turmoil.

In addition, a little-publicized Canadian study of over 70,000 women found that mammograms done between ages 40 and 50 actually did not increase the breast cancer detection rate! The researchers attributed this finding to the fact that women's breast tissue is denser between ages 40 and 50 (after age 50 breast tissue "thins out" due to menopause). Even though this study is well-known among medical "authorities" in these United States—and has never been refuted—these same "authorities" rarely mention it, and continue to recommend annual mammograms to all women over the age of 40.

But besides the general lack of accuracy, there's an even darker side to mammography. It involves radiation, which (if repeated) actually contributes to breast cancer risk. In fact, each mammogram increases risk of breast cancer by 1 percent. So if you follow the "expert" recommendation to get a mammogram every year after you turn 40, by the time you're 50, you'll already have increased your chance of getting breast cancer by 10 percent.

And a follow-up to the Canadian study mentioned above disclosed that the women in the 40 to 50 year age group who'd had annual mammograms actually had a slightly higher death rate from cancer than women who only underwent manual breast exams.

Certainly doesn't seem like a very good trade off!

All this probably leaves you wondering if there isn't something else you can do to detect breast cancer—especially early cases. We've been wondering the same thing for a long time! Fortunately, there is equipment that can do the job.

Detect cancer without increasing your risk

In the 1950s it was discovered that cancerous tissue maintains a steady temperature independent of cooling or heating the surrounding tissue—and the concept of thermography for breast cancer screening was born. Thermography has been researched since then, gaining FDA "approval" in 1982 (the same year "regular" mammography was approved, incidentally). Many versions of thermography (with variable reliability) have existed, leading up to this latest version, called infrared thermography, which has proved to be very reliable: It only misses 5 to10 percent of cancers and the number of false positives is equally low.

Infrared thermography detects differences in heat given off by the body (in this case, the breasts) by precise measurement of infrared frequency wavelengths. These wavelengths are very close to visual frequencies, and measuring them doesn't involve radiation like what is used in mammography, x-ray, CAT scans, and other tests. So thermography won't increase cancer risk, since nothing is "beamed" into or at the body.

In addition to not using radiation, thermography has other advantages too. First of all, there is no compression of the breasts, which is good news for at least three reasons: 1.) It's painless; 2.) Women with implants can relax; and 3.) It eliminates the concern that preexisting cancer will be spread by the compression of the tissue.

Another benefit of thermography is that it's very likely—although not yet proven—that it's more accurate for women ages 40 to 50, since breast tissue density makes no difference to heat emissions.

Thermography can also tell you and your doctor other important things about your breast health in addition to assessing the possibility of cancer. It's also possible for it to identify fibrocystic breast disease and hormone imbalances.

Of course, the goal is always to prevent breast cancer.

Prevention is even more important than detection—even early detection—and thermography can help with that, too. In contrast to mammography, which detects only anatomical changes in the breasts, thermography detects functional changes in breast tissue. It finds areas of abnormally increased or decreased blood flow. This is a huge advantage, since cancer takes approximately 5 to10 years to reach a size detectable with mammography or physical exam. With thermography, we're able to monitor functional changes associated with very early breast cancer and possibly even changes which precede breast cancer. Although it's too soon to say for certain, it's very possible that appropriate treatment may reverse those risk-associated changes.

So with the goal of prevention in mind, I now recommend that women have a yearly breast thermogram starting at age 40, or age 30 if you have a family history of breast cancer.

What to expect from the breast thermography "experience"

To make sure thermography is as accurate as possible, temperature reading is the "name of the game," so the procedure is performed in a room kept at 68° F. You sit in this cool temperature wearing the infamous "examination gown" (definitely not Dior!) for 15-20 minutes while your breast health history is reviewed. After you've acclimated to the temperature, a set of three pictures is taken—one frontal and two oblique (an angle between front and side)—followed by a one-minute "autonomic nervous system stress test" and another set of three images.

The autonomic system stress test involves placing your hands in cold water for exactly one minute. This challenge tells your body to send all the available heat via the blood from the surface of the body, inward. Any breast tissue that isn't functioning properly will not be able to do this and will then be highlighted on the second set of images.

Your appointment is finished with a manual breast exam, the findings of which are included in the notes that are sent with the thermographic images to be interpreted. (All thermographic images are sent electronically via the Internet to a qualified expert in thermographic image interpretation.)

Buyer beware

Although thermography is FDA "approved" it is still in the early stages of organization, so the facilities offering it may or may not have kept up with the many advances in thermographic technology. A high quality thermographic imaging facility should at least include the following four things:

- **Temperature-controlled room:** This is a must, since you're measuring temperatures! If the room is too hot, the results won't be accurate.

- **High-definition radiometric camera:** This kind of camera measures actual temperatures, not temperatures calculated from colors on the image or averaged temperatures from a video card. With this type of camera, temperature measurement is much more accurate and can be repeated and compared with even more accuracy.

- **Autonomic challenge test:** As I mentioned above, the autonomic challenge is usually done by having the client place her hands in cold water for 60 seconds. Although it's not the most pleasant experience, it's vital to a complete infrared thermogram and greatly increases the accuracy. Without it, the number of abnormal results are often much higher than they actually should be and cause unnecessary follow-up testing and considerable worry. (As a side note, non-radiometric cameras will not be able to detect the changes caused by the autonomic challenge test.)

- **Quantitative and qualitative interpretation:** This is the most up-to-date interpretation scoring system at this time. It includes both "qualitative" data—including hot spots, cold spots or irregular vascular patterns, along with "quantitative" data, which includes temperature readings from each of the 76,000 "pixels" recorded by the radiometric camera.

At present, there are many more practitioners offering mammograms than infrared thermograms, but the number of certified thermographers is growing. To find a certified thermographer near you, go to the International Association Of Certified Thermographers (IACT) website: www.iactthermography.org.

To read more about the thermography research discussed above, please refer to the following study:

Kuhl CK. "The 'coming of age' of non-mammography screening for breast cancer." *JAMA* 2008; 299(18): 2,203-2,205

I am very grateful to Olivia Franks, N.D., C.T.T (Certified Thermographic Technician) for much of the information contained in this chapter.

Chapter 5:

The natural secret to great sex after menopause

Over the years, it seems that much more attention has been paid to male sexual health and satisfaction than it has to female. Contrary to what the mainstream medical community might want to believe, that women are interested in having fulfilling sex lives too—yes, even after menopause. But sometimes it just physically isn't that easy. Atrophic vaginitis can make sex downright unpleasant for many women. This condition is very common and includes symptoms like vaginal dryness, itching or burning, painful sexual intercourse, light bleeding after intercourse, and sometimes incontinence.

You may have all of these symptoms or just a few. But, since the usual treatment for this problem is hormone replacement therapy (HRT), you may have decided to "just live with it," rather than face the risks that have recently surfaced regarding synthetic hormone replacement.

Keep in mind you can take hormone replacement safely with all-natural, identical-to-human HRT, but there may be an even simpler solution—all-natural ginseng.

Decades ago, a British researcher found that Panax ginseng can be used effectively to treat atrophic vaginitis. Women with a history of vaginal dryness and painful intercourse were asked to volunteer for biopsies of the vaginal mucosa. When examined microscopically, the biopsy specimens showed typical atrophy, with a thinner skin and little to no mucous production. Physical examination prior to biopsy showed the same changes.

The women were asked to take Panax ginseng for two to three months. Repeat biopsies showed significantly thickened mucosa with more normal surface mucous. Physical examination showed the same types of changes, and women reported disappearance of vaginal dryness and painful intercourse.

I usually advise 100 milligrams of a standardized Panax ginseng extract three times daily. After comfort has returned and symptoms have diminished, you can usually lower your dosage of ginseng to an appropriate maintenance level that works for you.

No one should have to give up hope, comfort, or great sex after menopause. If any of the symptoms listed above apply to you, Panax ginseng is certainly worth a try. It's available in almost any natural food store, as well as many pharmacies and supermarkets.

Chapter 6:

Breast cancer—stop the most feared disease among women from happening to you

It's no wonder that breast cancer is the biggest fear of so many women. All you hear about these days are the dismal odds: Currently, researchers expect one in eight women—that's 17 million—to be diagnosed with the disease. And the treatment options are nothing short of barbaric: Surgery that leaves you disfigured, radiation that leaves you swollen and tender, and chemotherapy that leaves you weak, bald, and nauseous.

Sure, there are a few brave women (like Suzanne Somers) who refuse the conventional recommendations and opt for alternative natural therapies. But even if they succeed in their fight against the disease, they have to endure the constant and critical questioning of their decision—not exactly the most supportive environment for a cancer patient (who needs it most).

But with all of the attention focused on breast cancer lately, I'm disappointed at how much of it is geared toward, basically, waiting until a woman actually has the disease and dealing with it then. Unfortunately, this has been the standard practice for years—though I'm sure you'd rather not become a part of that "standard." So why not focus on preventing breast cancer before it ever happens?

Most mainstream doctors would probably say that we just don't know enough about the causes of breast cancer to focus on prevention. That's partially true: Not all of the causes of the disease have been identified, so you can't completely eliminate the risk. But we do know about enough causes and risk factors to make it possible for you to cut your risk way back. First you have to determine just how at risk you are.

Measuring your levels of various estrogens is a simple technique to help predict if you're at higher risk for certain types of cancer (especially breast and uterine). Then, once you have that information, supplementing with the right kind of estrogen (along with other supplements and a diet rich in certain foods) can reduce your risk of ever getting those cancers—or possibly even help treat existing cases.

But since not all estrogen is created equal, let's take a few minutes to go over some of the intricacies.

Five estrogen metabolites you need to know about

The term estrogen doesn't actually describe a single molecule; instead, it's a "group word" covering two dozen or more molecules all built on a common framework. Since these molecules are transformed (metabolized) one into another into another, they're also all called estrogen metabolites.

The "early days" of estrogen research focused mostly on three estrogen metabolites called estrone, estradiol, and estriol.

Over the last three decades, with improved analytic techniques and evolving research interest, attention has turned to some of the other estrogen metabolites, including "good" and "bad" estrogens. The technical terms for these are 2-hydroxyestrogen (good) and 16a-hydroxyestrogen (bad), and together they make up what's known as the 2/16 ratio. High 2/16 ratios generally mean a lower risk of estrogen-related cancers (like breast, uterine, and ovarian). Low 2/16 ratios mean higher risk of these same cancers. (I've also observed an unusual number of low 2/16 ratios in men with newly diagnosed prostate cancer, and men with a strong family history of cancer.)

The good news is, testing your own 2/16 ratio couldn't be easier. You don't even have to leave home to do it. Some changes in the actual testing equipment have made the process a lot easier. In fact, the testing kits can be mailed to you at home, where you'll collect a urine specimen in the container provided. If you're pre-menopausal, try to collect the urine specimen during days 19 to 23 of your 28-day cycle, and be sure to note the cycle day and time, in case you need to take a repeat test or two. When you've collected your sample, just mail it back to the lab.

Once you send your sample back to the lab, it generally takes about two to three weeks to get your results.

Eat your way to a breast cancer-free future

You definitely want more "good" (2) estrogen than "bad" (16) estrogen—substantially more if possible. So when you get your results, check the proportion of these two substances: Any ratio below 1.0 is unfavorable. Although there's no consensus on an ideal ratio number, I recommend 2.0 or greater if possible.

If your 2/16 ratio is less than 1.0, there's a good chance you'll be able to boost it just by eating a few specific foods. Start with Brassica (or mustard family) vegetables. These include cabbage, broccoli, cauliflower, bok choy, Brussels sprouts and many others. You can also eat freshly ground flaxseed, 1 tablespoonful daily. You don't need to go overboard with Brassica vegetables. I know it seems odd to be warning you not to eat too many vegetables, but it is possible for Brassicas to cause suppressed thyroid function and even goiter if you eat a lot of them on a daily basis. Three to four servings a week is a good general range.

In a lot of cases, just eating these foods will bring a low 2/16 ratio to 1.0 or above in just four to six weeks without any other specific supplementation. But if you find you're still not getting sufficient improvement, you can also take di-indolylmethane (DIM) supplements to boost it even further. DIM is actually a substance found in Brassica vegetables, but it's also available in most health food stores in supplement form. If you need some extra help, take 60 milligrams three times daily, and check your 2/16 ratio again in another four to six weeks.

Should you or shouldn't you?
An answer to the soy question

When soy became a big-ticket item for American business giants, we were hit with an enormous wave of pro-soy promotion. Some of it is actually true. For example, in Asian countries where soy products are eaten regularly, the incidence of breast cancer is definitely lower.

But there's also been a "research backlash," including a recent study showing that former breast cancer patients who ate soy had a higher rate of cancer recurrence than a control group that ate no soy.

Despite the negative soy research, I'm not completely anti-soy. There is also a good deal of research about soy's health benefits. And incorporating soy products (tofu, tempeh, soy milk, etc.) into your diet is a good option for boosting 2/16 ratios. A little goes a long way though, and two or three servings a week is plenty.

Another do-it-yourself breast cancer risk test

There's another estrogen ratio that's just as important as the 2/16 for estimating your risk of estrogen- related cancer. It's called the estrogen quotient, or EQ.

As I mentioned above, early estrogen research focused mostly on three estrogen metabolites: Estrone (also labeled E1), estradiol (E2), and estriol (E3). Although it's only present in small quantities in the body, estradiol is the most "potent" estrogen, responsible for most of the feminizing changes of puberty. Unfortunately, estradiol and its nearby metabolite estrone were both found to be carcinogenic. Researchers found that the body treats these two hormones with extreme care, rapidly converting them to estriol. As far as anyone could tell, estriol didn't have any carcinogenic tendencies.

With all of this in mind, Henry Lemon, M.D. (a women's cancer specialist), came up with an equation that, like the 2/16 ratio, can estimate a woman's risk of breast cancer. He called this idea the estrogen quotient, or EQ, and formally it's the amount of estriol divided by the sum of the amounts of estrone and estradiol. In mathematical terms, it looks something like this: $EQ = E3 / (E1 + E2)$.

If a woman's EQ is low, her risk of breast cancer is higher. Basically, the higher the EQ, the better.

Sounds too easy to be true, but time after time the EQ proved itself. Take a look at some of Dr. Lemon's EQ research:

In 34 women with no signs of breast cancer, Dr. Lemon found the EQ to be a median of 1.3 before menopause and 1.2 afterward. The picture was quite different in 26 women with breast cancer. Their median EQ was 0.5 before menopause and 0.8 afterward.

In another study, Dr. Lemon found that women with higher EQs survived significantly longer after cancer surgery than women with lower EQs.

So, knowing that women need more estriol to boost their EQs, Dr. Lemon also tried using estriol treatments for breast cancer. He asked a small group of women with untreatable breast cancer (because it had metastasized to bones) to take a large dose of estriol. By the end of the study, an astounding 40 percent of these women had their cancers go into remission.

Less estriol, more cancer

Of course Dr. Lemon's EQ and estriol findings met with their share of criticism, and some researchers did publish claims disputing Dr. Lemon's results. But there was also plenty of additional evidence supporting him. For example:

• In one study of 150 close relatives (sisters and daughters) of breast cancer patients, researchers found that the majority had lower levels of estriol and higher levels of estrone and estradiol than women without a family history of the disease.

- American women (who have higher levels of breast cancer) have lower levels of estriol than Asian women (who have lower levels of breast cancer). Asian women living in Hawaii had levels of estriol midway between American women and Asian women living in Asia…and their levels of breast cancer were also midway between American and Asian women.

- Estriol enhances the ability of white blood cells to consume viruses, bacteria, and cancer cells.

- Women who have had children have significantly lower risk of breast cancer than women who have never had a child. During pregnancy, estriol levels climb enormously—by 1,000 times or more. Even after childbirth, estriol levels usually remain higher than they were before pregnancy.

This last bit of "pro-estriol" evidence concerning pregnancies leads me to some recent estriol research, which is once again reviving the "more estriol, less cancer" hypothesis.

A one-time boost can protect you for up to 40 years

In this one, 15,000 women were studied during a pregnancy occurring between 1959 and 1967. Invasive breast cancer cases or deaths from breast cancer were tabulated through 1997. What makes this study so remarkable is the fact that it looked ahead so far into the future of such a large group of women. Prospective studies like this are considered much more reliable than retrospective studies (ones that look back on information after it has occurred). And the results of this particular prospective study make it even more impressive:

The researchers found a clear protective effect based on the amount of estriol the women produced during their pregnancies: More estriol, less cancer later in life. Women in the uppermost 25 percent of estriol production during pregnancy had 58 percent less breast cancer over the next 30 to 40 years than women with the lowest 25 percent of estriol.

The authors concluded (cautiously, of course—they'd be laughed out of their lab coats by mainstream medical "experts" if they didn't downplay findings that nature might know best after all): "If confirmed, these results could lead to breast cancer prevention or treatment regimens that seek to block estradiol estrogen action using estriol, similar to treatments based on the synthetic anti-estrogen, tamoxifen."

After a decade or two of neglect, the EQ and the "estriol hypothesis" of estrogen-related cancer prediction and prevention (and maybe even treatment, like Dr. Lemon's unpublished research) are back. And some researchers are even starting to admit that maybe, just maybe, estriol in its natural form might work as well as (or even better than) synthetic drugs like tamoxifen.

What's your EQ?

Dr. Lemon tested estriol along with estrone and estradiol by having women collect their urine for 24 hours, then measuring the hormone levels in the specimens. It's still done the same way, and, like the 2/16 ration test, you can have a kit mailed to you at home, which makes things much more convenient, since you'll need to collect all your urine for a 24-hour period (only a small portion of the total collected amount is actually mailed in for testing, though).

If you haven't gone through menopause yet, and you have a menstrual cycle that follows the typical 28-day pattern, pick a 24-hour period between days 19 and 23 of your cycle (day 1 being the first day of menstrual bleeding) to collect your sample. If you've already gone through menopause, you can collect your sample anytime.

Again, once you send your sample back to the lab, it generally takes about two to three weeks to get your results.

The virtually fail-safe EQ-booster:
You may only need one drop a day

When your results arrive in the mail, you'll see all of your different hormone levels listed. The ones we're most concerned with for determining breast cancer risk via the EQ are estriol, estrone, and estradiol. Remember, it's not the absolute amount of estriol that appears to be the most important number but the relative amount of estriol compared with the sum of estradiol and estrone. Again, the equation looks like this: EQ= E3 / (E2 + E1).

The lab report might already have your EQ calculated and listed. Some labs today consider EQs of 0.4 to 0.6 as normal. But when Dr. Lemon did his research back in the 1960s and 1970s, he found that women need an EQ of at least 1.0 (this level or above was considered favorable; the further below 1.0, the more unfavorable). So was Dr. Lemon wrong?

Well, let's put it this way: If women only need an EQ of 0.4, why has breast cancer risk gone up? Not only do I think you still need an EQ of at least 1.0, as Dr. Lemon found 40 years ago, but in today's environment, with the amount of estrogen-mimicking carcinogens increasing dramatically, it's more important than ever to keep your level of estriol as high as possible. So I don't see any reason why we shouldn't still follow Dr. Lemon and shoot for an EQ of 1.0 or above.

If your EQ is below 1.0, there's a simple, almost fail-safe solution: SSKI. SSKI is a solution that combines iodine and potassium. It's the iodine that works to boost the EQ: Iodide (and iodine) reliably promote the metabolism of estrone and estradiol into estriol.

Take six to eight drops of SSKI mixed in several ounces of water daily for two to three months. Then repeat your test, doing the 24-hour urine collection at the same time of the month as your first one. More likely than not, your follow-up EQ will be above 1.0—sometimes considerably above. If it is, try tapering down the SSKI to the smallest amount that helps you maintain your EQ at 1.0 or above. Some women find that they only need one drop a day, though others need more.

Although SSKI is safe for the overwhelming majority of people, there are individuals who are very sensitive to it. On rare occasion, long-term use of larger quantities of SSKI may cause thyroid suppression. Thyroid blood tests always pick up on this if it occurs.

Start today to make sure you're cancer-free tomorrow

There's no reason to just wait and hope that you're not that one woman in eight who gets breast cancer. The 2/16 ratio and the EQ provide two easy ways to estimate your own risk of breast, uterine, and other estrogen-related cancers.

For more information on these tests, contact a physician-member of The American College for Advancement in Medicine (ACAM) at (800)532-3688 or www.acam.org or the International College for Integrative Medicine at (419)358-0273 or www.icimed.com.

If your risk factor calculations are unfavorable, or even if they're just OK, there are things you can do yourself—starting today—to lessen your breast cancer risk. Cancer is a frightening thing, but don't let that fear paralyze you: Do something about it—and pass the information along to your daughters and granddaughters, too!

Part XI

Men's Health

Chapter 1:

Become "King of the Bedroom" again! Powerful three-part combo helps reverse erectile dysfunction

Nothing messes with a man's head more than an episode of erectile dysfunction (ED). It can make even the most confident guy start to question his manhood.

ED can be an upsetting—and embarrassing—topic for men and their doctors. Which is why many health experts (including me) believe that research estimating that 10 percent of the world's population suffers from ED is way too low.

The fact is, if you're a senior suffering from ED, you're not alone. When you're in your 20s you have around a 6.5 percent chance of experiencing ED. But as your age rises your risk for ED jumps right along with it. By the time you reach 75 (and beyond) that risk will have climbed up to 77.5 percent.

If there's one piece of good news about ED it's that you don't need some pricey and dangerous prescription drug to get your sex life rolling again. In fact, I've found that three all-natural supplements may be all it takes to banish your bedroom woes for good.

But first let me explain what's *really* causing your ED.

From diabetes to drugs… ED has many triggers

Carrying around extra pounds, smoking and diabetes will all raise your risk of experiencing erection issues. In some studies, about half of the men with diabetes report having erectile dysfunction. Add that to that the number of men who have ED due to heart disease, and that accounts for 70 percent of all cases of the disorder.

But the most overlooked—and perhaps easily correctable—cause of erectile issues is prescription medications. ED is a stunningly common side effect of a whole slew of popular drugs.

Using the SIDER 2, an online side effects resource tool, I've counted no fewer than 84 prescription drugs that list erectile dysfunction as a side effect! Some of the main culprits are:

- **Antidepressants and antianxiety agents.** That's a huge problems because many doctors wrongly assume ED issues are psychological and prescribe these drugs.

- **Cardiac medications.** Calcium channel blockers, angiotensin II antagonists and non-selective beta blockers have all been linked to ED. All three classes are widely used to treat heart disease and hypertension, making it likely that much of the ED attributed to heart disease is actually a side effect of these drugs.

- **ED meds like Viagra and Cialis.** Believe it or not, these pills can actually worsen heart disease (and ED associated with heart disease), and can create a dangerous situation when combined with certain cardiac drugs.

Tackle erectile dysfunction with this triple threat

Fortunately, my research has led me to a natural three-part combo that safe… that's been proven to help restore erectile function… and could give you your bedroom mojo back in a hurry.

In a breakthrough study published in the World Journal of Pharmacy and Pharmaceutical Sciences, researchers found that a combination of l-arginine, Pycnogenol and Red ginseng may help successfully treat erectile dysfunction in most guys.

Better blood flow means stronger erections

L-arginine has many roles in the body, but its main uses are tied to its ability to form a substance called nitric oxide (NO). One of NO's primary functions is to relax blood vessels, including those located in the muscles of the corpus callosum, the channels of the penis that engorge with blood during sexual arousal.

When there's more NO present there's greater blood flow into the penis resulting in a stronger erection.

In fact, drugs like Viagra work by enhancing the effect of nitric oxide on the penis—but they still need L-arginine to produce the NO.

A number of studies, including some double-blind placebo controlled crossover studies, have confirmed L-arginine's unique ability to relieve ED. But combining it with Pycnogenol and Red ginseng seems to supercharge its effects.

Bark leads to dramatically increased blood flow

Pycnogenol, extracted from the bark of French pine trees, is a potent antioxidant and anti-inflammatory.

The extract is one case in which the whole really does exceed the sum of its parts. When studied separately the individual flavonoids and other organic acids found in Pycnogenol don't do very much for ED.

But together they form a powerful synergistic response. Pycnogenol dramatically increases overall blood flow, especially to the sexual organs.

Combo leads to over 90% improvement!

In one recent study, 40 men ages 25-45 with documented ED were given oral L-arginine for a month. The dose was relatively low, but the researchers did record a mild positive effect.

In the second month, 40 mg of Pycnogenol was added twice a day. The results were incredible… the men had a nearly 80 percent improvement.

But the researchers didn't stop there. They bumped up the dose of Pycnogenol in the third month and the improvement skyrocketed to over 90 percent!

Red ginseng, the third component of this "magic" ED formula, is no slouch either. Sometimes called Korean ginseng, Panax ginseng or Asian ginseng—and abbreviated KRG—Red ginseng is traditionally used in Chinese medicine to increase stamina, strength and virility in men.

And research reveals why.

KRG is very effective and exceptionally safe

Several studies have confirmed that KRG can be used to both treat, and prevent, male sexual dysfunction. In one double-blind, placebo-controlled study—published in the Asian Journal of Andrology—80 men with documented ED were given either 1,000 mg of KRG or a placebo. The results were uniformly positive.

In another study, published in the British Journal of Clinical Pharmacology, researchers poured over 28 studies on the use of KRG to treat ED. They identified seven which were of high enough quality to include in their meta-analysis.

The analysis revealed that not only did KRG perform significantly better than a placebo, but that the herbal remedy was also exceptionally safe to use.

Keeping it real with Korean ginseng

Korean Red ginseng (also known as Panax or Asian ginseng) shouldn't be confused with Siberian ginseng. The Siberian variety doesn't contain the ginsenosides that scientists believe are the active, and therapeutic, ingredients found in the other ginsengs. So be sure to read the label to make sure you're getting the right kind.

In fact, one great thing about this combination of L-Arginine, Pycnogenol and Red Ginseng for male sexual dysfunction is its safety record. And this is essential in an ED remedy, since the potential side effects of Viagra, Cialis and other common ED drugs aren't tolerated well by many men, and are dangerous to some.

Chapter 2:

This dangerous sleep disorder could be the real reason for your "overactive bladder"

As a guy approaches the age of 50, along with the sudden desire to buy a sports car he can expect to start hearing some complaints from his prostate.

It's basically a rite of passage, which is probably why I have so many bleary eyed men stumble into my office convinced that their prostate is to blame for their frequent nighttime trips to the bathroom. Many are shocked when I explain their prostate is fine, but then ask them if they snore.

It may seem like a strange question to ask a guy who comes in for trouble with an overactive bladder, but it's a question more doctors should be asking. Because frequent overnight urination is often caused by something *far* more sinister than a swollen prostate... and that's sleep apnea.

It's a connection that far too few doctors make, but if you're getting up more than twice a night to pee sleep apnea could be the cause.

A recent study published in October 2015 found that 84 percent of patients with sleep apnea suffered from frequent nighttime urination. But once that apnea was treated those round trips to the toilet dropped off significantly.

I'll connect the dots between sleep apnea and frequent urination in a moment, but first let's take a quick look at what sleep apnea actually is.

Sleep apnea comes with serious dangers

When you ask if they snore, for some reason most people laugh. But it's far from a laughing matter because sleep apnea and poor sleep are literally hazardous to your health.

Sleep apnea is far more than "just snoring." It's a serious condition that can have life-threatening health consequences. In one 2008 study published in the journal *Sleep*, researchers linked the condition to early death.

Sleep apnea causes you to literally <u>stop breathing</u> for short periods of time over and over again throughout the night. Your body reacts to this emergency by sending out a surge of adrenaline into your blood stream to jolt you awake to so you don't die.

And while those adrenaline surges save your life they cause *other* problems.

And it's not just fatigue that's a problem. Sleep apnea has been tied to pretty much every major killer in the industrialized world including high blood pressure, heart failure, atrial fibrillation, stroke, depression, obesity and car accidents. The bottom line is the worse you sleep the earlier you die.

Those adrenaline surges are *also* linked to that frequent nighttime urination I mentioned earlier.

You see, each surge of adrenaline diverts blood from your heart to your brain and this sudden shift increases production of a hormone called atrial natriuretic peptide (ANP). It's the ANP that makes your body produce more urine.

Racking up frequent flyer miles

The trouble is many people who suffer from sleep apnea have no idea they even have the condition, as a study published in the journal *Archives of Internal Medicine* illustrates perfectly.

The study was conducted in a sleep lab and a total of 80 patients were eventually observed by researchers. Whenever a subject woke up the researchers recorded what caused the patient to awaken... such as loud snoring or, most often, sleep apnea. The patient was then asked what he believed had caused him to wake up.

According to the researchers, the vast majority of the volunteers who woke up because of sleep disorders such as apnea attributed their waking to the pressure to urinate. Only five percent of the participants correctly identified the *real* reason they woke up.

Not really a surprise since were always asleep when apnea occurs so it's easy to not even know it's happening. And although heavy snoring *can* accompany sleep apnea, it doesn't always, so even those with a spouse may be unaware of the issue.

But since most folks *are* often able to recall how often they have to drag themselves out of bed for a bathroom run, racking up frequent flyer miles running back and forth to the bathroom night after night s can be an important clue to an undiagnosed sleep disorder. In fact, there's even been some research done which revealed that asking a patient how many times he urinates a night could be *as* reliable a predictor of sleep apnea as some of the *other* current testing methods used to diagnose the condition.

Misdiagnosis can leave you drowsy and drugged

Sleep apnea is shockingly common with an estimated 22 million Americans suffering from this dangerous condition. Twenty percent of adult men and nine percent of adult women will experience some form of sleep apnea in their adult life. Yet 80 percent of those cases go undiagnosed.

And it's not just the apnea alone that's dangerous, misdiagnosis leads to people being prescribed heavy-duty meds that they don't even need.

In fact, I just recently took one of my own patients off his prostate medication after I successfully treated his sleep apnea. And he's far from alone. Countless men end up on prostate shrinking or artery dilating meds they shouldn't be taking... and saddled with the disturbing side effects that go with them including dizziness, fatigue, impotence, decreased sex drive and even breast growth.

While many women end up on unneeded bladder-drying medications that deliver some serious side effects of their own including dry mouth and severe dizziness that can lead to devastating falls.

Even worse, far too many rushed-doctors respond to a patient's complaint of "trouble sleeping" by prescribing a sleep drug that not only may mask the problem but could turn a bad situation into a deadly one. The drugs can leave you unable to awaken from the snoring and apnea.

Putting a stop to sleep apnea

If you find yourself waking up multiple times a night, if you snore or if you find you get very sleepy during the day you should ask your doctor about sleep monitoring. Some insurances pay for a sleep study in your own home, and others will pay for an overnight sleep test in a clinic or hospital. Trying to sleep hooked up to a bunch of wires, or in a strange bed isn't the most comfortable way to spend a night, but it can help firm up a diagnosis.

If you're diagnosed with sleep apnea your doctor will most likely want to prescribe a device called a Continuous Positive Air Pressure machine, or CPAP for short. CPAP is a mask that you wear that continuously pushes air through your nose to keep your airway open so you don't stop breathing. CPAP is very effective. However the mask can be cumbersome and takes some getting used to, and as a result many people stop using them.

A more permanent solution is to lose weight. People who are carrying around some extra pounds are more prone to sleep apnea, but studies show that shedding the extra weight can help. In a 2000 study researchers found that for every 10 percent of weight lost sleep apnea decreases an impressive 26 percent.

While you work on losing the weight temporary fixes such as an anti-snoring mouth piece from your dentist or Breathe-Right-Nasal strips may help. And since sleep apnea typically occurs when sleeping on your back, learning to be a side sleeper can help.

Chapter 3:

Was your last testosterone number dead wrong? Here are the 4 tests that give you the real story

A couple weeks ago, a successful and fairly health-conscious 62-year-old man walked into my office with a problem I hear a lot: he couldn't build any muscle or strength.

He wasn't fatigued—far from it. He had a busy job and exercised like a demon every day. But he always ended up feeling physically weak, like he hadn't been exercising at all.

On top of that, here are some of the other symptoms he was experiencing:

- loss of sexual desire

- an inability to maintain erections like he did a few years ago

- extra breast tissue

- skin tags on his neck

- excess weight in his gut, but not his hips
  (so, a high "waist-to-hip ratio").

When I asked him whether his physicians had measured his hormones, he gave the answer I'd come to expect: "Yes, and they said my testosterone level was normal for my age."

Unfortunately, lots of guys are hearing from their doctors that their testosterone levels are OK—and, in many cases, that information is dead wrong. That's because many physicians aren't doing much more than some superficial lab tests and a whole lot of guess work.

But if you want to restore your testosterone levels—and get your energy, strength, and sex life back—you need to know what's really going on in your body with this critical hormone. And I've developed a four-test protocol that can help you do just that.

It's not about how much you've got— but how much of it you can use

The first test I conduct is for free testosterone. Testosterone in the body is largely bound to a protein called "sex hormone binding globulin" (SHPG). While testosterone is bound, it's not active in the body. However, when the testosterone is unbound—or, "free"—it's able to be active.

As we age, our SHPG levels increases, which binds up more testosterone. And that leads to a decrease in free testosterone for our bodies to use. Without ample free testosterone, we don't get the full effect of this hormone on our metabolism, energy, circulation, and sexual function.

When we only measure total testosterone, as was done in my patient, we're looking at both the free and bound testosterone together, and not getting the full picture of what the problem is.

Too much of the wrong hormone could be stifling your manhood

The second test that I do for patients is for estradiol, a form of estrogen. Now we normally think of that as a female hormone—but both men and women have it, and this delicate balance between testosterone and estrogen has a lot to do with human sexuality.

We know, for instance, that testosterone is critical in women for libido, sexual sensitivity, and response. Less well-known is that estrogen, particularly estradiol, is necessary for male sexual response.

This stands to reason, since we know that estrogen receptors are abundant in the male brain, testes, and penis—and receptors mean that the body is expecting them to be stimulated.

Receptors for estrogen in the penis are predominantly in the neurovascular bundles of the erectile tissue, and so estrogen affects erectile function regardless of how much testosterone is in the body.

Estrogen is produced in the male brain in areas most important for sexual desire, and estrogen can make guys more fertile by playing a critical role in sperm production.

But its role in regulating the male reproductive system doesn't mean that estradiol necessarily *stimulates* it. In fact, it frequently can suppress male sexuality.

In general, the higher the estradiol in the body of a man, the less active the free testosterone is. And the body has pathways to actually convert testosterone into estradiol, so measuring testosterone without measuring estradiol is foolish. Men with the same testosterone levels but with varying levels of estradiol will experience very different health issues from each other.

I can't tell you how many patients on testosterone creams come to me with adequate levels of blood testosterone but without having experienced the benefits of testosterone therapy. When I examine them, they exhibit subtle signs of increased estrogen, like extra breast tissue and diminished size of the testicles. When I measure their estradiol levels, they are through the roof—because the testosterone is just converting into estradiol and negating itself.

The final puzzle pieces are in your blood... and your brain!

The last two tests I performed on my patient may surprise you.

The third is called the glycohemoglobin test, also known as HbA1c, and it tests the amount of sugar that's bound to the hemoglobin in your red blood cells over the course of three months (which is exactly the life span of a red blood cell).

You see, high blood sugar is associated with high blood pressure, high blood lipids, and a number of physical findings including skin tags around the neck and a big belly. And increasing belly fat raises the level of the enzyme that helps break testosterone down into estradiol...resulting in high estrogen levels...and low testosterone.

This association of belly fat with low testosterone has been demonstrated multiple times. In a study published in the *European Journal of Epidemiology*, researchers took over 1,500 men in a Norwegian town and measured their hormone levels, waist-to-hip ratio, and lifestyle factors. The most predictive factor for low testosterone, amazingly, was the circumference of the man's waist.[1]

And the final test measures a hormone secreted by the pituitary gland, which tells the testes to make more testosterone. Much like other pituitary hormones (like TSH or ACTH), the Luteinizing hormone or LH goes up in response to a low testosterone, in an effort to stimulate the production of more of it. If the testosterone is low and the LH is ALSO low, we know that the pituitary is exhausted, or isn't being stimulated by the hypothalamus, or is missing a key nutrient such as zinc or manganese. That's what makes testing LH so important.

When you need more than one test, you need more than one remedy

Now, my patient's total testosterone level was *technically* in the normal range, but it was at the low end of normal. His free testosterone, on the other hand, was clearly below normal, even for a man his age.

To make matters worse, his estradiol level was above the laboratory upper limit of 39 picograms per milliliter (pg/mL)—and in my office, we consider any estradiol level above 25 pg/mL to be suspect.

While his blood sugar wasn't in diabetic range at 5.8 percent, it certainly could be considered high enough for an increased risk of diabetes and well above the range associated with good health.

Finally, his LH was at the upper range of normal, which would be appropriate for someone who had a functionally low testosterone level.

As a result of my findings from these four tests, I put my patient on a custom compounded cream including a bioidentical form of testosterone as well as a herb called chrysin, which naturally inhibits the conversion of testosterone into estradiol.

I also put him on a boron supplement, which helps boost the production of testosterone, and the herb berberine to help control blood sugar. In addition, I used a medical food designed to enhance insulin sensitivity and weight loss.

Finally, I put him on a Paleo-style diet, which does wonders in terms of both weight loss and insulin/glucose management.

And you know what? Just two months later, my patient was thinner, more powerful than ever, and ready to take on the world!

Sometimes their "normal" isn't right for you

Gentlemen, if you've already come up "normal" on a traditional testosterone test...but still feel like something is not quite right...ask your doctor to do a little more digging. He should be able to run a full hormone panel blood test that includes free testosterone, estradiol, and LH—or, at least, send you to a specialist in endocrinology who can do it.

The HbA1c test, although widely available, is usually only run on diabetes patients in conventional medical practices, so your mainstream doctor may be puzzled why you'd ask for it. Even if he orders one for you, he may not know how to properly interpret the results, especially in relation to the findings from the other three tests.

So whether or not you've had your testosterone tested, your best bet is to find a holistic doctor who can look at the "big picture" of your hormonal imbalances and prescribe a whole body approach to getting everything back where they should be.

If you're in the Boston area, you can make an appointment to see us at The Rothfeld Center for Integrative Medicine www.rothfeldcenter. com. If you're not, you can find a well-qualified doctor of holistic medicine through the American College for Advancement in Medicine www. acam.org, of which I am a proud member.

Chapter 4:

Turn back the hands of time with testosterone. Powerful hormone helps you lose weight, lower blood sugar, and build strength... in and out of the bedroom!

One of the most effective treatments I offer in my practice is bioidentical hormone replacement—for both men and women.

It's remarkable to see how these treatments rejuvenate my patients' brains, muscles, bones, and sex lives—and they start noticing the difference quickly.

And there practically no hormone out there that produces better or faster results than testosterone.

I ask my male patients to remember what it was like when they were in their late teens and early 20s, and they always get a big smile on their faces. Their hormones were raging, they felt like Superman, and they never worried about getting sick.

It's not a stretch to think that their health was so amazing *because* of their high testosterone levels...and as their testosterone levels dipped, their health started to dwindle as well.

There's lots of scientific data that support this link between testosterone levels and good health. And keeping a male's testosterone level in the normal-to-optimal range is the goal of almost all integrative doctors.

But unfortunately, this therapy took a "hit" in the beginning of 2014 when the FDA placed an official warning on it.

So I'd like to take this opportunity to explain what happened...why the FDA responded as they did...and how they got it wrong.

No matter what you may have read or heard elsewhere, testosterone is safe and effective. And the latest research—a study you can *trust*, from a *reliable* source with *real* results—confirms it.

But first: a little background.

Two bad apples spoiled the bunch

In 2013 and 2014, testosterone replacement was at an all-time high. The pharmaceutical industry had poured a decent chunk of money in to advertising and educating the public about "Low T"...which was the one time those TV ads ever did more good than harm.

But testosterone therapy hit a big roadblock when two different published studies implicated testosterone therapy in an increased risk of heart attacks and strokes.

The FDA subsequently issued a black box warning[1]—and, within weeks, lawyers started to circle like bloodthirsty sharks, striking fear into patients, their spouses, and their children. The calls started to pour in to my office. Worried patients wanted to know if they should stop their testosterone therapy.

This was shocking information to me, because at that point I'd already treated many men with testosterone without ever seeing anything to make me cautious about giving it to them.

But, trying to be a responsible physician, I delved into the two nefarious studies—and what I found was shocking. I instantly noted that there were gaping holes and problems with both studies—especially the most damning one, published in the heralded *JAMA* magazine.[2]

I was outraged at the poor science being used in these studies—and, fortunately, I wasn't the only one.

In response to the shoddy studies, an organization called The Androgen Study Group immediately formed to make sure that the public and the medical community could be properly educated...with real facts... that would be accurately reported.

ASG organized 25 major medical societies[3] as well as over 160 distinguished medical experts from around the world to petition the FDA to reconsider issuing a black box warning on testosterone therapy.[4] While the FDA didn't accept the petition, they did eventually soften their stance on testosterone replacement.[5]

The medical experts of the ASG were so passionate and confident in the mistakes that had been made that they did something else, too— something that had never been done before. They petitioned *JAMA* to remove the study and print a full retraction from their prestigious and influential magazine, stating that "the quality and magnitude of these errors indicate gross data mismanagement and contamination, to a degree that the reported results are no longer reliable."[6]

JAMA was forced to issue two retractions to the erroneous and misleading study to boot.[7,8]

Of course, by then, the damage had already been done.

The Androgen Study Group Chairman Dr. Abraham Morgentaler perhaps put it best when he was quoted as saying, "*JAMA* has violated the public trust...and *JAMA*'s continued support of this discredited study, defying the worldwide community of experts, represents medical literature malpractice."[9]

Bad science can spread like a virus

But something good did come out of this debacle. The outrage caused hundreds of doctors to do what I did, and dig down into the studies. Like me, they found some serious flaws.

The craziest mistake was that the researchers behind the study published in *JAMA* mistakenly included WOMEN in their data![10] They didn't even realize it until the ASG brought it to their attention.[11]

And then, shockingly, the authors of the *JAMA* study didn't disclose their egregious errors for two whole months[12][13]—just enough time for the press to take this bombshell study and run with it, plastering their pages with headlines that testosterone therapy was harmful.

The cat was let out of the bag.

Now, the only reason that this study was picked apart was because it was about a therapy that people are passionate about: hormones. Most people and doctors are not passionate about their diabetes or hypertension drugs!

So, if the researchers made such embarrassing errors—and *JAMA* editors missed them—that begs the question: What other studies have been loaded with errors and falsehoods?

And how have these flaws shaped the way that we practice medicine, because of a resulting firestorm of negative press?

I wonder what other beneficial therapies have been wounded by the same calamity—and which dangerous therapies have managed to squeak by unnoticed.

A study that was designed to fail (but didn't)

But now, there's a new study that's good enough to start to shift the public perception of this amazing therapy that's been dragged through the mud.

Earlier this year, a new study out of the Intermountain Medical Center Heart Institute in Utah directly addressed and REFUTED the FDA warning, showing that testosterone therapy is not only safe in elderly men...but actually *protects their hearts*![14]

Of course, this data about testosterone prolonging the lives of men with heart problems isn't really revolutionary—there have already been studies that have shown that testosterone replacement can add years to your life.[15]

But the great part of this study is that these researchers didn't take the easy way out and rig the system to make sure that the results ended up in their favor. Instead, they had the guts to up the stakes and enroll patients who had the *highest* risk of having a stroke or a heart attack.

The study followed 750 men between 58 and 78 years old—all with severe coronary artery disease—for three years. They gave some of the patients very high-dose testosterone therapy via injection, but the study showed no increased risk in cardiovascular events (stroke, heart attack, or death).

Not only that, but it actually showed a reduced risk. The researchers compared their results to an aged-matched group of cohorts and found that the patients who didn't receive testosterone had a whopping 80 percent greater risk of stroke, heart attack, or death.

What a difference from thinking that testosterone is the cause of heart disease!

The unrefuted research speaks for itself

One of the silver linings from the attacks on testosterone is that they prompted the Androgen Study Group to amass ALL of the data about testosterone therapy over the last 70 years, which you can read all about on their website www.androgenstudygroup.org. And one of the major takeaways is that this new study is just the tip of the iceberg of amazingly positive studies supporting the benefits of testosterone therapy.

Even more studies show that raising your low T levels can reduce your cardiovascular risk factors such as obesity, fat mass, waist circumference, blood pressure, and glycemic control.

Based on the literature, however, there is clear, absolute risk of having a LOW level of testosterone. The data shows that low testosterone levels are associated with atherosclerosis, osteoporosis, cardiovascular risk factors, and even early death.

Between the abundance of studies that have shown a positive outcome...as well as the scarcity of data that show that this therapy is dangerous...I really wonder how in the world the FDA issued a black box warning on this therapy in the first place.

Are you ready to get back in the saddle?

Gentlemen, there are some "side effects" of testosterone therapy that you'll want to watch out for...and warn your wives of: better sex drive, energy, memory, and stronger erections. Taking testosterone can help you feel younger, stronger, and more vital—both in and out of the bedroom.

It can help you turn back the hands of time!

If your current doctor doesn't want to go down this path with you, please find an integrated doctor to work with who will.

Chapter 5:

Feeling fat? Irritable? No sex drive? "Female" hormone is wrecking your health—here are 3 ways to beat it

Doesn't it feel sometimes like we're seeing an explosion of health conditions that you practically never heard of a generation ago?

I'm talking about obesity, depression, diabetes, hormone disorders, and even a growing epidemic of sexual dysfunction. It's easy to blame all the processed foods we eat or our sedentary lifestyles.

But there's something else going on—and if you want to protect your health, you need to know about it.

We are swimming in a sea of estrogen.

Estrogen is an amazing hormone that both female and male bodies need. But these days we're being exposed to way too much of it—and too much estrogen can be a VERY dangerous thing.

Elevated levels of estrogen can cause a host of deleterious medical issues that range from breast cancer (or any female cancer) to prostate cancer[1] all the way to erectile dysfunction, low libido and irritability.

And guys, if you've noticed that you're growing breasts, your penis is shrinking, or you've been getting more emotional than you used to be, then I'll bet that excessive estrogen is getting in the way of your health and wellbeing.

This topic is so important—yet so broad—because hormones effect every aspect of the human body. They are absolutely crucial for optimal health. When your hormones are out of balance, to put it bluntly... nothing good is going to happen!

You may be swimming in estrogen, but you don't have to drown in it—because I'm here to throw you a lifeline. Just hang on, and I'll show you how easy it can be to normalize your levels once again.

The estrogen dominance double whammy

The problem ~~with~~ ~~estrogen~~ is that it's coming from both inside and outside our bodies. It's a real double whammy!

In fact, we're getting hit with estrogen from two different sources that are colliding to form the "perfect storm" in the human body.

The first tidal wave of estrogen is coming from our own fat cells! This is a definite case of the body rebelling against us and creating self-sabotage.

The most amazing fact about obesity and fat is that fat is alive. What I mean is that the fat cells (adipose tissue) that are inhabiting any part of your body are basically another "organ" that is active and secreting things that you do not want in your body.

In men and women, these fat cells secrete inflammatory hormones and produce estrogen. Because this production and secretion of estrogen is irrespective of a female's ovaries or adrenals, it creates way too much estrogen for most females' livers to process.

In men, the amount of estrogen that is being secreted from fat cells is disastrous at many levels. It's basically turning men into women.

Now, I'm not saying that a man should have NO feminine qualities, but the level of estrogen that is created by these fat cells is wreaking havoc. This level of estrogen floating in a man's bloodstream is growing breasts ("man boobs"), shrinking penises, and creating fat, mood swings, infertility, and erectile dysfunction.

The second tidal wave of estrogen is coming from outside sources in the form of "xenoestrogens." *Xeno* means "foreign"—and this means that our bodies are being influenced and invaded from a source outside of the human body (like chemicals) that actually imitates or mimics our own hormones.

The main source of the xenoestrogens from chemicals comes from BPA. BPA is the one of the main chemicals in plastics (plastic water bottles, plastic containers, and plastic food packaging are the main sources) and it is inevitably leached out into the food and drink we consume. A study of over 2,000 people found that more than 90 percent of them had BPA in their urine. Traces have also been found in breast milk, the blood of pregnant women, and umbilical cord blood.[2,3]

These chemical xenoestrogens have become so ubiquitous that they have also polluted our waterways. Some bodies of water around the world are so polluted with these xenoestrogens from plastics and chemicals that some fish and frogs are turning from male to female and becoming sterile.[4,5]

BPA is such a known hormone disruptor (more aptly-named endocrine disruptor)[6,7] that even the FDA admits that newborns shouldn't be exposed to it and have removed BPA from almost all baby bottles[8] (it will say BPA Free on it).

A few countries have completely banned it! In fact, in 2008 Norway banned BPA from all consumer products.[9]

The bad news is that many other chemicals (such as pesticides and herbicides) have similar xenoestrogenic effects—and they're also inevitably contributing to this sea of estrogen.

The other source of xenoestrogens is from non-organic meat products. It's routine to use hormones on chickens and cattle in this country to make them grow bigger, more quickly. These hormones stay in the meat products after packaging, shipping, and even after cooking—and when you eat them, you are getting a dose of hormones!

This is why you see all the ads about chicken being "hormone-free" as well as why many health conscious people flock (pun intended) to stores such as Whole Foods to get organic meat that comes from animals that are not exposed to hormones.

Don't try to fix estrogen problems with more estrogen

Excessive estrogen plays a huge role in almost every female health disorder— ranging from PMS to fibroids, endometriosis, infertility, and breast cancer. In fact, the media made fun of singer Sheryl Crow when she alluded to plastic water bottles being the culprit for her breast cancer, but it's not a stretch to think that excessive exposure to xenoestrogens could have been a contributor.

When you understand that our own fat cells make estrogen irrespective of what the ovaries make, then it is not a shock that obesity is being proven to be a high risk factor for many female-specific disorders including breast cancer.[10]

Thus, weight loss and the use of supplements to lower excess estrogen are at the top of the list of many of my female patients' protocols.

Believe it or not, the combination of obesity and xenoestrogens is speeding the development of the young girls in this country so much that they had to rewrite the medical textbooks in for when little girls start to get their periods.[11]

The real amazing fact about excess estrogen in a female and the phrase "estrogen dominance" is that many OB-GYN's do not believe in this phenomenon. Almost 90 percent of the female patients who walk in to my office are estrogen dominant and suffer from excessive estrogen... but when my patients tell their OB-GYN's this they poo-poo the idea and just offer them more and more birth control pills.

This is such a tragedy because those oral contraceptives are just loaded with more estrogen—and therefore, they further perpetuate the problem. The only good news about the birth control pill and why some women feel better with them is because the steady dose of estrogen with progesterone eliminates the swings and discrepancies between the estrogen and progesterone ratio.

BUT... the fact remains that the liver and the body still to process even MORE estrogen.

Lady hormones can be a man-killer

I am very familiar with estrogen and estrogen levels, and I take this hormone very seriously in my office.

You see, I'm a big fan of using testosterone therapy for men for hormone optimization, and I check and follow estrogen (estradiol) levels in all of my hormone replacement patients. In my opinion, if you are using testosterone therapy in any form (gel, shots, or pellets)... and your doctor is not checking your estrogen level... then you are not getting the most out of this costly therapy.

You could even be hurting your body.

To illustrate this, I recently had an obese man come to me for hormone help because his testosterone cream was "not working." He said that he felt better with the cream for the first week and then it "quit" working.

The bad news is that he had continued it for another year before finding me.

His primary care physician had determined that testosterone was the culprit of his fatigue and lack of sex drive—and he told him that because his "levels" were better, he should keep using the cream. He said the reason the patient didn't feel "well" was because he was overweight.

I, however, promptly checked his estrogen level, and guess what? It was very elevated.

We switched him to a Paleo Diet, got him on some supplements that would lower the estrogen level, and changed his testosterone dosage a bit—and within a few short months, his estrogen was normal, he lost 20 pounds, and his energy and sex drive were tons better.

Unfortunately, this is a very common story that's occurring to many men throughout the world using testosterone cream. Unfortunately, it's basically giving testosterone therapy a bad reputation.

Tons of men have used testosterone creams and have stopped because they really do not feel different on the cream and it is too expensive and cumbersome (rubbing the cream on) to keep using it without any rewards for their labor.

The sad news is that if the estrogen were addressed, they could be reaping the multitude of amazing benefits of their hormone replacement therapy.

3 steps to beating back estrogen

For most of my patients, when I use testosterone replacement therapy, we can keep the estrogen levels in check with supplements such as DIM, I3C, or chrysin.

In some patients (especially if they are doing testosterone shots), however, these supplements are not strong enough to keep the estrogen levels in the "safe" range, and I have to use a breast cancer drug (called anastrazole) to keep their levels in check.

The drug is very effective for males, and we only have to use it once a week (it only comes in one dose).

But before you start any kind of drug regimen, I recommend a three-pronged approach to reducing your estrogen exposure and levels in your body naturally:

1. Limit your exposure to xenoestrogens. Buy organic meats, and limit the amount of plastic that you use. Don't microwave in plastic, don't reuse plastic water bottles, and don't use a plastic water bottle if it is has been left out in the heat too long.

2. Lose fat and adipose tissue. Less fat will make less extra estrogen. As you are well aware, I'm a fan of the Paleo diet, and I strongly encourage you to adopt this amazing lifestyle that will transform your life.

3. Reduce estrogen in your bloodstream. The two best supplements that accomplish this goal, DIM and I3C, are both extracts from cruciferous vegetables (such as broccoli, Brussels sprouts, cabbage, etc).

A doctor well-versed in integrative medicine can check all of your hormone levels and work with you on a plan to lose weight and get everything back in balance.

Chapter 6:

Detect and reduce your prostate cancer risk with these simple steps

Of course, prostate cancer is the worst case scenario of prostate problems. But there's plenty you can do to prevent it from happening to you. You can determine your own risk of prostate cancer by testing yourself for two major risk factors. And if your test results aren't as favorable as you'd like, you can make a few simple diet changes and take certain supplements to lower your risk.

You need to know your 2/16 ratio too

The first step in reducing your prostate cancer risk is actually one of the same steps women can take for breast cancer: The 2/16 ratio test.

Recently, the journal *Cancer Causes and Control* published a study that directly examined the 2/16 ratio/ prostate cancer relationship. Researchers compared 113 men with prostate cancer to 317 men without prostate cancer. They reported that "…elevated 2-hydroxyestrone urine levels suggested a reduced prostate cancer risk…Conversely, elevated 16 alpha-hydroxyestrone levels were associated with an increased risk of prostate cancer…finally, the [2/16] ratio was associated with a reduced risk of prostate cancer."

This wasn't the first clue that the 2/16 ratio might be relevant for prostate cancer. A few years ago, another study showed some intriguing results. Researchers "followed" the diets of several thousand men for several years and found that men who ate at least three 1/2-cup servings of Brassica vegetables per week had a 41 percent reduction in prostate cancer risk. (Brassica vegetables include cabbage, cauliflower, broccoli, Brussels sprouts, bok choy, and others.) Since these vegetables raise the 2/16 ratio, it seemed reasonable to guess that at least some prostate cancer is related to the 2/16 ratio. Now the new study mentioned above confirms that guess.

The good news is, testing your own 2/16 ratio couldn't be easier. You don't even have to leave home to do it. Some changes in the actual testing equipment have made the process a lot easier. In fact, the testing kits can be mailed to you at home, where you'll collect a urine specimen in the container provided. When you've collected your sample, just mail it back to the lab.

Once you send your sample back to the lab, it generally takes about two to three weeks to get your results.

You definitely want more "good" (2) estrogen than "bad" (16) estrogen—substantially more if possible. So when you get your results, check the proportion of these two substances: Any ratio below 1.0 is unfavorable. Although there's no consensus on an ideal ratio number, I recommend 2.0 or greater if possible.

If your 2/16 ratio is less than 1.0, there's a good chance you'll be able to boost it just by eating a few specific foods. Start with Brassica (or mustard family) vegetables. These include cabbage, broccoli, cauliflower, bok choy, Brussels sprouts and many others. One thing to keep in mind: It is possible for Brassicas to cause suppressed thyroid function and even goiter if you eat a lot of them on a daily basis, so three to four servings a week is a good general range.

The natural cancer-fighting substances in these vegetables—isothiocyanates and indoles—help regulate and improve the 2/16 hydroxyestrogen ratio. In essence, a normal 2/16 ratio means less cancer risk.

You might find that you only need to incorporate one of these foods into your diet to raise your 2/16 ratio, but sometimes it takes a combination to make a big difference. In a lot of cases, just eating these foods will bring a low 2/16 ratio to 1.0 or above in just four to six weeks without any other specific supplementation. But if you find you're still not getting sufficient improvement, you can also take di-indolylmethane (DIM) supplements to boost it even further. DIM is actually a substance found in Brassica vegetables, but it's also available in most health food stores in supplement form. If you need some extra help, take 60 milligrams three times daily, and check your 2/16 ratio again in another four to six weeks.

Of course, it's also important to note that the 2/16 ratio is only one risk factor for prostate cancer, and while fixing this problem definitely lowers cancer risk, it doesn't eliminate it. And, unfortunately, once cancer has started, lowering the amount of "bad" estrogen is not likely to cure the cancer—but it is very likely to slow the progression.

Is your testosterone turning into estrogen?

By now you might be wondering why a test that predicts estrogen-related cancer risk also works for evaluating prostate cancer risk. Well, even the manliest men produce some estrogen. In fact, your body actually turns testosterone into estrogen. This process is called aromatization.

If everything is functioning properly, only a small fraction of your total testosterone becomes estrogen. Unfortunately, as men get older, there's a tendency for this process to speed up, turning more and more testosterone into estrogen. (This is called excess aromatization.) With excess aromatization, your body makes more estrogen than is good for your prostate—and it leaves too little testosterone behind. This raises your risk of both prostate enlargement and prostate cancer.

Excess aromatization is rare before age 40 to 45 (although it is possible). So if you're in that age bracket, you might want to have your aromatization checked—especially if there's a history of prostate cancer in your family.

The excess aromatization test involves collecting your urine for 24 hours. You only need to mail a small amount of the total sample to the laboratory for testing, and, if you want, the 2/16 test can be done on the same specimen. If you have trouble getting your doctor to order these test kits for you, contact a physician-member of The American College for Advancement in Medicine (800)532-3688; www.acam.org or The International College of Integrated Medicine (419)358-0273; www.icimed.com.

Boost your manhood with a flower?

When your test results arrive in the mail, look at your total estrogen and testosterone levels. If your total estrogen exceeds the "normal" range listed for men, or if your testosterone level is way too low (less than your estrogen level), that indicates excess aromatization.

If your lab results show excess aromatization, chrysin, a flavonoid derived from passionflower, can slow it down to normal again. Take 500 milligrams of chrysin three times daily. (The brand of chrysin containing a very small amount of diadzein, an isoflavone, appears to be more effective.) Then take another test in four to six weeks.

In the majority of cases, a follow-up test shows more testosterone and less estrogen, which means that the excess aromatization has been slowed. I definitely recommend trying chrysin first. But if it doesn't seem to work for you, the only alternative available right now is a patent medication called Arimidex. Carefully adjusted fractional doses of Arimidex will effectively slow aromatization. If you end up needing to take Arimidex, please work closely with a physician who can help you take the smallest dose necessary to do the job.

Make a different sort of "date"

There you have it: Two simple tests for figuring out your prostate cancer risk—and a few easy solutions to lower it if it's too high. In fact, since so many of these steps are similar to breast and cervical cancer risk testing, you and your wife may want to consider ordering your test kits at the same time. Then, if you need to take steps to lower your risks, you'll be able to help each other through the process.

You should still continue to take as many other protective measures as you can—including taking 200 to 300 micrograms of selenium, 20 to 30 milligrams of lycopene, and 3 milligrams of boron per day: The more you protect yourself, the better!

PART XII

Essential Health Secrets

Chapter 1:

Keep killer stress at bay for mere pennies a day using this one simple vitamin secret

It's the Rodney Dangerfield of conditions. No one gives stress the respect it deserves. When we're suffering from it we've been taught if we just ignore it, it will go away. (It doesn't, of course.) Even worse, it's seldom taken seriously by those in the medical profession, the very people who ought to know what a threat to your health it actually is.

Yet, astoundingly, at least 60 percent of all doctor's visits can be linked back to stress, according to a 20 year study by the Kaiser Permanente Medical Group. Other clinical studies estimate that stress-related visits may run as high as 75 percent!

We know that stress can increase blood sugar levels, raise blood pressure, suppress digestion and alter your immune system response. Chronic stress can eventually lead to a number of health issues including weight gain, heart disease, memory issues, sleep problems and depression.

Yet the only treatments that your conventional doctor has to offer are heavy-duty—and potentially addictive drugs—such as the benzodiazepine Xanax or the antidepressant Prozac. And that's if he takes your complaint seriously enough to even bother with a prescription.

Far too many patients are given a condescending pat on the head and are told they just need to learn to relax. As a result many people turn to "self-treatment" with alcohol or marijuana to cope. But those "solutions" come with harmful side effects of their own.

There is another option, however. It's one you'll never hear about in any conventional doctor's office. But it's so effective that it tops my personal list of preferred treatments for stress relief and overall mental well-being.

Vital vitamin complex key to stress relief

I'm talking about B vitamins, otherwise known as a B complex.

In one randomized, double-blind placebo-controlled study published in the journal Human Psychopharmacology: Clinical and Experimental patients were given a high-dose B complex vitamin. After three months, the group that got the B vitamins reported significantly less stress in their workplace.

And there's a good reason for that; B vitamins, and in particular folic acid and B12 and B6, play a critical role in mood and mental function. Without adequate levels of B on board your body is unable to properly utilize amino acids such as tryptophan and tyrosine to form the brain chemicals, or neurotransmitters, which are necessary to deal with stress including serotonin, dopamine, norepinephrine and epinephrine.

Drive down stress with a NATURAL antidepressant

If a B complex alone doesn't drive down your stress and lift your mood you may want to talk with a doctor skilled in natural medicine about the natural antidepressant Deplin (www.deplin.com). Deplin is a powerful activated form of folic acid that, like a traditional B complex, can also be used in tandem with an antidepressant.

Antidepressant failure often caused by low B

In fact, a lack of building block B nutrients lies at the heart of why many re-uptake inhibiting antidepressants fail. When you don't have enough B vitamins available and your neurotransmitter levels drop, antidepressants that are designed to recirculate your available brain chemicals end up having very little to recirculate. This means, of course, that you aren't getting any of the drug benefits, but you're still facing all of the risks and side effects.

Unfortunately, when an antidepressant drug fails far too many docs will simply switch the drug without ever considering that the nutritional well may simply have run dry. But a quality B complex could keep you from ever needing the drug in the first place.

I've found that the majority of stressed patients respond incredibly well to a B complex. A quality supplement will typically only run you pennies a day, and if you're battling stress yourself I encourage you to consider giving one a try.

Chapter 2:

Hidden heavy metal exposure could be killing you!

Lead paint poisoning isn't something we think about much these days. After all, lead was removed from gasoline and paint way back in 1978. But lead was recently thrust back into the headlines when we learned that Freddie Gray, who tragically died in Baltimore in April 2015, was repeatedly exposed to the heavy metal as a child.

Still lead poisoning isn't something most of us have to worry about anymore, right? It's been gone from our lives for more than 30 years now.

The truth is lead exposure is still an issue. In fact, if you were born before 1978, chances are YOU have entirely too much lead in your body right now. Let's take a look at how your own early life exposure may be impacting you.

A look at the link between lead and health

High levels of lead in the blood can harm developing brains and bodies leading to organ damage, decreased cognitive function, aggression and even death. A child who is poisoned by lead starts out life at a distinct disadvantage. But even when your own lead levels don't reach the sky high levels that are considered "poisoning" by today's mainstream medicine standards, there can be very real consequences to lower levels of lead exposure over time.

You see, unlike conventional medicine doctors, holistic physicians recognize that simply being exposed to lead... as you surely were in your younger years, and may still be today... can have a dire impact on health, even if a victim isn't technically "poisoned" by mainstream medicine's standards.

That's because the lead is essentially ferreted away in many nooks and crannies throughout your body, but mostly in your bones. Meaning that every time that you exercise, or even walk, some of that lead is squirted into your bloodstream. And that can have tragic... and even deadly... consequences.

"Low" levels of lead kill

For example, a study published in the journal Circulation in 2006 revealed that even a blood lead level as "low" as between 3.6 and 10 micrograms per deciliter was associated with 25 percent higher risk of death from any cause, a 55 percent higher risk of death from cardiovascular disease, an 89 percent higher risk of death from heart attack and two and a half times the risk of death from stroke.

Another study, published in 2010, followed nearly 10,000 patients with slightly elevated lead levels when they were over 40 years old. Researchers found that having a lead level between 5 to 9 micrograms per deciliter was clearly associated with an increased risk of death from all causes, cardiovascular disease and cancer.

If you want to know what your own lead level is ask your physician for a blood lead test. If you have access to an integrative medicine physician, ask for a hair test or a urine provocation challenge to test for heavy metals.

Keep in mind that there shouldn't be ANY lead in your blood. So even if your count comes back within the so-called "normal range," any number above zero should be seen as a potential problem. If this is the case talk with doctor about chelation and other strategies for bringing your number down to zero.

Chapter 3:

Soothing solutions for anxiety

For some people, caffeine can be a hidden source of anxiety. Caffeine-induced anxiety, or "caffeinism," occurs most often in individuals from families with blood sugar problems. Eliminating your intake of refined sugar is likely to reduce your anxiety, and, of course, eliminating caffeine will help too.

Vitamin and mineral supplements can also be sources of relief. Niacinamide, a form of vitamin B3, helps most people with anxiety and, to some degree, depression (especially for individuals whose family has a history of blood sugar problems). I usually recommend taking 500 to 1,000 milligrams a day along with a good B-complex vitamin supplement. The B-complex helps "back up" the niacinaminde, and it also helps settle anxiety on its own.

Herbal remedies like ginkgo (40 milligrams of a standardized extract, three times a day) and Siberian ginseng (100 to 200 milligrams, three times a day) can also be a big help.

Chapter 4:

No more needles, no more waiting... Four life-saving health tests you can do at home!

Let's face it. By the time you call for an appointment and drag yourself to your doctor's office, you're already sick as a dog.

The next thing you know, your doctor is ordering a whole battery of tests and you're stuck waiting by the phone for days to get the results.

Imagine how much simpler life could be if you could catch these illnesses early—before they became serious—right from the comfort of your own home.

Here are four easy-to-do tests that could help detect an underlying condition that could lead to heart disease, diabetes, and even cancer.

Home Test #1: Thyroid Function

How well your thyroid works can determine how likely you are to end up overweight or suffering from serious illnesses, like heart disease and diabetes.

There's a very simple way of measuring thyroid function that I've been recommending to patients for many years —the ***Underarm Basal Body Temperature Test***.

This test is the brainchild of Dr. Broda Barnes, a physician and researcher who studied the effects of thyroid exhaustion on metabolism. It was Dr. Barnes who first wrote that people can still be suffering from functional hypothyroidism, even if their TSH test results come back fine.

Take your underarm body temperature (use an analog thermometer, not a digital one) as soon as you wake up in the morning, keeping the thermometer in place for 10 minutes. For premenopausal woman, choose the second or third day of your cycle.

If your temperature is under 97.8, you may have low thyroid function—particularly if you're showing symptoms like weight gain, fatigue, constipation, and dry skin. Talk to your doctor about treatment. I have my patients follow Dr. Barnes' protocol, which is to take Armour Thyroid and other desiccated thyroid preparations.

Home Test #2: Adrenal Exhaustion

The ***Pupil Dilation Test*** is so easy, you can do it without getting up out of your chair. And it can tell you a lot about your adrenal health.

I learned about this test from the writings of Dr. James Wilson, who has written extensively about adrenal exhaustion.

Like the thyroid, the adrenal gland is easily worn out, especially in response to stress. You've probably heard of the "fight or flight" response that activates our adrenal glands. But one of the things that happens at the same time is that our pupils dilate.

So testing your pupils is actually an easy way to see how your fight-or-flight response—and adrenals—are functioning.

Just look in the mirror, and shine a strong light into one of your eyes (without blinding yourself). If your adrenals are functioning perfectly, your pupil should contract from the light and stay small until the light is removed.

However, if your adrenals are exhausted, your pupil will contract for less than 30 seconds, and sometimes only for a few seconds before dilating again. This is a rough sign of adrenal exhaustion.

Sometimes your pupil might not even be able to make up its mind, and it will alternately constrict and dilate despite that bright beam of light being aimed straight for it. It's as if you can't decide whether to put up your dukes, run for the hills, or lay down and play dead.

If you find yourself wide-eyed—even in the face of a blinding beam of light—call your doctor. For more than just a rough estimate of function, he can order a saliva test to measure your levels of cortisol. If it's high, that's a big waving red flag that your body is stressed out and you have adrenal fatigue.

Home Test #3: Cell Acidity

Your urine is a good reflection of what's actually going on in your cells—especially after six or more hours of rest. That's why you should take the *Urine Acid Test* first thing in the morning.

This test has an impressive pedigree, having been pioneered by kidney doctor Dr. Julian Seifter and Dr. Russell Jaffe, an innovator in functional medicine. According to their research and practice, metabolism tends to make your body's cells acidic. When everything is running smoothly, that acidity is buffered by the alkaline foods you eat and by minerals like potassium and magnesium.

Measure the acid and alkaline balance of your urine using pH paper that you can find at any pharmacy. A pH reading of less than 6.5 is considered a type of "metabolic acidosis"—and it's harmful to your cells.

Toxins will linger in your body for much longer than normal, literally poisoning your cells. You'll get sick and feel fatigued if you don't get your acidity back in balance.

If your morning pH is less than 6.5, eat a more alkaline diet—and that means getting more vegetables and less animal protein into your system.

Home Test #4: Gut Health

The time it takes food to pass through your system and be eliminated is called "transit time," and it's a good indicator of intestinal health. You can measure it easily with the *Transit Time Test*.

The quicker the transit time, the less likely you are to develop digestive tract cancers, hemorrhoids, varicose veins, and a number of other conditions. When your transit time is slower—say, up to five to six times slower—toxins linger in your digestive tract and do their damage in a leisurely manner.

Measure your own transit time by taking 1.5 to 3 g of activated charcoal tablets. You can get them at any health store, and you should drink a large glass of water with them, preferably right after a bowel movement. As you subsequently go to the bathroom, pay attention to what the stool looks like and look for the appearance of the black, crumbly tablets. Your transit time should ideally be in the 12- to 18-hour range—from the time you swallow something (in the case of the test, the charcoal) to the time you eliminate it. If it takes longer than 18 hours for the charcoal to come out, add some roughage to your diet and test again. If your transit time isn't reduced by a high-fiber diet, consult your doctor.

You don't have to wait for your doctor to order tests like these. And if he's not a holistic doc, he might not even know about them.

But if your condition isn't severe, you may be able to improve your health on your own—by just changing what you eat or adding simple supplements.

For more information on Dr. Barnes and his work, visit www.BrodaBarnes.org.

For more on Dr. Wilson and his writings on hormone fatigue, visit www.adrenalfatigue.org.

To explore more of Dr. Jaffe's findings, visit www.drrusselljaffe.com.

Chapter 5:

That supplement or detox may be making you miserable— but don't panic! Power through the darkest hours to get to the dawn of good health

Have you ever started taking a supplement—or even an antibiotic—and had a bad reaction?

That is, in the first few days of taking it, you just felt "off"… almost flu-like… with headaches, fever, and body aches?

Maybe you even thought you might be allergic to it!

Well, this type of reaction is commonplace with the use of certain supplements and medications—and, believe it or not, although you may feel even *worse* than you did before, it could actually be a good thing.

Because usually, that kind of reaction means that your body is going through some form of cleansing or detoxification.

This is a classic example of having to feel worse before you feel better—because, as the proverb says, "The darkest hour is just before the dawn."

But while you might be tempted to quit the natural therapy or the treatment protocol immediately... thinking that something has gone terribly wrong... often, you just have to give it time.

You have to let the bad out to make room for the good. And all that "bad" stuff coming up to the surface doesn't always feel so good.

Don't let sleeping dogs lie

You see, when this happens, supplements are killing infections that are lurking in the human body... and these bugs (and the human body) are not "happy" when we try to escort them off of the premises.

These unpleasant reactions occur when the body releases chemicals (called cytokines) in response to internal toxins (endotoxins) that have been released into the bloodstream, liver, and lymphatic system.

Basically, some supplements and medications awaken a "sleeping dog" inside the body and the body gets "irritated" when these by-products are released.

And the more by-products that need to be released, the worse you'll feel.

This detoxification reaction may be a necessary evil in the quest for wellness, but it's tricky to figure out whether you're experiencing:

What's in a name?

"Herxheimer reaction" is a bit of misnomer. Its official name in medical textbooks is the "Jarisch-Herxheimer reaction," after the two European dermatologists who discovered it while actually treating syphilis with mercury and then antibiotics.

Because of the confusion that using the "Herx" moniker causes— as well as some funny looks—I prefer the term "detoxification reaction," regardless of whether it's from a true antibiotic or one of the germicidal nutraceuticals.

---

1. a *real* allergic reaction (see sidebar)

2. a classic detoxification reaction, or

3. an intensified version of what is called a "Herxheimer reaction." (see sidebar)

In the case of the Herxheimer reaction (or "Herx" for short), someone might feel quite poorly after starting a round of antibiotics because of the amount and type of infection that's being killed off.

In those cases, it could be that the antibiotic was just what their body needed—and if they could just keep taking it and "get over the hump," then they could say goodbye to their health woes.

However, the reaction may instead show us that the meds are too strong for this particular patient. Their lymphatic system and/or liver may be too sluggish for this level of treatment. And the same goes for supplements.

The more your body fights detox, the more you need it!

The amazing part of my job is seeing every day how certain very common supplements act as natural "bug"-killers—or, "natural antibiotics," if you will—that they will create this detoxification reaction.

If you ask me, these nutraceuticals should really be called natural "germicides"—because they're killing not just bacteria, but also certain parasites, yeast, or even viruses.

This can happen with an array of different supplements, including chlorella and cilantro (which are often paired together for a detox regimen).

Some of the other common herbs and over-the-counter supplements that could provoke these responses include garlic, oil of oregano, olive leaf extract, berberine, grapefruit seed extract, and cat's claw. I've even seen it occur from herbs—like milk thistle—that work directly on the liver.

But I've seen it occur most consistently with curcumin, an amazing herb with a dizzying array of benefits for the human body.

One of the reasons that it works so well for such a myriad of health issues is that it so thoroughly detoxifies the human body... which then provokes a detoxification reaction. With curcumin, the symptoms can include those aforementioned flu-like symptoms, as well as headaches and even rashes—all of which that seem so similar to an allergic reaction.

But in reality, if your body is responding in such a way to curcumin, it desperately needs to figure out how to tolerate this treatment—because it could be a big boon for your overall health.

If the detoxification reactions are too intense for a patient at my clinic, sometimes we'll abandon the treatment protocol and go "back to the drawing board." Then, we'll use protocols to support and cleanse the liver and the lymphatic system.

And then we start anew, with a stronger system that's hopefully able to handle the disease-fighting treatment.

Things may get worse before they get better

This apparent "worsening" of a condition is such a common occurrence in the integrative medical world that sometimes I forget that the general public and mainstream doctors don't understand what's happening—or even believe in this phenomenon. But I'm certain that this is occurring many times every day... around the world... to a host of unsuspecting people.

Don't be one of them. If it happens to you, there are ways of dealing with the detoxification reaction that can come in handy and help you power through the tough times.

First of all, a safe move would be to stop the treatment for a day or two... restart at half the dose that provoked the response... and then see how you do.

But there are a couple of other natural, drug-free "tricks" you can try to get through the "dark" period when your symptoms are getting worse before they get better.

One of the most helpful ones out there is good old-fashioned baking soda. Some doctors recommend the easy-to-use, plop-plop-fizz-fizz remedy Alka-Seltzer—but, specifically, the "Gold" version, which is aspirin-free and basically just baking soda. It can balance out the acidity of your body, helping your system detoxify more quickly.

And finally, even though it's nothing fancy, drinking a lot of water is a tried-and-true way of flushing the toxins out of your body. You can drink it from a bottle or from the tap—just make sure it's been filtered and isn't one of those fashionable "waters" that have added sugar and other flavorings.

Chapter 6:

Stop marinating in your own toxins! Cleanse your system ... and look and feel better... with this crazy bedroom trick

We spend a third of our lives in bed—and yet, to be honest, I'm not sure the mainstream medical world knows much about sleep.

Believe it or not, the way that we sleep can cause a range of medical ailments ranging from baggy eyes to Alzheimer's. But it turns out that changing *how* we sleep can also improve many conditions and even our overall quality of life.

A few years ago, one of my patients came in for a follow-up appointment with me and looked so much better than he usually did. He was bright and lively, and told me that he'd been sleeping better.

What was his secret to better sleep and more energy?

"I sleep with the head of my bed raised six inches," he said.

I was a bit taken aback. He then explained that he'd heard about something called "Inclined Bed Therapy" and decided to give it a try.

Lo and behold, it worked right away. Right from the very first morning, he'd woken up with loads more energy.

In fact, it's made such a difference that he hasn't slept flat ever since.

This was a surprising and somewhat shocking discovery for me, but it turns out that the practice is rooted in ancient medicine. Inclined beds were even found in Egyptian tombs... raised to the height of about six inches!

Inclined Bed Therapy may seem a bit radical, but once you see the science behind it—and the difference it can make in your health—I think you'll be convinced to give it a try.

Simple sleep system delivers major health benefits

I was intrigued enough that when I got home from work that day, I started to research this interesting method of sleep therapy.

It turns out that one Englishman starting thinking outside the box (which you know I like to do), and came up with an ingenious and potentially life-saving way of altering our sleep habits.

The man credited for this medical breakthrough, Andrew Fletcher, has no medical background or training. But in my opinion, that is good news!

He's actually an engineer, and engineers think about solving complex issues much more rationally than a medical researcher would. Instead of trying to invent a drug that would circumvent or band-aid a symptom, Mr. Fletcher used common sense.

Recognizing that plants and trees use the force of gravity to get water and sap to the top of their leaves, he realized that humans also have a similar system of ducts and tubes in their bodies that move fluids through the limbs (which are like our "branches").

Putting two and two together, he figured out that elevating the head of our beds would create a similar suction-like pressure and elevator-effect in the human body during sleep that would create a constant flow of fluids throughout the night.

Lying flat, on the other hand, creates a stagnant pond of bodily fluids that leads to a host of health issues.

By now, most people know that sitting on the couch all day is an unhealthy habit. So why should that same type of stagnation be any healthier while we're asleep?

NASA even studied the hazardous health consequences of space travel by having study subjects lie flat in bed for prolonged periods of time.

Keeping our bodily fluids moving while we sleep is essential for good health. And we're learning that Inclined Bed Therapy promotes this movement, and is a useful tool for fighting a variety of serious health conditions.

Use gravity to beat pain, skin disease, and more

Inclined Bed Therapy accomplishes so many cool and amazing things because it's not just your blood that gets circulated while you sleep. The "suction" that's created from forcing the head to be raised about six inches also moves your lymphatic and cerebrospinal fluid (the special fluid that recirculates from our brains to the bottom of our spinal cords).

The movement of blood, lymph, and cerebrospinal fluid while sleeping has the potential to heal and aid in a number of health conditions.

The movement of the lymph is essential for healthy living. It can help move the "trash" in and out of the body, which is crucial for detoxification.

The lymphatic flow in the body influences many diseases, as we discussed in the last issue, but Inclined Bed Therapy has also been said to help many skin issues such as psoriasis and eczema, as well as any form of sinus and head/neck congestion.

On top of that, Inclined Bed Therapy also forces the cerebrospinal fluid to be recirculated at a faster rate and helps to keep the brain from marinating in its own toxins. In fact, the movement of cerebrospinal fluid has led to a number of dramatic success stories with neurological disorders such as Alzheimer's, stroke, Multiple Sclerosis, seizures, and spinal cord injuries.

Finally, a researcher in Micronesia did a small study that showed that Inclined Bed Therapy improved blood sugar by a significant amount in 6 of the 7 patients studied. Interestingly, at the beginning of the study all of the participants had reported also experiencing issues with back pain, edema, difficulty sleeping, frequent night urination, snoring, morning light headedness, and pain in joints. But after sleeping with their heads elevated, all participants reported that these problems improved by the end of the study.[1]

The obvious gravitational drainage produced by Inclined Bed Therapy can also eliminate morning headaches and reduce those bags under your eyes. Not only can it help your face look better, but it's also been shown to improve varicose veins and leg edema!

Here's how to try Inclined Bed Therapy

With Inclined Bed Therapy, you need to get your head raised about six inches above your feet, which can be accomplished a few different ways.

Some people like to start with a sleeping wedge, but most people find it a bit too cumbersome. Others just like to use large or multiple pillows, but sleeping in that position may create some neck discomfort.

The best way that I have found is to get bed risers from a store such as Bed Bath & Beyond and use only two of the four that come in the set to lift the bed frame legs at the headboard end of the bed. These risers are usually used to create storage space under the bed, so they're very sturdy and secure.

Just don't use satin sheets—because you might slide right out of the bed!

The good news is that most people feel the difference in the first few nights of sleep. Some people, however, can experience a "detox reaction" within the first two weeks. I tell my patients to try to stick with it for at least two weeks, and then the body will get to the other side of the healing process.

Everyone knows that sleep is an incredibly important part of our health and wellbeing. We spend such an extraordinary amount of time sleeping and it makes a lot of sense to try to optimize this precious part of our lives.

I think Mr. Fletcher's out-of-the-box thinking with Inclined Bed Therapy is just brilliant—and I believe it can help just about anyone, regardless of any medical conditions they may be struggling with.

Check out his website www.inclinedbedtherapy.com and give a serious attempt at sleeping with your bed inclined.

Some brilliant ideas can sometimes be so simple!

Chapter 7:

Send UTIs packing with this simple sugar secret

If you've ever had a urinary tract infection (UTI), you know just how painful it can be—especially when you go to the bathroom.

And let's face it—when you have a UTI, you *always* seem to be running to the toilet.

In some cases, symptoms can come and go—or you might not even realize you have a UTI at all.

But UTIs are a serious risk to your health. They cause more than 8 million visits to doctors and hospitals every year.[1] And although they're more common in women, men are far from immune—especially if they have swollen prostates.

If you've been treated for a UTI, you were probably given a course of powerful antibiotics (which comes with serious risks of their own). Or maybe someone told you to try an old kitchen cure—cranberry juice.

But believe it or not, there's a potent, natural sugar called D-mannose that can cure even the worst UTIs packing, without antibiotics.

It's derived from the humble cranberry—but it's far more powerful and effective than anything you'll pick up at the supermarket.

Flush out the bad bugs— and ONLY the bad bugs

I saw a patient recently who mentioned that her bladder was "weak." Her gynecologist had recommended a drug to "dry up" her bladder, but luckily she hadn't started taking it.

Those drugs not only dry the bladder up, but they also usually dry up the patients' brains—causing memory loss, dry mouth, and dizziness.

When I tested her urine and it came back showing some small amount of white blood cells, I told her to take D-mannose twice a day. A week later, she called the office to say that the symptoms she'd been struggling with for 20 years had VANISHED without taking ANY antibiotics.

The latest scientific findings support what my patient experienced personally. In fact, there's a great study that was done in 2014 that showed that D-mannose could provide _the exact same benefit_ as an antibiotic— while having almost no side effects and no damage to the flora of the gut lining (which is a common hazard with antibiotics).[2]

Think about the amount of antibiotics that could be avoided by the use of this almost zero-risk "good for you" sugar molecule!

Now, D-mannose will only help prevent and treat the type of bacterial UTI caused by _Escherichia coli_ (E. coli)—but, fortunately, that covers 90 percent of all UTIs.

D-mannose works because it sticks to the E. coli and actually blocks the little buggers' tentacles from binding to the walls of the urinary system. With nowhere to anchor, the bacteria get flushed out of your body with the rest of the debris in your urine.

And, unlike antibiotics that clear the good with the bad out of your system, with D-mannose, you get to keep all your good flora intact.

Skip the sugary drinks and get right to the powerful sugar molecule

Since drug companies can't make money off of this natural substance, there's been no real push to validate and standardize this amazing treatment.

The conventional medial community doesn't exactly poo-poo the use of D-mannose for the prevention of UTIs per se, but they haven't taken it as seriously as they should.

Now, as I said, you can find D-mannose in cranberries. But trying to use actual cranberries in the prevention and treatment of UTIs is like using a teeny fly swatter to kill a bear.

D-mannose is more like an anvil. To put it in perspective, when D-mannose is isolated and extracted from the berry, it can be 25 to 50 times more powerful than cranberry juice.

Besides, you don't want to use store-bought cranberry juice—even if it's unsweetened—for UTI treatment or prevention because of its high sugar content (in the form of fructose), which can be upwards of 30 grams per eight-ounce serving.[3]

Even though D-mannose itself is a sugar molecule, only a small portion of it gets metabolized in the intestines, so it doesn't raise your blood sugar.

Fortunately, you can easily get D-mannose as a natural supplement in pill form at your local vitamin store or health food shop.

If you think you may have a UTI, you should call your doctor—but it won't hurt to start taking the D-mannose right away, while you wait to get into his office and for your urine culture results to come back from the lab. In just those couple of days of waiting, your infection could move to your kidneys and send you into the hospital.

To relieve simple urinary tract discomfort, the recommended dose of D-mannose is about 2,000 mg for adults and 1,000 mg for children, four to five times a day. Once the symptoms disappear, you should continue with that same dosage for another two days or so.

Now, the recommended dose for *preventing* infections would be 500 mg to 1,000 mg twice a day or 2,000 mg once a day. Since intercourse can cause a UTI, taking 2,000 mg of mannose an hour prior to sex and another 2,000 mg right after is also an option.

Chapter 8:

Medical foods: The natural health revolution that even the mainstream can buy into

You can be sure that Big Pharma didn't intend any of this—but, believe it or not, one of the biggest boons to my practice has been all these drug commercials they're running around the clock.

Just the other night I was watching TV and saw commercials for everything from an antipsychotic to a chemotherapy drug for lung cancer. I don't know how these ads are even legal!

But by the time they're done listening to commercial announcers rattle off lists of dangerous side effects, lots of patients end up combing through the Internet or Yellow Pages looking for holistic doctors like me. They want to treat their serious health conditions—but without all the risks of prescription drugs.

In fact, even some mainstream doctors are starting to hear the same thing.

The good news is that there are many safe, natural remedies on the market today called medical foods that are changing the way that lots of docs like me practice medicine.

You won't see medical foods advertised on television. But they can be just as powerful as those prescription meds...without the ridiculously long list of dangers.

Finally—a natural remedy that the mainstream can get behind

Medical foods are good "middle of the road" options for some of your most serious medical conditions. They are totally natural, yet so "strong" that they necessitate a prescription.

They can be a huge help to someone who's open-minded and is looking for alternatives.

These medical foods are basically supplements with superpowers. Technically, because they require a prescription, you could call them a "drug," but they're actually the opposite of a drug—because they use natural ingredients to treat the root cause of many illnesses. Or, in some cases, they at least provide sound nutritional support for these diseases.

For example, there's Limbrel, a medical food used to treat arthritis. But there are lots of others on the market, like:

- Oxepa (for lung problems);
- Suplena (for kidney failure); and
- Ultrase (for various pancreatic diseases).

These souped-up supplements have FDA oversight but, like regular supplements, are not FDA approved. The FDA defines them as:

"a food which is formulated to be consumed or administered enterally under the supervision of a physician and which is intended for the specific dietary management of a disease or condition for which distinctive nutritional requirements, based on recognized scientific principles, are established by medical evaluation."[1]

This paragraph is very intriguing because it is basically the FDA admitting that certain diseases CAN be managed with a supplement—or, even more importantly, that a nutrient deficiency has been scientifically proven as the root cause of some diseases.

I know that I'm reading between the lines a bit, but to me, this is HUGE. There are a fair number of these medical foods popping up, and it's exciting to read the literature on these drugs...all the studies out there that prove that nutrient deficiencies can cause severe disease and that repletion of these nutrients can reverse the problem.

To take the conversation full circle, this also shines light on the fact that the non-medical foods (non-natural drugs) are actually just covering up disease and "band-aiding" the true medical issue.

This is an instance when the FDA helps us bridge the gap between "conventional" and "alternative" medicine. That's because your local doctor can look these medical foods up and feel safe about prescribing them—because the FDA recognizes these medical foods as a sound medical decision backed by plenty of science.

The companies that make these medical foods actually have "vitamin" reps that come and call on my office like the other drug companies try to do; but when these reps come by, I smile when I see them because they usually bring me free samples that I'm excited to give to my patients.

The great news is that these reps are going to ALL the doctors that they can get in to see—and as you would expect, the majority of them are conventional doctors. Therefore, you can hope that your local doctor has listened to them, and at least read the literature that's been dropped off at his office.

Be the change you wish to see in your own health

If you can't find a doctor like me in your area, you can safely broach the option of these medical foods with your own family physician. These medical foods can be the lynchpin for him to practice some medicine that takes an offensive approach against disease—rather than a defensive approach against your symptoms.

And, believe it or not, even some doctors that are about as opposed to natural health as you can get—and never recommend supplements to their patients—are often comfortable letting you give medical foods a try.

And, hopefully, as more of these doctors see how well medical foods perform, they'll become more comfortable recommending other natural remedies as well.

A guy can dream, can't he?

I'm proud to be writing things like this to be part of the movement that changes the way that medicine is practiced—and how people can use alternatives to drugs to stay healthy and prosper as they age.

Medical foods are sparking a bona fide revolution in natural health. And I'm looking forward in future issues to making you aware of the latest remedies that show the most promise.

Chapter 9:

Send those winter blues packing with this amazing vitamin cure

As a holistic doctor practicing on the East Coast, I dread this time of year. And it's not because I'm some "Scrooge."

It's because as the days get shorter—and there's less sunlight—I watch my patients' health take a nosedive.

Too little sunlight exposure can pose a serious hazard to your health. You might feel depressed, despondent, fatigued, and even hungry all the time.

This malady is a real disease, and it's called Seasonal Affective Disorder (also known as SAD). It affects 10 percent of the entire population, and although it can be quite disabling, it's an elusive phenomenon.

The hidden cause behind Seasonal Affective Disorder

We can't test for SAD, and we haven't developed any treatments for it—besides exposing those affected to more light or treating their depression with prescription meds and psychotherapy.

But lots of docs like me have known for a long time the real cause of the condition—too little vitamin D, which your body makes from sunlight.

How do we know that these SAD patients don't have enough vitamin D? Because they feel a whole lot better when they DO get enough.

To prove my point: last year, a husband and wife that I have been treating for many years finally decided to "snow bird" down to Florida after suffering through New England winters for too long.

When they returned north in the spring to come in and see me, we were all astounded—their health had improved RADICALLY compared to appointments around the same time in previous years. They had more energy, better moods and even better blood sugars, cholesterol and of course vitamin D levels.

Of course, it helps that vitamin D is linked to the production of the incredibly important "feel good" brain chemicals of dopamine and serotonin.[1]

Without that glorious sun exposure, our vitamin D levels take a nosedive–bringing our mood down with it.

It's no shocker—vitamin D makes us healthy AND happy

You have to understand that in reality, vitamin D is really a hormone—NOT a vitamin—and it affects every major organ in our bodies.

We holistic doctors know how important optimizing the vitamins, minerals, and hormones in the body is. In fact, I consider the level of vitamin D equally as important as the levels of thyroid, cortisol, human growth hormone, and estrogen, progesterone and testosterone.

The human body has an amazing mechanism to make vitamin D, and sitting out in the sun helps it produce its own natural supply. When the Ultraviolet B form of sunlight (UVB) hits your skin, your body harvests it and converts a cholesterol molecule (7-dehydrocholesterol) into vitamin D, which then travels through the liver and kidneys in order to be fully activated and utilized by the body in the form of *calcitriol*, which has been shown to be a powerful cancer-fighter.[2]

Yes, I said a cholesterol molecule! Meanwhile, conventional doctors are trying to lower this valuable resource at every opportunity they get with statin drugs!!

The calcitriol (the active version of vitamin D) that circulates around the human body does way more than just help your bones. There are physiological links of vitamin D's role in many different organs and vital bodily functions, and it has a huge influence over the immune system and the brain, mood, and brain chemistry.

A good supply of vitamin D boosts your brain function and immunity AND reduces inflammation—and that means it can reduce your risk of congestive heart failure, inflammatory bowel disease, COPD, respiratory infections, severe allergic reactions, and gum disease.[3]

You can drink milk 'til the cows come home, but it won't give you enough D

Vitamin D is one of the most common nutrient deficiencies among men and women.[4] It's running rampant because most of us aren't even getting outside enough ANY time of year—not to mention during the winter, when we're all nervous about getting sick or slipping on ice and snow.

But staying indoors...under all those artificial lights...is only making us prime candidates for SAD.

Those of us who do manage to go outside have been programmed to block the sun's rays by wearing sunscreen or a hat, but this sun "protection" has shut out your body's access to the sun's life-saving and uplifting effects. It's truly a calamity—it's almost like we are TRYING to get SAD!

And as we cower in the shadows, waiting for spring to hit, not even changing our diets can boost our levels of D enough to make a difference.

The weird truth is: There are very few foods that naturally have vitamin D in them.

A great article published in the 2004 edition of the *American Journal of Clinical Nutrition* goes so far as to claim that there's NO WAY that milk and food can get us to where we need to be. We are not getting enough vitamin D even from the foods that are FORTIFIED with it![5]

If you think you're getting a bountiful helping of vitamin D from drinking milk, you'll be shocked to find out that even cow milk is not loaded with natural vitamin D. The government mandated that cow milk be fortified with vitamin D starting in 1933, so the version of D that you've been pouring on your oatmeal is actually synthetic.

I'm not a big fan of dairy anyway, because cow's milk has been adulterated through pasteurization and homogenization—not to mention the use of growth hormones and antibiotics on cattle.

Get three times the oomph from bioidentical vitamin D supplements

It's encouraging that a fair percentage of conventional doctors are actually checking vitamin D levels, but they are prescribing a synthetic form of vitamin D, called *ergocalciferol,* that comes from the irradiation of a kind of mushroom.

Synthetic vitamin D replacement (D_2) doesn't measure up to sun exposure OR the over-the-counter natural version of vitamin D, called vitamin D_3 or *cholecalciferol.* In fact, the synthetic vitamin D_2 is only a third as potent as bioidentical D_3, and according to an amazing study published in the *Journal of Clinical Endocrinology and Metabolism* in 2013, and it also stops working much sooner.[6]

And you can be sure that D_3 doesn't come from fungus. It comes from the wool of sheep (lanolin) or from the skin or livers of fatty fish (salmon, tuna, or cod). There's a reason why your mother or grandmother used to force the cod liver oil down your throat when you were young!

How much D do you need?

Most doctors don't usually come up with a long-term plan for their patients' vitamin D. Conventional doctors will prescribe one large dose (50,000 units) once a week for a month or two—without any refills!

But a one-time replenishment of this vitamin does not cure your deficiency in one fell swoop!

The truth is: If vitamin D levels are not checked regularly, or if you don't get vitamin D from some other source, then your levels will surely drop back down to a suboptimal level.

Holistic doctors like me actually shoot much higher than the standard levels of "normal" when evaluating a patient. In the effort to optimize patients, I aim for vitamin D levels way above the standard 30 ng/ml—ideally, more like from 50 to 70.

Dedicate yourself to vitamin D in EVERY season

No matter what the season, make sure that your doctor is regularly checking your vitamin D level, and if it's low, take the over-the-counter natural D supplement. Better yet, try the bioidentical version of vitamin D, vitamin D_3. You can only get it at a health food store, and it's not appropriate for vegetarians or vegans.

Finally, try to get at least 10 minutes of direct sunlight every day. Unfortunately, depending on where you live and the time of year, that sunlight might not even be available to you. So if you are still experiencing the "winter blues," consider getting a natural light lamp to brighten your days—and your mood.

Alternative Health Resources

American Academy of Environmental Medicine (AAEM)
Phone: (316)684-5500; www.aaemonline.org

American Association of Naturopathic Physicians
Phone: (866)538-2267; www.naturopathic.org

American College for Advancement in Medicine (ACAM)
Phone: (888)439-6891; www.acam.org

International College Integrative Medicine
Phone: (419)358-0273; www.icimed.com

Nutrition & Healing
www.nutritionandhealing.com

.

References

Part I: Cancer

Toss your sunscreen and step out of the shadows!
You can prevent skin cancer and still enjoy time the sun this summer

[1] Wang Z et al.. Ultraviolet irradiation of human skin causes functional vitamin A deficiency, preventable by all-trans retinoic acid pre-treatment. *Nature Medicine* 1999; 5(4): 418-422

The cancer-fighting mineral you can't afford to ignore

[1] Eskin BA, Shuman R, Krouse T, Merion JA. Rat mammary gland atypia produced by iodine blockade with perchlorate. *Cancer Res.* 1975 Sep;35(9):2332-9.

[2] Aceves C, Anguiano B, Delgado G. Is iodine a gatekeeper of the integrity of the mammary gland? *J Mammary Gland Biol Neoplasia* 2005 Apr;10(2):189-96.

[3] Shrivastava A, et al. Molecular iodine induces caspase-independent apoptosis in human breast carcinoma cells involving the mitochondria-mediated pathway. *J Biol Chem.* 2006 Jul 14;281(28):19762-71

[4] Arroyo-Helguera O, Anguiano B, Delgado G, Aceves C. Uptake and antiproliferative effect of molecular iodine in the MCF-7 breast cancer cell line. *Endocr Relat Cancer.* 2006 Dec;13(4):1147-58.

[5] Tretsch D, et al. Acute iodide intoxication with cardiac irritability. *Arch Int Med* 1074;134:760-762

The "unimportant" molecule curing cancer: Do-it-yourself tips for boosting your levels—without Big Pharma's help

[1] Tinley TL, Leal RM, Randall-Hlubek DA, et al. "Novel 2-methoxyestradiol analogues with antitumor activity." *Cancer Research* 2003; 63: 1,538-1,549

[2] Pribluda VS, Gubish ER Jr., Lavallee TM, et al. "2-methoxyestradiol: an endogenous antiangiogenic and antiproliferative drug candidate." *Cancer Metastasis Rev* 2000; 19(1-2): 173-179

[3] Golebiewska J, Rozwadowski P, Spodnik JH, et al. "Dual effect of 2-methoxyestradiol on cell cycle events in human osteosarcoma 143 B cells." *Acta Biochemica Polonica* 2002; 49(1): 59-65

[4] Drissa A, Bennani H, Giton F, et al. "Tocopherols and saponins derived from Argania spinosa exert an antiproliferative effect on human prostate cancer." *Cancer Invest* 2006; 24(6): 588-592

[5] Mueck AO, Seeger H, Huober J. "Chemotherapy of breast cancer-additive anticancerogenic effects by 2-methoxyestradiol?" *Life Sci* 2004; 75(10): 1,205-1,210

[6] Gomez LA, de Las Pozas A, Reiner T, et al. "Increased expression of cyclin B1 sensitizes prostate cancer cells to apoptosis induced by chemotherapy." *Mol Cancer Ther* 2007;6(5): 1,534-1,543

[7] Schumacher G, Hoffmann J, Cramer T, et al. "Antineoplastic activity of 2-methoxyestradiol in human pancreatic and gastric cancer cells with different multidrug-resistant phenotypes." *J Gastroenterol Hepatol* 2007; 22(9): 1,469-1,473

[8] Mueck AO, Seeger H, Wallwiener D, Huober J. "Is the combination with 2-methoxyestradiol able to reduce the dosages of chemotherapeutics in the treatment of human ovarian cancer? Preliminary in vitro investigations." *Eur J Gynaecol Oncol* 2004; 25(6): 699-701

[9] Golebiewska J, Rozwadowski P, Spodnik JH, et al. "Dual effect of 2-methoxyestradiol on cell cycle events in human osteosarcoma 143 B cells." *Acta Biochemica Polonica* 2002; 49(1): 59-65

[10] Shogren KL, Turner RT, Yaszemski J, Maran A. "Double-stranded RNA-dependent protein kinase is involved in 2-methoxyestradiol-mediated cell death of osteosarcoma cells." *J Bone Miner Res* 2007: 22(1): 29-36

[11] She MR, Li JG, Guo KY, et al. "Requirement of reactive oxygen species generation in apoptosis of leukemia cells induced by 2-methoxyestradiol." *Acta Pharmacologica Sinica* 2007; 28(7): 1,037-1,044

[12] Fong YC, Yang WH, Hsu SF, et al. "2-methoxyestradiol induces apoptosis and cell cycle arrest in human chondrosarcoma cells." *J Orthop Res* 2007; 25(8): 1,106-1,114

[13] Miller KD, Haney LG, Pribluda VS, Sledge VW. "A phase I safety, pharmacokinetic and pharmacodynamic study of 2-methoxyestradiol (2ME2) in patients with refractory metastatic breast cancer." *Proceedings of the American Society of Clinical Oncology* 2001; 170: 20-43a

[14] Davoodpour P, Landstrom M, Welsh M. "Reduced tumor growth in vivo and increased c-Abl activity in PC3 prostate cancer cells overexpressing the Shb adapter protein." *BMC Cancer* 2007; 7: 161

[15] Ho A, Kim YE, Lee H, et al. "SAR studies of 2-methoxyestradiol and development of its analogs as probes of anti-tumor mechanisms." *Bioorg Med Chem Lett* 2006; 16(13): 3,383-3,387

[16] Tinley TL, Leal RM, Randall-Hlubek DA, et al. "Novel 2-methoxyestradiol analogues with antitumor activity." *Cancer Research* 2003; 63: 1,538-1,549

[17] "Drug found effective in treating, preventing breast cancer," Science Daily (www.sciencedaily.com), 11/4/07

[18] Cicek M, Iwaniec UT, Goblirsch MJ, et al. "2-methoxyestradiol suppresses osteolytic breast cancer tumor progression in vivo." *Cancer Res* 2007; 67(21): 10,106-10,111

[19] Miller KD, Haney LG, Pribluda VS, Sledge VW. "A phase I safety, pharmacokinetic and pharmacodynamic study of 2-methoxyestradiol (2ME2) in patients with refractory metastatic breast cancer." *Proceedings of the American Society of Clinical Oncology* 2001; 170: 20-43a

[20] Miller KD, Haney LG, Pribluda VS, et al. "A phase I study of 2-methoxyestradiol (2ME2) plus docetaxel in patients with metastatic breast cancer." *Proceedings of the American Society of Clinical Oncology* 2002; 21: 111a.

[21] Dahut W, Lakhani NJ, Gulley JL, et al. "Phase I clinical trial of oral 2-methoxyestradiol, an antiangiogenic and apoptotic agent, in patients with solid tumors." *Cancer Biology & Therapy* 2006; 5(1): 22-27

[22] Sweeney C, Liu G, Yiannoutsos C, et al. "A phase II multicenter, randomized, double-blind, safety trial assessing the pharmacokinetics, pharmacodynamics, and efficacy of oral 2-methoxyestradiol capsules in hormone-refractory prostate cancer." *Clinical Cancer Research* 2005; 11: 6,625-6,633

[23] Salama SA, et al. "Estrogen metabolite 2-Methoxyestradiol induces apoptosis and inhibits cell proliferation and collagen production in rat and human leiomyoma cells: a potential medicinal treatment for uterine fibroids." *J Soc Gynecol Invest* 2006; 13: 542-550

Part II: Heart

Could a stroke steal your future?

[1] Keli S et al. Dietary flavonoids, antioxidant vitamins, and incidence of stroke: the Zutphen Study. *Arch Int Med* 1996;156(6) 637-642

[2] Joshipura KJ et al. Fruit and vegetable intake in relation to risk of ischemic stroke. *JAMA* 1999;282(13):1233-1239

[3] Khaw KT, Barrett-Connor E. Dietary potassium and stroke-related mortality: a 12-year prospective population study. *NEJM* 1987;316(5):235-40

[4] Liu S et al. Whole grain consumption and risk of ischemic stroke in women: a prospective study. *JAMA* 2000;284;(12):1534-1540

[5] Bone K, Mills S. Hawthorn. In Principles and Practice of Phytotherapy. Churchill Livingstone, London, 2000. pp. 439-447

[6] ibid, pp. 404-417

[7] Murray M. Gotu Kola. in The Healing Power of Herbs, Prima Publishing, Rocklin, California, 1995. pp. 173-183

[8] Bone K, Mills S. Hawthorn. In Principles and Practice of Phytotherapy. Churchill Livingstone, London, 2000. pp. 439-447

[9] Sumi H et al. A novel fibrinolytic enzyme (nattokinase) in the vegetable cheese natto, a typicl and popular food in the Japanese diet. *Experientia* 1987;43:1110-1111

[10] Sumi H et al. Enhancement of the fibrinolytic activity in plasma by oral administration of nattokinase. *Acta Haematol* 1990;84:139-145

Part IV: Diabetes

Do-it-yourself pain relief for diabetic neuropathy: Even the "last resort" is natural and side-effect-free!

[1] Jamal GA, et al. "Gamma-linolenic acid in diabetic neuropathy," *Lancet* 1986; 1: 1098

[2] Ziegler D, et al. "Treatment of symptomatic diabetic neuropathy with the anti-oxidant alpha-lipoic acid," *Diabetologica* 1995; 38: 1,425-1,433

[3] Ruhnau KJ, et al. "Effects of 3-week oral treatment with the antioxidant thioctic acid (alpha-lipoic acid) in symptomatic diabetic polyneuropathy," *Diabet Med* 1999; 16: 1,040-1,043

[4] Hixson JR. "Hot stuff for diabetic neuropathy:capsaicin," *Med Tribune*, 9/14/89, pages 12-13

[5] Lee P, Chen R. "Vitamin D as an analgesic for patients with Type 2 diabetes and neuropathic pain," *Arch Intern Med* 2008; 168(7): 771-772.

Get your type 2 diabetes under control... without a single drug

[1] Yin, J., H. Xing, et al. (2008). Efficacy of berberine in patients with type 2 diabetes mellitus. *Metabolism* 57(5): 712-7.

[2] Zhang, Y., X. Li, et al. (2008). Treatment of type 2 diabetes and dyslipidemia with the natural plant alkaloid berberine. *J Clin Endocrinol Metab* 93(7): 2559-65.

[3] Turner, N., J. Y. Li, et al. (2008). Berberine and its more biologically available derivative, dihydroberberine, inhibit mitochondrial respiratory complex I: a mechanism for the action of berberine to activate AMP-activated protein kinase and improve insulin action. *Diabetes* 57(5): 1414-8.

[4] Lee, Y. S., W. S. Kim, et al. (2006). Berberine, a natural plant product, activates AMP-activated protein kinase with beneficial metabolic effects in diabetic and insulin-resistant states. *Diabetes* 55(8): 2256-64.

[5] Ma, X., T. Egawa, et al. (2010). Berberine-induced activation of 5'-adenosine monophosphate-activated protein kinase and glucose transport in rat skeletal muscles. *Metabolism.*

[6] Hwang, J. T., D. Y. Kwon, et al. (2009). AMP-activated protein kinase: a potential target for the diseases prevention by natural occurring polyphenols. *N Biotechnol* 26(1-2): 17-22.

[7] Zhang, H., J. Wei, et al. (2009). Berberine lowers blood glucose in type 2 diabetes mellitus patients through increasing insulin receptor expression. *Metabolism* 59(2): 285-92.

[8] Kong, W. J., H. Zhang, et al. (2009). Berberine reduces insulin resistance through protein kinase C-dependent up-regulation of insulin receptor expression. *Metabolism* 58(1): 109-19.

[9] Chen, C., Y. Zhang, et al. (2010). Berberine inhibits PTP1B activity and mimics insulin action. *Biochem Biophys Res Commun* 397(3): 543-7.

[10] Yu, Y., L. Liu, et al. (2009). Modulation of glucagon-like peptide-1 release by berberine: in vivo and in vitro studies. *Biochem Pharmacol* 79(7): 1000-6.

[11] Al-masri, I. M., M. K. Mohammad, et al. (2009). Inhibition of dipeptidyl peptidase IV (DPP IV) is one of the mechanisms explaining the hypoglycemic effect of berberine. *J Enzyme Inhib Med Chem* 24(5): 1061-6.

[12] Ni YX (1988) Therapeutic effect of berberine on 60 patients with type II diabetes mellitus andexperimental research [article in Chinese]. *Zhong Xi Yi Jie He Za Zhi* 8:711–713.

[13] Wei J, Wu J, Jiang J, Wang S, Wang Z (2004). Clinical study on improvement of type 2 diabetesmellitus complicated with fatty liver treatment by berberine [article in Chinese]. *Zhong Xi Yi JieHe Ganbing Za Zhi* 14:334–336.

[14] Xie P, Zhou H, Gao Y 2005 The clinical efficacy of berberine in treatment of type 2 diabetes mellitus [article in Chinese]. *Chin J Clin Healthcare* 8:402–403.

Part V: Digestion

Age and antacids—a double whammy against your body's optimal health

[1] Reference cited in Wright JV and Lenard L, Why Stomach Acid Is Good for You, Natural Relief From Heartburn, Indigestion, and GERD, Chapter 5.. M. Evans and Company, New York City, 2001

[2] Dial S, Delaney JA, Barkun AN, Suissa S. Use of gastric acid-suppressive agents and the risk of community-acquired Clostridium difficile-associated disease. *JAMA* 2005 Dec 21;294(23):2989-95.

[3] Yang YX, Lewis JD, Epstein S, Metz DC. Long-term proton pump inhibitor therapy and risk of hip fracture. *JAMA* 2006 Dec 27;296(24):2947-53.

[4] Laheij RJ, et al. Risk of community-acquired pneumonia and use of gastric acid-suppressive drugs. *JAMA* 2004 Oct 27;292(16):1955-60.

[5] Clemons TE, Milton RC, Klein R, Seddon JM, Ferris FL 3rd; Age-Related Eye Disease Study Research Group. Risk factors for the incidence of Advanced Age-Related Macular Degeneration in the Age-Related Eye Disease Study (AREDS) AREDS report no. 19. *Ophthalmology* 2005 Apr;112(4):533-9.

[6] Age-related Eye Disease Study Group (AREDS). Risk factors associated with Age-related macular degeneration, *Ophthalmology* 2000:107:2224-2232.

[7] Henry EB, Carswell A, Wirz A, Fyffe V, McColl KE. Proton pump inhibitors reduce the bioavailability of dietary vitamin C. *Aliment Pharmacol Ther.* 2005 Sep 15;22(6):539-45.

[8] All references cited in Wright JV and Lenard L, Why Stomach Acid Is Good for You, Natural Relief From Heartburn, Indigestion, and GERD, Chapter 5. M. Evans and Company, New York City, 2001

Part VI: Immune System

5 ways to make sure you've had your last bout with the common cold: And 3 cures you never knew could work so well

[1] "Listing of the ISTERH/NTES/HTES '07 Scientific Program," International Society for Trace Element Research in Humans website (http://www.angelfire.com/nd/isterh/2007conference/glimpse.html), accessed July 28, 2007

[2] Prasad AS, Fitzgerald JT, Bao B, Beck FW, Chandrasekar PH. "Duration of symptoms and plasma cytokine levels in patients with the common cold treated with zinc acetate. A randomized, double-blind, placebo-controlled trial," *Ann Intern Med*;133(4): 245-252

[3] Eby GA, Davis DR, Halcomb WW. "Reduction in duration of common colds by zinc gluconate lozenges in a double-blind study." *Antimicrob Agents Chemother* 1984;25(1): 20-24

[4] "History of Zinc Lozenges in Treating and Curing Common Colds" George Eby Research website (http://george-eby-research.com/html/history.html), accessed July 28, 2007

Part VII: Women's Health

Forget your annual mammogram! New tool offers better, earlier breast cancer detection (and it's pain-free, too!)

[1] Kuhl CK. "The 'Coming of age' of non-mammography screening for breast cancer." *JAMA* 2008; 299(18): 2,203-2,205

[2] Miller AB, Baines CJ, To T, Wall C. "Canadian National Breast Screening Study: 1. Breast cancer detection and death rates among women aged 40 to 49 years." *CMAJ* 1992; 147(10): 1,459-1,476

[3] Miller AB, To T, Baines CJ, Wall C. "The Canadian National Breast Screening Study-1: breast cancer mortality after 11 to 16 years of follow-up. A randomized screening trial of mammography in women age 40 to 49 years." *Ann Intern Med* 2002; 137(5 Part 1): 305-312

[4] Miller AB, Baines CJ, To T, Wall C. "Canadian National Breast Screening Study: 2. Breast cancer detection and death rates among women aged 50 to 59 years." *CMAJ* 1992;147(10):1477-88

[5] Warner E, Plewes DB, Hill KA, et al. "Surveillance of BRCA1 and

BRCA2 mutation carriers with magnetic resonance imaging, ultrasound, mammography, and clinical breast examination." *JAMA* 2004; 292(11): 1,317-1,325

[6] Leach MO, Boggins CR, Dixon AK, et al; MARIBS study group. "Screening with magnetic resonance imaging and mammography of a UK population at high familial risk of breast cancer: a prospective multicenter cohort study (MARIBS)." *Lancet* 2005; 365(9,473): 1,769-1,778

[7] Tilanus-Linthorst M, Verhoog L, Obdeijn IM, et al. "A BRCA1/2 mutation, highbreast density and prominent pushing margins of a tumor independently contribute to a frequent false-negative mammography." *Int J Cancer* 2002; 102(1): 91-95

[8] Lehman CD, Isaacs C, Schnall MD, et al. "Cancer yield of mammography, MR and US in high-risk women: prospective multi-institutional breast cancer screening study." *Radiology* 2007; 244(2): 381-388

[9] Sardinelli F, Podo F, D'Agnolo G, et al. "Multicenter comparative multi-modality surveillance of women at genetic-familial high risk for breast cancer (HIBCRIT study): interim results." *Radiology* 2007; 244(2): 698-715

Part VIII: Men's Health

Drop the finasteride!

[1] Hart JP, Cooper WL. Vitamin F in the treatment of prostatic hypertrophy. Report Number 1, Lee Foundation for Nutritional Research, Milwaukee, Wisconsin, 1941.

[2] Bush IM, et al. Zinc and the prostate. Presented at the annual meeting of the American Medical Association, Chicago, 1974

[3] Fahim MS, Fahim Z, et al. Zinc treatment for reduction or hyperplasia of the prostate. *Fed Proc* 1976;35:361

[4] Thompson IM, Goodman PJ, Tangen CM, Lucia MS, Miller GJ, Ford LG, Lieber MM, Cespedes RD, Atkins JN, Lippman SM, Carlin SM, Ryan A, Szczepanek CM, Crowley JJ, Coltman CA. The influence of finasteride on the development of prostate cancer. *N. Engl. J. Med.* 2003 Jul 17;349(3):215-24

[5] De Stefani E, Deneo-Pellegrini H, Boffetta P, et al. Alpha-linolenic acid and risk of prostate cancer: a case-control study in Uruguay. *Cancer Epidemiol Biomarkers Prev* 2000;9:335-8.

[6] Ramon JM, Bou R, Romea S, et al. Dietary fat intake and prostate cancer risk: a case-control study in Spain. *Cancer Causes Control* 2000;11:679-85.

[7] Pandalai PK, Pilat MJ, Yamazaki K, et al. The effects of omega-3 and omega-6 fatty acids on in vitro prostate cancer growth. *Anticancer Res* 1996;16:815-20.

[8] De Toit PJ, van Aswegen CH, du Plessis DJ. The effect of essential fatty acids on growth and urokinase-type plasminogen activator production in human prostate DU-145 cells. *Prostaglandins Leukot Essent Fatty Acids* 1996;55:173-7.

[9] Leitzmann MF, Stampfer MJ, Wu K, Colditz GA, Willett WC, Giovannucci EL. Zinc supplement use and risk of prostate cancer. *J Natl Cancer Inst.* 2003 Jul 2;95(13):1004-7.

[10] Imamov O, Lopatkin NA, Gustafsson JA. Estrogen receptor beta in prostate cancer. *N. Engl. J. Med.* 2004 Dec 23;351(26):2773-4.

Part IX: Anti-Aging, Memory, Hearing, and Vision

Five ways to avoid that hearing aid

[1] Ochi K, Kinoshita H, Kenmochi M, Nishino H, Ohashi T. Zinc deficiency and tinnitus. *Auris Nasus Larynx.* 2003 Feb;30 Suppl:S25-8.

[2] Arda HN, Tuncel U, Akdogan O, Ozluoglu LN. The role of zinc in the treatment of tinnitus. *Otol Neurotol.* 2003 Jan;24(1):86-9.

The mineral breakthrough helping terminal patients defy death: And why you should be taking a little of it, too

[1] Moore G J, et al. "Lithium-induced increase in human brain grey matter." *Lancet* 2000; 356: 1,241-1,242

[2] Chuang DM, Hashimoto R, Kanai H., et al. "Lithium stimulates progenitor proliferation in cultured brain neurons." *Neuroscience* 2003; 117(1): 55-61

[3] Nonaka S, Chuang DM. "Neuroprotective effects of chronic lithium on focal cererbral ischemia in rats." *Neuroreport* 1998; 9(9): 2,081-2,084

[4] Manji HK, Chen G, Moore GJ. "Lithium at 50: Have the neuroprotective effects of this unique cation been overlooked?" *Biological Psychiatry* 1999; 46(7): 929-940

[5] Chuang DM. "Lithium exerts robust neuroprotective effects in vitro and in the CNS in viv Therapeutic implications." *Neuropsychopharmacology* 2000; 23(S2): S39

[6] Takashima A, Murayama M, Murayama O, et al. "Lithium inhibits amyloid secretion in COS7 cells transfected with amyloid precursor protein C100." *Neuroscience Letters* 2002; 321(1-2): 61-64

[7] Diaz-Nido J, Alvarez G, Avila J, et al. "Lithium protects cultured neurons against beta-amyloid-induced neurodegeneration." *FEBS Letters* 1999; 453(3): 260-264

[8] Zhong J, Lee WH. "Lithium: a novel treatment for Alzheimer's disease?" *Expert Opin Drug Saf* 2007; 6(4): 375-383

[9] Schrauzer GN, Shreshta KP. "Lithium in drinking water and the incidence of crimes, suicides, and arrests related to drug addiction." *Biological Trace Elements Research* 1990; 25: 105-113

[10] McMillan TM. "Lithium and the treatment of alcoholism: a critical review." *British Journal of Addiction* 1981; 76: 245-258

[11] Fornai F, Longone P, et al. "Lithium delays progression of amyotrophic lateral sclerosis." *Proc Natl Acad Sci USA* 2008; 105(6): 2,052-2,057

Part X: Essential Health Secrets

Vitamin K: What's it good for?

[1] *J Dent Res* 1948;27:235-241

[2] *J Canad Dent Assoc* 1943;9(8):359-356

[3] Merkel RL. The use of menadione bisulfite and ascorbic acid in the treatment of nausea and vomiting of pregnancy. *Am J Ob Gyn* 1952;64(2):416-418

[4] Kubovic M et al. Analgesic effect of vitamin K. *Proc Soc Exp Biol Med* 1955;90:660-662

[5] Hart JP et al. Circulating vitamin K levels in fractured neck of femur. *Lancet* 1984;2:283

[6] Hart JP et al. Electrochemical detection of depressed circulating levels of vitamin K1 in osteoporosis. *J Clin Endocrinol Metab* 1985;60:1268-1269

[7] Tomita A. Post-menopausal osteoporosis: 47Ca study with vitamin K2. *Clin Endocrinol* (Japan) 1971;19:731-736.

[8] Knapen MHJ et al. The effect of vitamin K supplementation on circulating osteocalcin (bone Gla protein) and urinary calcium excretion. *Ann Intern Med* 1989;111:1001-1005

[9] Bouckaert JH Said AH. Fracture healing by vitamin K. *Nature* 1960;185:849

[10] Seyuma Y et al. Comparative effects of vitamin K2 and vitamin E on experimental arteriosclerosis. *J Vit Nutr Res* 1999;69(1):23-26

[11] Jie K-SG et al. Vitamin K status and bone mass in women with and without aortic atheroclerosis. *Calcif Tiisue Int* 1996;59:352-356

[12] Mitchell T. Vitamin K. Life Extension (magazine) 2000;6(2):32-38

1 program, 2 months, lasting relieffrom almost any symptoms—And the older you are, the better it works

[1] James Breneman, James, M.D., Basics of Food Allergy, Springfield (IL): Charles C. Thomas Publisher, 1978

Send even the most stubborn infections—cold sores, toenail fungus, and more—into hiding for good

[1] Buck DS, Nidorf DM, Addino JG. "Comparison of two topical preparations for the treatment of onychomycosis: Melaleuca alternifolia (Tea Tree) oil and clotrimazole." *J Family Practice* 1994; 38(6): 601-605

[2] Bassett IB, Pannowitz DL, Barnetson RS. "A comparative study of tea-tree oil versus benzoyl peroxide in the treatment of acne. Medical Journal of Australia." *Med J Australia* 1990; 153(8): 455-458

[3] Satchell AC, Saurajen A, Bell C, et al. "Treatment of interdigital tinea pedis with 25% and 50% tea tree oil solution: a randomized, placebo-controlled, blinded study," *Australas J Dermatol* 2002; 43(3): 175-178

[4] Belaiche P. "Treatment of vaginal infections of Candida albicans with the essential oil of Melaleuca alternifolia." *Phytotherapy* 1985; 15: 13-15

[5] Pena EF. "Melaleuca alternifolia oil. Its use for trichomonal vaginitis and other vaginal infections," *Obstet Gynecol* 1962; 19: 793-795

[6] Wölbling RH, Rapprich K: *Der Deutsche Dermatologe* 1983; 10(31): 1,318-1,328

[7] Wölbling RH, Milbradt R. *Therapiewoche* 1984; 34: 1,193-1,200

[8] Koytchev R, Alken RG, Dundarov S. "Balm mint extract (Lo-701) for

topical treatment of recurring herpes labialis," *Phytomedicine* 1999; 6(4): 225-230

⁹ Saller R, Buechi S, Meyrat R et al. "Combined herbal preparation for topical treatment of Herpes labialis," *Forsch Komplementarmed Klass Naturheilkd* 2001; 8(6): 373-382

Harnessing the healing power of light
Part 1: What you need to know about UV rays—beyond sunburn

¹ Miner AL, Losina E, Katz JN, et al. "Infection control practices to reduce airborne bacteria during total knee replacement: a hospital survey in four states." *Infect Control Hosp Epidemiol* 2005; 26(12): 910-915

² Kujundzic E, Matalkah F, Howard CJ, et al. "UV air cleaners and upper-room air ultraviolet germicidal irradiation for controlling airborne bacteria and fungal spores." *J Occup Environ Hyg* 2006; 3(10): 536-546

³ Ritter MA, Olberding EM, Malinzak RA. "Ultraviolet lighting during orthopaedic surgery and the rate of infection." *J Bone Joint Surg Am* 2007; 89(9): 1,935-1,940

⁴ Miner AL, Losina E, Katz JN, et al. "Infection control practices to reduce airborne bacteria during total knee replacement: a hospital survey in four states." *Infect Control Hosp Epidemiol* 2005; 26(12): 910-915

⁵ Kujundzic E, Matalkah F, Howard CJ, et al. "UV air cleaners and upper-room air ultraviolet germicidal irradiation for controlling airborne bacteria and fungal spores." *J Occup Environ Hyg* 2006; 3(10): 536-546

⁶ Ritter MA, Olberding EM, Malinzak RA. "Ultraviolet lighting during orthopaedic surgery and the rate of infection." *J Bone Joint Surg Am* 2007; 89(9): 1,935-1,940

⁷ Koek M, Buskens E, Steegmans P, et al. "UVB phototherapy in an outpatient setting or at home: a pragmatic randomized single-blind trial designed to settle the dispute. The Pluto study." *BMC Med Res Methodol* 2006; 6: 39

⁸ Silva SH, Guedes ACM, Gontijo B, et al. "Influence of narrow-band UVB phototherapy on cutaneous microbiota of children with atopic dermatitis." *Journal of the European Academy of Dermatology and Venereology* 2006; 20(9): 1,114-1,120

⁹ Marshall S. "Technology insight: ECP for the treatment of GvHD – can we offer selective immune control without generalized immunosuppression?" *Nature Clinical Practice Oncology* 2006; 3: 302-314

[10] Edelson R, Berger C, Gasparro F, et al. "Treatment of cutaneous T-cell lymphoma by extracorporeal photochemotherapy. Preliminary results." *NEJM* 1987; 316: 297-303

[11] Kumar V, Lockerbie O, Keil SD, et al. "Riboflavin and UV-light based pathogen reduction: extent and consequence of DNA damage at the molecular level." *Photochem Photobiol* 2004; 80: 15-21

[12] Edelson R, Berger C, Gasparro F, et al. "Treatment of cutaneous T-cell lymphoma by extracorporeal photochemotherapy. Preliminary results." *NEJM* 1987; 316: 297-303

[13] Vowels BR, Cassin M, Boufal MH, et al. "Extracorporeal photochemotherapy induces the production of tumor necrosis factor-? by monocytes: implications for the treatment of cutaneous T-cell lymphoma and systemic sclerosis." *Journal of Investigative Dermatology* 1992; 98: 686-692.

[14] Potashov LV, Cheminava RV. "Reinfusion of the patient's own irradiated blood in surgical patients." *Vestn Khir Im II Grek* 1980; 125(10): 144-146

[15] Boudurov N, Filipov ZH. "Effect of ultraviolet ray-irradiated autogenous blood on hematological indices in horses." *Vet Med Nauki* 1976; 13(10):11-19.

[16] Ivanov EM, Shakirova OV, Zhurayskaia NS. "Use of auto-transfusion of UV-irradiated blood in chronic bronchitis." *Klin Med* (Mosk) 2002; 80(6): 21-25

[17] Paleev NR, Vetchinnikov ON, Plaksina GV, Brucheeva IS. "The efficacy of the extracorporeal ultraviolet irradiation of autologous blood in the treatment of chronic nonspecific lung diseases." *Vestn Ross Akad Med Nauk* 1993; 3: 3-6

[18] Kuvshinchikova VN, Shmelev EI, Mishin VI. "Effectiveness of extracorporeal ultraviolet blood irradiation in treatment of chronic obstructive bronchitis in pulmonary tuberculosis." *Probl Tuberk* 1998; 3: 48-50

[19] Isaev IuV, Dzhangirova GM, Padenko AV, Lipikin AA. "Use of UV autologous blood irradiation for preventing the occurrence of tracheobronchitis during tracheostomy." *Vestn Khir Im II Grek* 1987; 138(4):116-118

[20] Alizade IG, Karaeva NT. "Experience in the use of auto-transfusions of laser-irradiated blood in treating hypertension patients." *Lik Sprava* 1994; May-Jun(5-6): 29-32

[21] McGlade JP, Gorman S, Zosky GR, et al. "Suppression of the asthmatic

phenotype by ultraviolet B-induced, antigen-specific regulatory cells." *Clinical & Experimental Allergy* 2007; 37(9): 1,267–1,276

[22] Bernstein JA, Bobbitt RC, Levin L, et al. "Health effects of ultraviolet irradiation in asthmatic children's homes." *Journal of Asthma* 2006; 43: 255-262

[23] Paleev NR, Cherniakov VL, Vetchinnikova ON. "Ultraviolet irradiation of the blood in the treatment of pyo-inflammatory complications in patients with terminal renal failure." *Vestn Akad Med Nauk* SSSR 1991; 3: 15-20

[24] Gaiseniuk LA. "Use of re-infusions of isolated irradiated auto-blood for the correction of hematopoietic disorders." *Med Radiol* (Mosk) 1987; 32(11): 15-18

[25] Hansen E, Knuechel E, Altmeppen J, Taeger K. "Blood irradiation for intraoperative auto-transfusion in cancer surgery: demonstration of efficient elimination of contaminating tumor cells." *Transfusion* 1999; 39(6): 608-615

[26] Hansen E, Bechmann V, Altmeppen J. "Intraoperative blood salvage in cancer surgery: safe and effective?" *Transfus Apher Sci* 2002; 27(2): 153-157

[27] Sawyer L, Hanson D, Castro G, et al. "Inactivation of parvovirus B19 in human platelet concentrates by treatment with amotosalen and ultraviolet A illumination." *Transfusion* 2007; 47(6): 1,062-1,070.

[28] Thai TP, Houghton PE, Campbell KE, Woodbury MG. "Ultraviolet light C in the treatment of chronic wounds with MRSA: a case study." *Ostomy Wound Manage* 2002; 48(11): 52-60

[29] Thai TP, Keast DH, Campbell KE, et al. "Effect of ultraviolet light C on bacterial colonization in chronic wounds." *Ostomy Wound Manage* 2005; 51(10): 32-45.

[30] Conner-Kerr TA, Sullivan PK, Gaillard J, et al. "The effects of ultraviolet radiation on antibiotic-resistant bacteria in vitro." *Ostomy Wound Manage* 1998; 44(10): 50-6.

[31] Phoenix DA, Harris F. "Light activated compounds as antimicrobial agents—patently obvious?" *Recent Patents Anti-Infect Drug Disc* 2006; 1(2): 181-99.

Harnessing the healing power of light
Part 2: Time-tested strategies for beating superbugs and more of today's deadliest health threats

[1] Douglass WC. Into the Light: Tomorrow's Medicine Today. Second Opinion Publishing, Inc, Dunwoody, GA 1995.

[2] www.Nobelprize.org

[3] Ude WH. *Journal of Surgery* 1943; 61(1)

[4] Knott EK. "Development of Ultraviolet blood irradiation," *American Journal of Surgery* 1948; 76: 165-171

[5] Hancock VK, Knott EK. "Irradiated blood transfusion in treatment of infections," *Northwest Medicine* 1934; 33: 200

[6] Miley G. *Archives of Physical Therapy* 1943; 23: 536

[7] Douglass WC. Into the Light: Tomorrow's Medicine Today. Second Opinion Publishing, Inc, Dunwoody, GA 1995.

[8] Rebbeck EW. "Ultraviolet irradiation of blood in the treatment of Escherichia coli septicemia," *Archives of Physical Therapy* 1943; 24: 158-167

[9] Rebbeck EW. "Ultraviolet irradiation of auto-transfused blood in the treatment of postabortional sepsis," *American Journal of Surgery* 1942; 55:476-486

[10] Miley GP. "Ultraviolet blood irradiation therapy in acute poliomyelitis," *Archives of Physical Therapy* 1946; 25: 651-656

[11] Miley G. *American Journal of Bacteriology* 1943; 45:303

[12] Edelson RL. "Photopheresis: a clinically relevant immunobiologic response modifier," *Annals of the New York Academy of Sciences* 1991; 636(1): 154-164

[13] Barr ML, Meiser BM, Eisen HJ, et al. "Photopheresis for the prevention of rejection in cardiac transplantation," *The New England Journal of Medicine* 1998; 339(24): 1,744-1,751

[14] Malawista S, Trock DH, Edelson R. "Treatment of rheumatoid arthritis by extracorporeal photochemotherapy: a pilot study," *Arthritis Rheum* 1991; 34: 646-654

[15] Ludvigsson J, Samuelsson U, Ernerudh J, et al. "Photopheresis at onset of type 1 diabetes: a randomized, double blind, placebo controlled trial," *Arch Dis Child* 2001; 85: 149-154

[16] Rostami AM, Sater RA, Bird SJ, et al. "A double-blind placebo-controlled trial of extracorporeal photopheresis in chronic progressive multiple sclerosism," *Neurology* 1990; 40(Suppl 1): 393-394

[17] Miley GP, Seidel RE, Christensen JA. "Preliminary report of results observed in 80 cases of intractable bronchial asthma," *Archives of Physical Therapy* 1943; 24: 533

[18] Miley GP, Seidel RE, Christensen JA. "Ultraviolet blood irradiation in apparently intractable bronchial asthma," Archives of Physical Medicine 1946; 27:24

[19] Douglass WC. Into the Light: Tomorrow's Medicine Today. Second Opinion Publishing, Inc, Dunwoody, GA 1995.

[20] Miley GP, Seidel RE, Christensen JA. "Ultraviolet blood irradiation in apparently intractable bronchial asthma," *Archives of Physical Medicine* 1946; 27:24

[21] Miley GP. "Efficacy of ultraviolet blood irradiation therapy in the control of Staphylococcemias," *American Journal of Surgery* 1944; 64: 313-322

[22] Miley GP, Christensen JA. "Ultraviolet blood irradiation therapy: Further studies in acute infections," *American Journal of Surgery* 1947; 73: 486-493

[23] Miley GP. "Present status ultraviolet blood irradiation (Knott technic)," *Archives of Physical Therapy* 1944; 25: 368-372.

[24] Miley GP, Rebbeck EW. "The Knott technic of ultraviolet blood irradiation as a control of infection in peritonitis," *Review of Gastroenterology* 1943; 10: 1

[25] Miley GP. "The Knott Technic of ultraviolet blood irradiation in acute pyogenic infections. A study of 103 cases with clinical observations on the effects of a new therapeutic agent," *New York State Journal of Medicine* 1942, 42(1): 38-46

[26] Miley GP, Christensen JA. "Ultraviolet blood irradiation therapy: Further studies in acute infections," *American Journal of Surgery* 1947; 73: 486-493

[27] ibid

[28] ibid

[29] Edelson R, Berger C, Gasparro F, et al. "Treatment of cutaneous T-cell

lymphoma by extracorporeal photochemotherapy. Preliminary results," *New England Journal of Medicine* 1987; 316: 297-303

[30] Gollnick K. "Chemical aspects of photodynamic action in the presence of molecular oxygen." In Nygaard OF (ed): Radiation Research: Biomedical, Chemical, and Physical Perspectives. New York: Academic Press, 1975, pp. 590-611.

[31] Olney RC. "Treatment of viral hepatitis with Knott technic of blood irradiation," *American Journal of Surgery* 1955; 90: 402-409

[32] Dougherty TJ, Kaufman JE, Goldfarb A, et al. "Photoradiation therapy for the treatment of malignant tumors," *Cancer Research* 1978; 39: 2,628-2,635

[33] McCaughton JS. "Overview of experiences with photodynamic therapy for malignancy in 192 patients," *Photochemistry and Photobiology* 1987; 46: 903-909

[34] McCaughton JS, Doughtery TJ. "Summary of clinical reports of photodynamic therapy," *Postgrad Gen Surg* 1989

[35] Miley GP. "The Knott Technic of ultraviolet blood irradiation in acute pyogenic infections. A study of 103 cases with clinical observations on the effects of a new therapeutic agent," *New York State Journal of Medicine* 1942, 42(1): 38-46

[36] Miley GP, Rebbeck EW. "The Knott technic of ultraviolet blood irradiation as a control of infection in peritonitis," *Review of Gastroenterology* 1943; 10: 1

[37] Miley GP, Christensen JA. "Ultraviolet blood irradiation therapy: Further studies in acute infections," *American Journal of Surgery* 1947; 73: 486-493

[38] Miley G, Christensen JA. "Ultraviolet blood irradiation therapy in acute virus-like infections," *Review of Gastroenterology* 1948; 15: 271-277

[39] Miley GP. "Ultraviolet blood irradiation," *Archives of Physical Therapy* 1942; 23: 536

[40] Miley GP. "Ultraviolet blood irradiation: Therapy in acute pyogenic infection at Hanhemann Hospital," *Hahnemannian Monthly* 1940

Killer appliances? 9 ways to protect yourself from the new pollution more deadly than lead poisoning

[1] Milham S, Morgan L. "New electromagnetic exposure metric: high frequency voltage transients associated with increased cancer incidence in teachers in a California school," *American Journal of Industrial Medicine* 2008; 51(8):579-586

[2] Havas M, Stetzer D. "Dirty electricity and electrical hypersensitivity: five case studies," World Health Organization Workshop on Electrical Hypersensitivity, October 25-26, Prague, Czech Republic. (Accessed at www.stetzerelectric.com)

[3] Wertheimer N, Leeper E. "Electrical wiring configurations and childhood cancer." *Am J Epidemiol* 1979; 109: 273-284

[4] Milham S, Morgan L. "New electromagnetic exposure metric: high frequency voltage transients associated with increased cancer incidence in teachers in a California school," *American Journal of Industrial Medicine* 2008; 51(8):579-586

[5] Ahlbom A, Cardis E, Green A, et al. "Review of the epidemiologic literature on EMF and health." *Environmental Health Perspectives* 2001; 109 (Suppl 6): 911-933

[6] Green LM, Miller AB, Villeneuve PJ, et al. "A case-control study of childhood leukemia in southern Ontario Canada and exposure to magnetic fields in residences." *Int J Cancer* 1999; 82: 161-170

[7] Greenland S, Sheppard AR, Kaune WT, et al. "A pooled analysis of magnetic fields, wire codes, and childhood leukemia." *Epidemiology* 2000; 11: 624-634

[8] Kheifets LI, Afifi AA, Buffler PA, Zhang ZW. "Occupational electric and magnetic field exposure and brain cancer: a metaanalysis." *J Occup Environ Med* 1995; 37: 1,327-1,341

[9] Kheifets LI, Gilbert ES, Sussman SS, et al. "Comparative analyses of the studies of magnetic fields and cancer in electric utility workers: studies from France, Canada, and the United States." *Occup Environ Med* 1999; 56: 567-574

[10] Blackman C, Blank M, Kundi M, Sage C. "BioInitiative report: A rationale for a biologically-based public exposure standard for electromagnetic fields (ELF and RF)." The BioInitiative, 8/31/07. (Accessed at www.bioinitiative.org)

[11] "The Health Consequences of Involuntary Exposure to Tobacco Smoke:

A Report of the Surgeon General." US Department of Health and Human Services (US DHHS), 2006. (Accessed at www.surgeongeneral.gov/library/secondhandsmoke)

[12] Hardell L, Carlberg M, Söderqvist F, et al. "Long-term use of cellular phones and brain tumours: increased risk associated with use for > or =10 years." *Occup Environ Med* 2007; 64(9): 626-632

[13] Lahkola A Tokola K, Auvinen A. "Meta-analysis of mobile phone use and intracranial tumors." *Scand J Work Environ Health* 2006; 32(3):171-177

[14] Kan P, Simonsen SE, Lyon JL, Kestle JRW. "Cellular phone use and brain tumor: a meta-analysis." *J Neurooncol* 2008; 86(1): 71-78

[15] Lowenthal RM, Tuck DM, Bray IC. "Residential exposure to electric power transmission lines and risk of lymphoproliferative and myeloproliferative disorders: a case controlled study." *Int Med J* 2007; 37(9): 614-619

[16] Stevens RG. "Electric power use and breast cancer: a hypothesis." *Am J Epidemiol* 1987; 125: 556-561

[17] Stevens RG, Davis S, Thomas DB, et al. "Electric power, pineal function, and the risk of breast cancer." *FASEB J* 1992; 6: 853-860

[18] Erren T. "A meta-analysis of epidemiologic studies of electric and magnetic fields and breast cancer in women and men." 2001. *Bioelectromagnetics* 2001; Suppl 5: S105-S119

[19] Havas M. "Dirty electricity elevates blood sugar among electrically sensitive diabetics and may explain brittle diabetes." *Electromagnetic Biology and Medicine* 2008; 27(2): 135-146

[20] Havas M, Stetzer D. "Dirty electricity and electrical hypersensitivity: five case studies," World Health Organization Workshop on Electrical Hypersensitivity, October 25-26, Prague, Czech Republic. (Accessed at www.stetzerelectric.com)

[21] Hakansson N, Gustavsson P, Johansen C, Floderus B. "Neurodegenerative diseases in welders and other workers exposed to high levels of magnetic fields." *Epidemiology* 2003; 14: 420-426

[22] Savitz DA, Checkoway H, Loomis DP. "Magnetic field exposure and neurodegenerative disease mortality among electric utility workers." *Epidemiology* 1998; 9: 398-404

[23] Blackman C, Blank M, Kundi M, Sage C. "BioInitiative report: A rationale for a biologically-based public exposure standard for electromagnetic fields (ELF and RF)." The BioInitiative, 8/31/07. (Accessed at www.

bioinitiative.org)

[24] ibid

[25] www.electricalpollution.com

[26] ibid

[27] ibid

[28] Havas M, Stetzer D. "Graham/Stetzer Filters Improve Power Quality in Homes and Schools, Reduce Blood Sugar Levels in Diabetics, Multiple Sclerosis Symptoms, and Headaches." Presented at the International Scientific Conference on Childhood Leukemias, 9/6/04. (Accessed at www.electricalpollution.com)

[29] "The health effects of electrical pollution." National Foundation for Alternative Medicine. (Accessed at www.stetzerelectric.com)

[30] Havas M, Stetzer D. "Graham/Stetzer Filters Improve Power Quality in Homes and Schools, Reduce Blood Sugar Levels in Diabetics, Multiple Sclerosis Symptoms, and Headaches." Presented at the International Scientific Conference on Childhood Leukemias, 9/6/04. (Accessed at www.electricalpollution.com)

[31] ibid

[32] "The health effects of electrical pollution." National Foundation for Alternative Medicine. (Accessed at www.stetzerelectric.com)

[33] Havas M, Illiatovitch M, Proctor C. "Teacher and student response to the removal of dirty electricity by the Graham/Stetzer Filter at Willow Wood School in Toronto, Canada." Presented at the 3rd International Workshop on the Biological Effects of Electromagnetic Fields, 10/4/04. (Accessed at www.emrpolicy.org)

[34] Havas M. "Electromagnetic hypersensitivity: Biological effects of dirty electricity with emphasis on diabetes and multiple sclerosis." *Electromagnetic Biology and Medicine* 2006; 25: 259-268

[35] www.electricalpollution.com

[36] Boyd EB. "Can you hear me now?" Conscious Choice, 9/08, p. 22